J. Klekamp · M. Samii Syringomyelia

Springer-Verlag Berlin Heidelberg GmbH

Jörg Klekamp   Madjid Samii

Syringomyelia

Diagnosis and Treatment

With Contributions by Cordula Matthies
to the Text on Neurophysiology

With 113 Figures in 456 Separate Illustrations,
Some in Colour, and 36 Tables

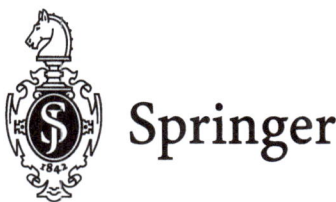

Springer

Privat-Dozent Dr. Jörg Klekamp
Professor Dr. Madjid Samii

Klinikum Hannover Nordstadt
Neurochirurgische Klinik
Haltenhoffstrasse 41
30167 Hannover, Germany

e-mail: JoergKlekamp@t-online.de

ISBN 978-3-642-62651-7

Library of Congress Cataloging-in-Publication Data
Klekamp, Joerg, 1958–
  Syringomyelia: diagnosis and treatment / Joerg Klekamp, Madjid Samii.
     p. ; cm.
  Includes bibliographical references and index.
  ISBN 978-3-642-62651-7   ISBN 978-3-642-56023-1 (eBook)
  DOI 10.1007/978-3-642-56023-1
  1. Syringomyelia. I. Samii, Madjid. II. Title.
  [DNLM: 1. Syringomyelia – diagnosis. 2. Syringomyelia – therapy. WL 400 K64s 2002]   RC406.S9 K565
  2002   616.8'3–dc21   2001042630

http://www.springer.de

© Springer-Verlag Berlin, Heidelberg 2002
Originally published by Springer-Verlag Berlin, Heidelberg New York in 2002
Sofecover reprint of the hardcover 1st edition 2002
The use of general descriptive names, registered names, trademarks, etc. in this publication does not imply,
even in the absence of a specific statement, that such names are exempt from the relevant protective laws
and regulations and therefore free for general use.
Product liability: The publishers cannot guarantee the accuracy of any information about the application
of operative techniques and medications contained in this book. In every individual case the user must
check such information by consulting the relevant literature.

Cover design: Erich Kirchner, Heidelberg, Germany
Typesetting: H. Stürtz AG, Würzburg, Germany

Printed on acid-free paper   SPIN 10837491   24/3130/SM   5 4 3 2 1 0

For Our Families

Preface

Syringomyelia has fascinated neurologists and neurosurgeons for decades, if not for centuries. The slowly progressing cystic cavitations of the spinal cord have led scientists and clinicians to various pathophysiological hypotheses and treatment strategies. Until recently, no clear concept existed as to what caused a syrinx and how and when a particular patient should be treated. The introduction of magnetic resonance imaging (MRI) has revolutionized our view of syringomyelia. For the first time, we are able to diagnose a syrinx before it produces clinical symptoms, and we can follow the course of the syrinx before and after surgical treatment with a noninvasive method. This has led to a huge amount of information not available to previous scientists. Nevertheless, pathophysiology and treatment are still controversial.

The aim of this book is to give a guideline on how to approach a patient with a syrinx. Based on clinical experience, we have modified our strategies repeatedly in an attempt to improve clinical results. We have developed a treatment concept, evolved out of 20 years of clinical and experimental work, which has proven to be a solid basis for our decision making. Clinical courses, surgical indications, techniques, and postoperative results are discussed for each of the different pathologies known to be associated with syringomyelia. In this manner, we hope to give a coherent overview on all aspects of syringomyelia, which should help physicians to counsel and treat patients with this fascinating but also potentially devastating disease.

Finally, we wish to acknowledge the tremendous impact that cooperation with Ulrich Batzdorf at the University of California in Los Angeles had on our work in this field over many years. Fruitful discussions and this ongoing cooperation helped to improve treatment strategies. Clinical and also experimental studies were performed together, which led to several publications. Most of the statistics of this book are based on the collaborative research of the Departments of Neurosurgery at the Klinikum Hannover Nordstadt and the University of California.

Hannover, June 2001

Jörg Klekamp
Madjid Samii

Acknowledgements. We wish to express our thanks to Dr. C. Matthies for her evaluation of neurophysiological results for patients with syringomyelia. Her protocol, outlined in Chap. 3.1.3., was of tremendous help during surgery. Drs. R.-H. Prawitz, A. Majewski, and Prof. B. Terwey provided excellent neuroradiological information for surgical planning and postoperative controls for our patients. Their expertise had a strong impact on our understanding of neuroradiological features of patients with an often malformed and severely altered anatomy. Prof. B. Terwey provided the excellent phase-contrast cine MRI studies.

Contents

General Information

Each chapter of this book has been written in a way that it can be read as a separate section without the need to go through previous ones. Pre- and postoperative neurological symptoms are analyzed according to a scoring system (Table 1) [3]. Additionally, the overall clinical condition is documented according to the Karnofsky score [2]. Success of treatment requires at least the stopping of a progressive neurological course. When a patient develops progressive neurological symptoms after surgery, this is defined as a clinical recurrence. Using clinical recurrences as an indicator for treatment failure, long-term results are documented with survival statistics [1]. Unlike the majority of publications on syringomyelia, which present only percentages of patients with postoperative improvement, stabilization, or deterioration, this method allows accounting for varying follow-up times and gives a much more realistic picture of postoperative results.

The overwhelming majority of operations illustrated in this book were performed in the prone position. All intraoperative photographs are oriented in the same fashion: cranial to the left, caudal to the right. When the semi-sitting positioning was used, this is mentioned in the figure legend and the photograph is presented according to the surgeon's view.

Table 1. Neurological scoring system

Score	Sensory dist., swallowing, pain, dysesthesias	Motor weakness	Gait ataxia	Bladder function	Bowel function
5	No symptom	Full power	Normal	Normal	Normal
4	Present, not significant	Movement against resistance	Unsteady, no aid	Slight dist., no catheter	Slight dist., control
3	Significant, function not restricted	Movement against gravity	Mobile with aid	Residual, no catheter	Laxatives, control
2	Some restriction of function	Movement without gravity	Few steps with aid	Rarely incontinent	Rarely incontinent
1	Severe restriction of function	Contraction without movement	Standing with aid	Often catheter	Often incontinent
0	Incapacitated function	Plegia	Plegia	Permanent catheter	Permanent incontinence

References

1. Kaplan EL, Meier P (1958) Nonparametric estimation from incomplete observations. J Am Stat Assoc 53:457–481
2. Karnofsky DA, Burchenal JH (1949) The clinical evaluation of chemotherapeutic agents in cancer. In: MacLeod CM (ed) Evaluation of chemotherapeutic agents. Columbia University Press, New York, pp 191–205
3. Klekamp J, Samii M (1993) Introduction of a score system for the clinical evaluation of patients with spinal processes. Acta Neurochir (Wien) 123:221–223

1 Introduction

1.1
Definitions of Cord Cavitations

Syrinx is the Greek name for a cavity of tubular shape. Ollivier D'Angers introduced this term in 1827 for cystic cavitations of the spinal canal [122]. Since then, the term "syringomyelia" has been applied to every kind of intramedullary cyst by some authors; others restrict its use to certain subtypes of cystic lesions and distinguish syringomyelia, hydromyelia, or myelomalacia as separate entities. Still other authors combine these terms into syringohydromyelia or hydrosyringomyelia.

For the purpose of this book it seems appropriate to define the term syringomyelia and to differentiate it from other cystic processes of the spinal cord:

▶ Syringomyelia is a cystic cavitation of the spinal cord, containing fluid that is identical or similar to cerebrospinal (CSF) and extracellular fluid (ECF). The cavity may be formed by dilatation of the central canal or lie within the parenchymal substance. It may be lined by ependymal cells or gliotic tissue. Syringomyelia is always associated with an underlying disorder that is characterized by obstruction of CSF flow (Fig. 1.1), tethering of the spinal cord (Fig. 1.2), or a spinal tumor (Fig. 1.3). A syrinx may expand slowly with the passage of time.

▶ Hydromyelia is a dilatation of the central canal associated with hydrocephalus, an obstruction of the Foraminae of Luschka and Magendie, and a communication between the fourth ventricle and central canal. The cavity is lined by ependymal cells and may expand secondarily into the cord parenchyma. The cavity may enlarge progressively with time.

▶ Myelomalacia is a cystic necrosis of the spinal cord and describes the final state of spinal cord damage due to trauma or ischemia. It is not of progressive character, clinically or radiologically. Extension and localization of the cyst depend on the type and severity of spinal cord damage. The cavities are lined by gliotic tissue. Initially, the cavity is filled with detritus. With the passage of time, the fluid is cleared of protein to resemble ECF (Fig. 1.4).

▶ Cystic neoplasms. This variety constitutes an entity where the entire cyst wall is formed by neoplastic cells. In most instances, the lining of such cysts will accumulate some gadolinium during magnetic resonance imaging (MRI). However, cystic neoplasms may be indistinguishable from syringomyelia using standard neuroradiological techniques. The cyst fluid contains a high amount of protein and resembles plasma filtrate (Fig. 1.5).

▶ Glioependymal cysts. The cyst wall of glioependymal cysts does not accumulate gadolinium during MRI. The etiology of these cystic formations is unclear. Mostly, they are located in the area of the conus medullaris. They are not associated with tumors, CSF flow obstruction, hydrocephalus, or spinal cord tethering (Fig. 1.6). As they contain ECF and are under high pressure once they produce neurological symptoms, fenestration or drainage appears to be the treatment of choice.

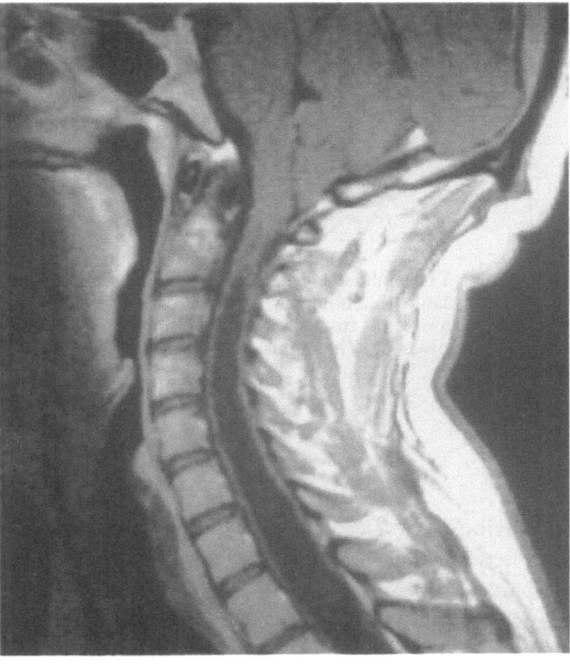

Fig. 1.1. T1-weighted sagittal MRI scan of a 49-year-old woman with a typical Chiari I malformation and syringomyelia. Subarachnoid space at the foramen magnum is obstructed by cerebellar tonsils obliterating the cisterna magna

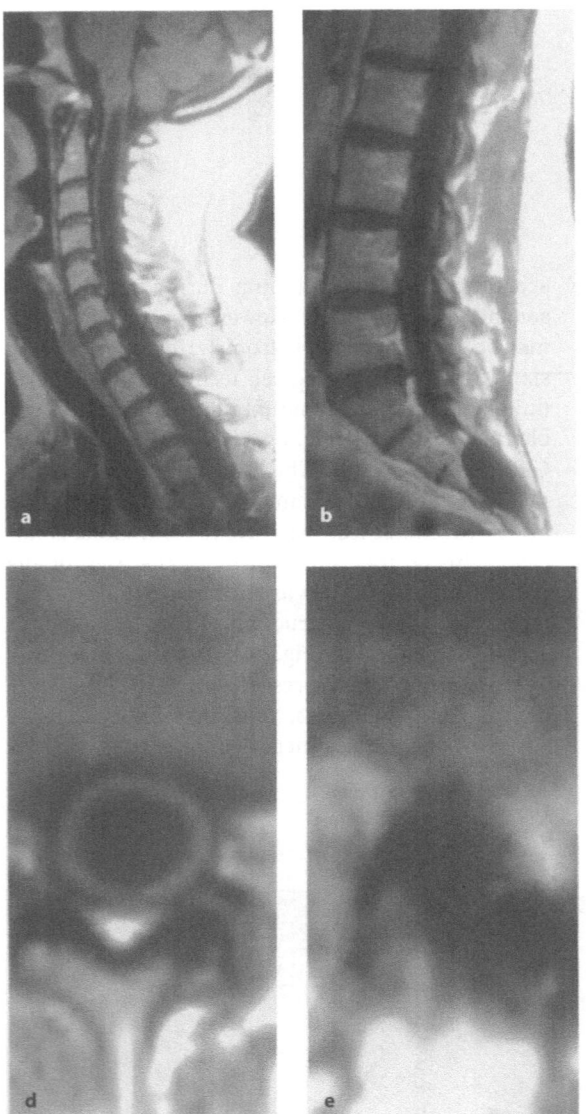

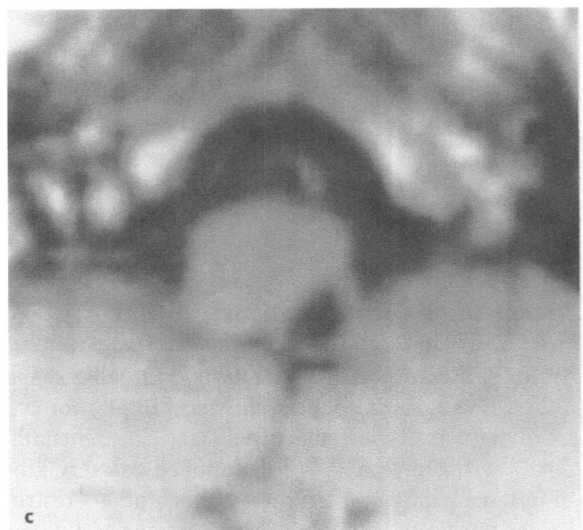

Fig. 1.2 a–e. T1-weighted sagittal and axial MRI scans of a 37-year-old woman with a holocord syrinx and a tethered cord (**a, b**). The syrinx extends from the medulla oblongata (**c**) down to the lumbar spine (**d**). The conus medullaris is tethered at the level of S2 (**e**)

Obviously, a clear-cut distinction between these different entities cannot be made in every patient. In patients with posttraumatic syringomyelia, for instance, myelomalacia and syringomyelia overlap in many cases. Nevertheless, we will use the terms as defined above throughout this text as they resemble different pathophysiological entities. Furthermore, depending on the type of cyst, different treatment strategies have to be implemented.

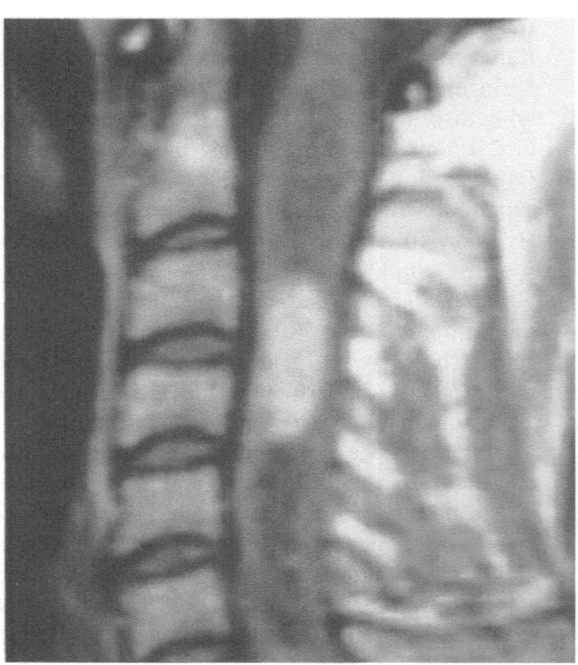

Fig. 1.3. T1-weighted sagittal MRI scan with gadolinium of a 35-year-old man with an intramedullary ependymoma at the C3 to C4 level. A syrinx has developed above and below the tumor

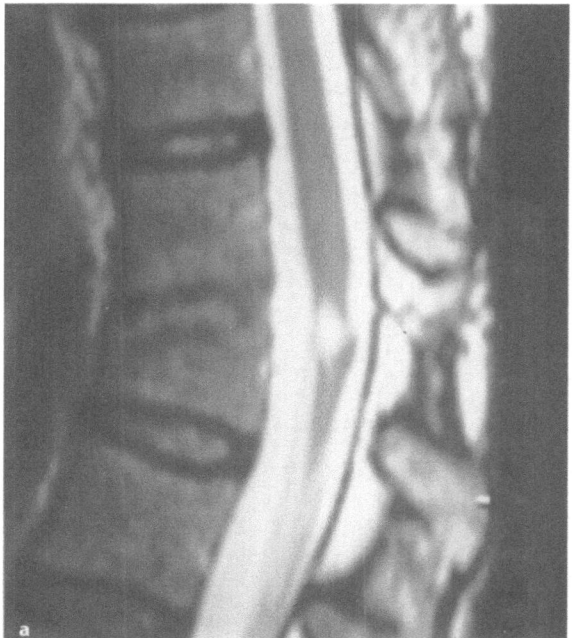
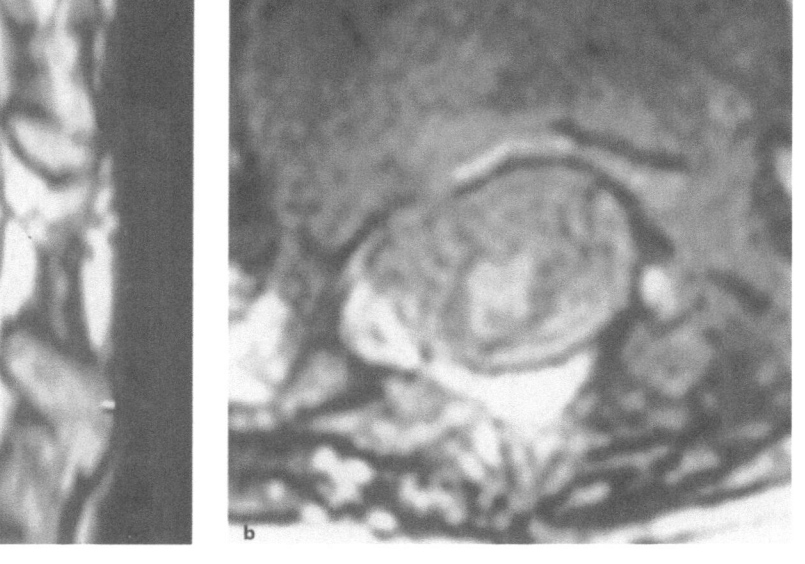

Fig. 1.4 a, b. T2-weighted sagittal (**a**) and axial (**b**) MRI scan of a 48-year-old woman with myelomalacia at the level of Th12. She suffered a compression fracture of Th12 and an incomplete spinal cord lesion. The MRI was taken 20 years after the accident as a routine control. The clinical situation had remained stable during this time

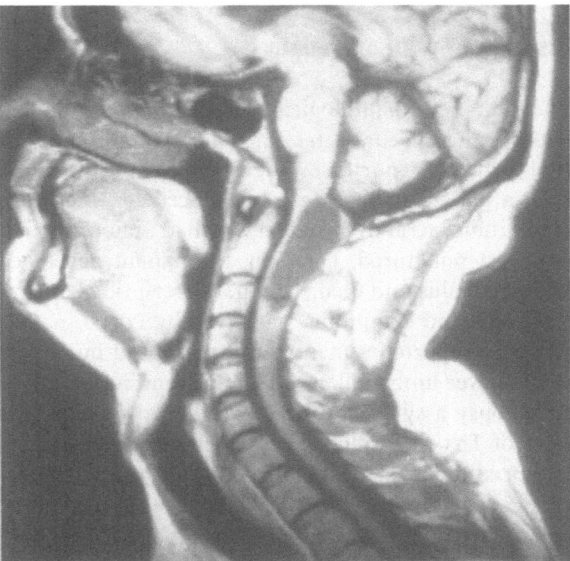

Fig. 1.5. T1-weighted MRI scan of a 47-year-old man with a cystic intramedullary astrocytoma of the craniocervical junction

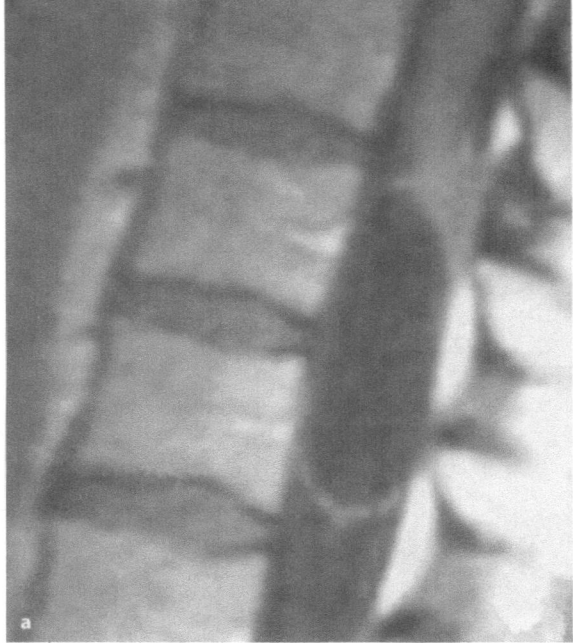 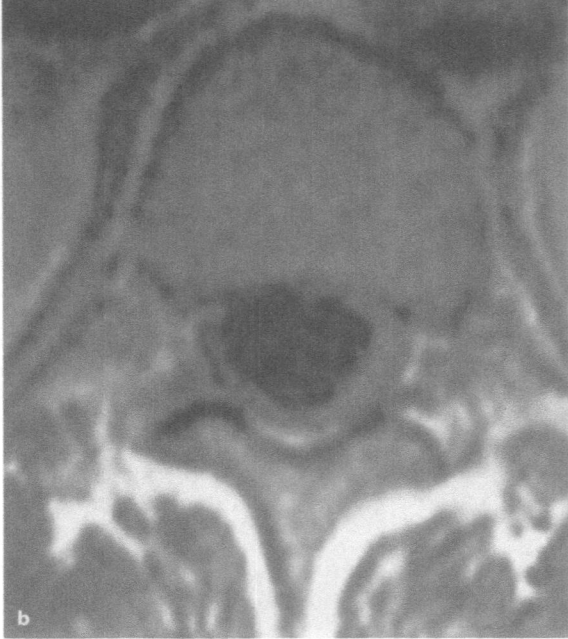

Fig. 1.6 a, b. T1-weighted MRI scans of a 45-year-old woman with a cyst of the conus medullaris. Sagittal (**a**) and axial (**b**) scans reveal the eccentric location of this cystic lesion. There was no enhancement of the cyst wall with gadolinium

1.2
History of Syringomyelia

The first neuropathological description of a patient with syringomyelia dates back to 1546 by Estienne [50]. Brunner reported on the first attempt of treating such a patient in 1700 [25]. He described a newborn with lumbosacral dysraphism who had an intramedullary cyst punctured. Later on, the patient developed hydrocephalus and died. The first descriptions of clinical signs and symptoms was given by Portal in 1804 [131]. He reported a man who experienced numbness of his lower limbs followed by an ascending paralysis. At autopsy a syrinx in the cervical cord down to the level of Th3 was found. Finally, Ollivier D'Angers introduced the term syringomyelia in 1827 [122]. He defined syringomyelia as a pure dilatation of the central canal. The first description of syringobulbia (Figs. 1.7, 1.8) is attributed to Spiller in 1908, who interpreted it as a cranial extension of a syrinx [150].

Diagnosis of syringomyelia was a major obstacle until the advent of MRI. At first, diagnosis was suspected clinically and later proven at autopsy. The first neuroradiological descriptions of syringomyelia date back to the 1920s, after Sicard and Forestier introduced lipidiol myelography [148]. Jirasek [83] in-

jected contrast directly into the syrinx in 1927. A less invasive method of imaging syringomyelia was described by Greenwald et al. in 1958 [63]. They injected air into the subarachnoid space (SAS) as a contrast agent. With changes of patient positioning, they tried to detect changes in spinal cord diameter to distinguish between a syrinx and an intramedullary tumor [63].

The modern era of imaging started with the combination of computer-assisted tomography (CT) and water-soluble contrast agents injected into the SAS [39, 40]. With this method, contrast accumulated inside the syrinx (Fig. 1.9). With the advent of MRI, a noninvasive method of even better quality became available [37, 119, 181]. Further insights into the nature of syringomyelia were obtained by studies of CSF flow with cardiac-gated cine MRI [166], which also allowed visualization of fluid flow inside the syrinx itself (Fig. 1.10).

The modern era of therapy started with Abbe and Coley in 1892 [1]. They described a patient who developed syringomyelia 4 years after an episode of meningitis. They punctured the cyst after a hemilaminectomy without producing any clinical benefit for the patient. The concept of cyst puncture and myelotomy was then continued by Elsberg [49] and Pousepp [132], with only a few patients operated on until the late 1920s. The first larger series of surgically treated patients was published by Peiper in 1931 [127]. He had collected 44 cases. Schaeffer reported on 50 patients from the literature 1 year later [143]. By 1936, reports appeared which suggested insertion of a stent into the syrinx in order to maintain communication between

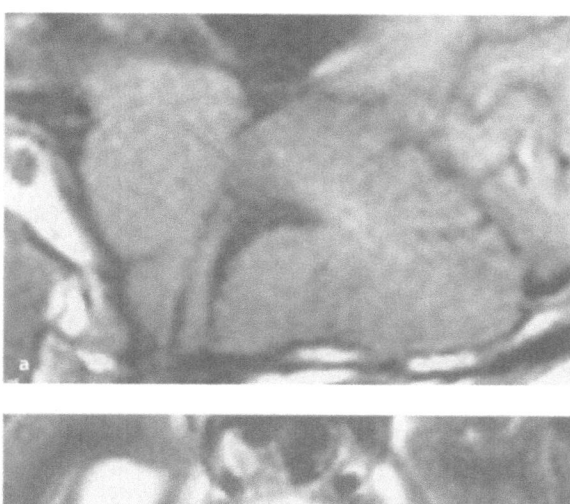

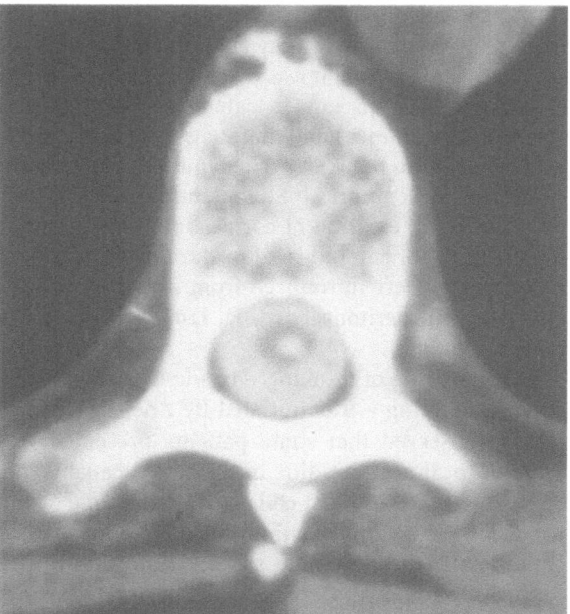

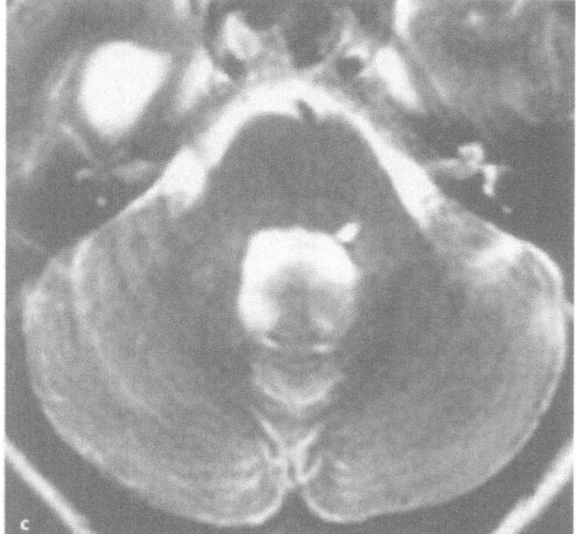

Fig. 1.7 a–c. T1-weighted sagittal (a) and T2-weighted axial (b, c) MRI scans of a 42-year-old woman with a Chiari I malformation and syringobulbia. The cleft-like cyst extends from the medulla oblongata (b) to the cerebellar peduncle (c) on the left side

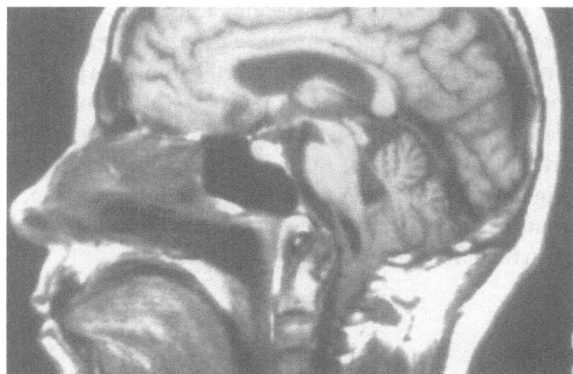

Fig. 1.8. T1-weighted MRI scan of a 58-year-old woman with a Chiari I malformation and syringobulbia of considerable size

Fig. 1.9. Postmyelographic CT of a 54-year-old patient with a posttraumatic syrinx. Intrathecal water-soluble contrast has accumulated inside the syrinx

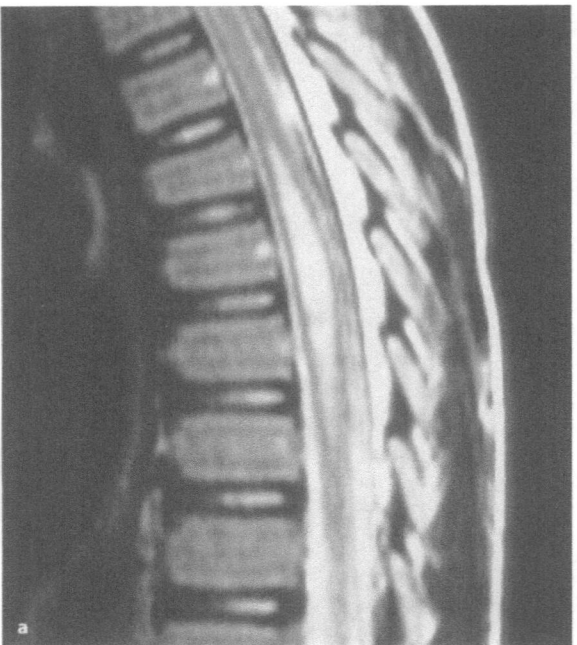 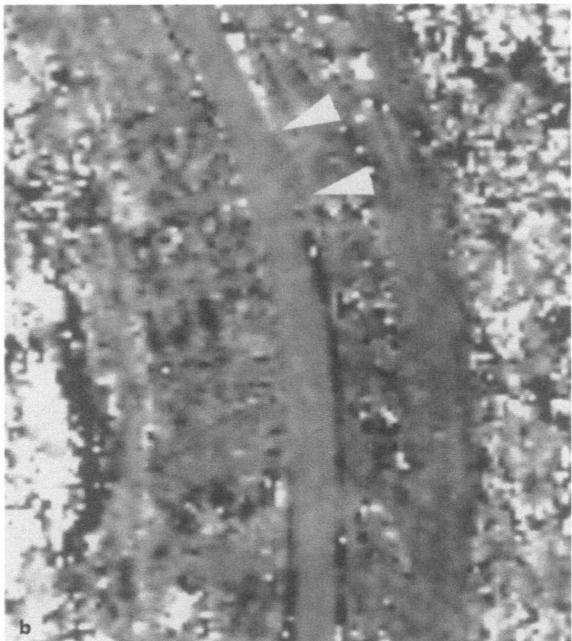

Fig. 1.10 a, b. a This T1-weighted MRI scan of an 11-year-old boy reveals a syrinx at Th7 to Th10. There was no history of trauma. The phase contrast cine MRI (**b**) shows absent flow signals above the syrinx (*arrows*), a constant finding throughout the entire cardiac cycle, indicating an area of CSF flow obstruction at this level in the posterior subarachnoid space

syrinx and SAS [56]. It turned out that many patients treated by simple myelotomy subsequently required a second operation, and it was discovered that the initial myelotomy was no longer patent. In the following years all sorts of ideas and materials were suggested to keep connection between syrinx and SAS patent: gutta percha [53], silk sutures [98], tantalum wire [87], silastic wicks [136], excision of cord tissue [127], suture of the pia to the arachnoid [110] or dura mater [112, 123]. Later, shunts were introduced from syrinx to SAS [91, 126, 139, 158], peritoneal [11, 92, 129, 130], or pleural cavities [177, 179].

A second line of thinking – trying to avoid myelotomy or shunting – was initiated by Adelstein in 1938 [3]. He observed that some patients presented with areas of focal arachnoiditis in the spinal canal. When he saw that the cord had collapsed by the time he had performed the dura opening and dissection of arachnoid scars, he no longer saw an indication to perform a myelotomy to evacuate the syrinx. He closed the wound and obtained satisfactory postoperative results for the first time without myelotomy and evacuation of the syrinx. He had treated the syringomyelia by improving CSF circulation.

The first surgical attempts at the foramen magnum for patients with syringomyelia and Chiari I or II malformation were performed in the 1930s. Russel and Donald [140] suggested in 1935 to decompress the foramen magnum in patients with Chiari II malformation to improve CSF circulation and hydrocephalus without knowing that Van Houweninge Graftdijk had already performed such an operation by 1932 [162]. Walter Penfield was the next in 1938 [128]. However, their patients had died from the procedure. The first surgical successes were reported by McConnell and Parker [101] in two out of five patients in 1938. The introduction of a surgical concept for these patients has to be attributed to Gardner in 1959 [60], after a first overview of the literature together with a review of their first 17 patients in 1950 [59]. The rather high mortality and complication rates [170] with what became known as the Gardner operation led Gardner himself to propose a second surgical strategy: terminal ventriculostomy [61]. He reported good results in 10 of 12 cases. In the following years, this procedure was utilized by others, particularly for patients who showed further clinical progression despite a foramen magnum operation. However, it soon became clear that terminal ventriculostomy was of no benefit for the majority of patients.

1.2.1
Review of Pathophysiological Hypotheses

Foremost, the history of syringomyelia is a history of pathophysiological hypotheses. Any analysis of clinical cases shows that syringomyelia may be associated with almost any disease of the spinal canal. The various associations are probably the reason for the large diversity of pathophysiological concepts which have been proclaimed in the last 100 years. Single cases were often taken as some sort of prototype for a hypothesis, which was then generalized for all patients with syringomyelia. Naturally, using such an approach to understand the pathophysiology of a disease which may be associated with a great variety of disorders is likely to fail. Nevertheless, we would like to give an overview of the pathophysiological concepts which have been published during these last 100 years.

1.2.1.1
Dysraphic Hypothesis

Brunner's description in 1700 marks the first attempt at treatment of dysraphism and syringomyelia [25]. Autopsy of the child revealed myelomeningocele, syringomyelia, and hydrocephalus. The hydrocephalus was probably related to a Chiari II malformation. Association of the syrinx with these malformations led to the conclusion that the syrinx either constituted a malformation in its own right or had to be seen as part of the lumbosacral malformation complex. Morgagni remarked in 1769 on the frequent association between spinal cord cysts and dysraphic malformations [111]. Olliver D'Angers also explained the syrinx on this basis [122]. He considered syringomyelia to be a developmental arrest of the spinal cord. Cleland described a case of hydrocephalus associated with spina bifida in 1883 [33], several years before Chiari published his papers on this subject [29, 30]. In this patient, Cleland observed a dilatation of the central canal without communication to the fourth ventricle and a downward displacement of the cerebellum and brainstem – a malformation to be later called Chiari II malformation. He thought that a primary dysgenesis of the brainstem was the key to this malformation leading to hydrocephalus and a dilated central canal and its rupture into the myelocele in the spinal canal.

Later it became clear that syringomyelia may be found without such gross deformities. Hinsdale [77] modified this concept and noted that syringomyelia constituted a developmental defect of ependymal and glial cells, i.e., the dysraphic basis of syringomyelia was transformed from the macroscopic to the microscopic level. Histological examinations of the spinal cord were thought to prove that a syrinx always started inside the central canal. Gliosis around the cyst

wall was interpreted as degeneration of glial cells and part of the same developmental problem that affected the ependymal cells [16, 75, 125, 149].

1.2.1.2
Neoplastic Hypothesis

The association between syringomyelia and intramedullary tumors led to a revision of this concept. Simon was the first to point out the association between spinal cord tumors and syringomyelia in 1875 [149]. Rethought, gliosis was then seen as degeneration of a low-grade glioma of the spinal cord [18, 24, 28, 53, 75, 76, 81, 124, 135, 144, 146, 149, 151, 161], either congenital or acquired postnatally. With the introduction of X-rays this concept gained a lot of popularity as this hypothesis not only seemed plausible but also offered a form of treatment – radiotherapy. Raymond reported in 1905 [134] of a 16-year-old patient with syringomyelia who experienced marked improvement of motor and sensory function after radiotherapy. A few years later, Sahatchieff published a series of 36 patients treated in this manner, with symptomatic improvement in 80% of them [141]. Until the 1930s, several similar reports appeared in the German, French, Italian, and Russian literature [35, 38, 62, 99]. In England and the USA, neurologists remained skeptical. Grinker [67] questioned this therapy in 1934. Several patients had shown neurological progression despite some relief of pain after radiotherapy. Tauber and Langworthy [159] pointed out that radiotherapy should be reserved for patients with neoplastic conditions associated with syringomyelia. For patients who developed a syrinx after meningitis or trauma, it had become clear that radiotherapy was not the appropriate treatment. Boman and Iivanainen [20] established in a study of patients treated from 1920 to 1965 that, compared with untreated patients, radiotherapy made no difference to the long-term course of syringomyelia.

Interestingly enough, the neoplastic hypothesis still had its proponents well into the 1960s. In 1967 a report on chemotherapy with nitrogen mustard for syringomyelia appeared in the literature. Borysowicz [23] reported on 50 patients who were treated in this manner; a great majority of these patients reported improvement of pain and sensory function and almost half of them reported an improvement in motor power. This publication, however, has remained the only report on chemotherapy for syringomyelia.

1.2.1.3
Inflammatory Hypothesis

In 1869, Hallopeau [74] described syringomyelia as an inflammatory process of ependymal cells which undergo sclerotic changes. Due to obstruction of the central canal, syringomyelia resulted. Recently, Milhorat et al. [109] revitalized this hypothesis on the basis of pathological analyses of the central canal in man. Like Alajouanine et al. [4], they thought of a viral spinal-cord inflammation affecting the ependyma. However, none of them produced any evidence of viral infection in patients with syringomyelia.

1.2.1.4
Ischemic Hypothesis

Another variant of the inflammatory hypothesis was supported by the association between syringomyelia and severe forms of meningitis. Charcot and Joffroy [28] and Joffroy and Archard [84] described autopsy cases of postmeningitic syringomyelia in 1869 and 1887, respectively, and concluded that syringomyelia was the result of ischemic spinal cord damage, due to venous obstruction and arterial thrombosis from inflamed meninges. This assumption was corroborated later by experimental evidence. In 1914, Camus and Roussy [26] injected a mixture of fatty acids, sodium nucleinate, and talc into the cervical SAS of 11 dogs to produce acute cervical meningitis. Histologically, they found spinal cord cavities with perivascular inflammatory cells and necrosis of spinal cord tissue. A similar study with comparable results was later performed by McLaurin et al. [103] in 1954. Hoffman et al. [79] injected a mixture of blood and pantopaque into the cisterna magna of dogs and positioned them on an inclined plane to ensure a spinal deposition of the material. The animals acquired severe spinal arachnoiditis with ischemia of the spinal cord predominantly in the cervical region. These studies had produced severe forms of necrotizing arachnoiditis and myelomalacia rather than syringomyelia.

Tatara [155] used a less traumatic method and performed a thoracic laminectomy to inject 0.1 ml of a 33% kaolin solution into the SAS of rabbits and 0.05 ml of a 16% kaolin solution in rats. Of these animals, 31.2% and 22.2%, respectively, developed a spinal cord cyst within 16 weeks postinjection.

Cho et al. [31] examined the contribution of spinal arachnoiditis on development of posttraumatic syringomyelia and injected a kaolin solution into the spinal SAS after inflicting trauma on the thoracic cord. Compared to animals with thoracic trauma but no additional arachnoiditis, which demonstrated a cavitation of the cord in 12.5% of cases, the animals with arachnoiditis presented a syrinx in 55% of animals. They concluded that arachnoiditis does play a significant role in the development of posttraumatic syringomyelia. However, both Cho et al. and Tatara attributed the syrinx to vascular factors, for lack of alternative explanations. Other studies have shown that syringomyelia may be caused by quite subtle arachnoid changes, which are not associated with ischemia [12, 82].

Apart from severe forms of meningitis, syringomyelia was thought to develop from obstruction of the anterior spinal artery at the foramen magnum in patients with a Chiari malformation [96]. Experimental studies performed as early as 1912 were able to produce intramedullary cavitations due to spinal cord compression [93]. Several investigators took up this model and considered these cavities to resemble syringomyelia [64, 65, 66, 153, 154, 160, 178]. In 1935, Tauber and Langworthy [159] were able to produce spinal cord cavities by ligature of the anterior spinal artery in cats. Apart from arterial obstruction, venous obstruction also may cause spinal cord cavitations [100], which can be interpreted as venous infarctions.

Netsky [115] noted the association between vascular changes and syringomyelia and reported that a syrinx formed, due to insufficient blood supply to central parts of the cord as a consequence of intramedullary vascular anomalies. McGrath observed in 1965 that a particular strain of dogs, Weimaraner dogs, developed intramedullary cysts associated with an autosomal recessive disorder characterized by marked skeletal deformities. These animals developed progressive paraplegia at the age of 4–6 weeks. Morphologically, he noted an abnormal angiogenesis of the spinal cord, so that the syrinx was attributed to chronic ischemia [102].

Vascular factors will certainly contribute to progressive myelopathy in patients with spinal cord compression or severe forms of arachnoiditis. However, progressive expansion of a syrinx over a period of years and the space-occupying effect of syringomyelia cannot be explained by ischemia and necrosis alone, i.e., syringomyelia must be distinguished from myelomalacia.

1.2.1.5
Hematomyelic Hypothesis

This hypothesis postulates that syringomyelia develops from an initial spinal cord insult associated with an intramedullary hematoma (hematomyelia). This assumption was mainly used to explain the origin of posttraumatic syringomyelia. In 1867, Bastian [13] was the first author to describe a posttraumatic syrinx. More attention was paid to a paper by Holmes [80] in 1915 on gunshot injuries to the spinal cord. The first experimental paper on this subject was published by Schmaus [145] in 1890, who described what he called a "commotio spinalis". Later, McVeigh [104] simply used his finger to crush the spinal cords of his animals in order to study spinal cord trauma. More standardized ways of inflicting spinal cord trauma used weights which were dropped onto the cord from a defined height [5, 6, 7, 34, 41, 45, 57, 105, 117, 118, 164, 165]. Even better standardized were models which used a clip applied to the spinal cord [52, 138, 156, 157]. Yezierski et al. [182] were able to produce necrotic cysts by injecting excitatory amino acids into the spinal cord; these amino acids are set free in the cord after trauma and are thought to play a significant role in the pathophysiology of posttraumatic events in the spinal cord. All of these models produced a lesion of the spinal cord which was invariably associated with a spinal cord cavity at the level of the trauma. The extent of the cavity was directly related to trauma severity. After resorption of the hematoma, the cyst filled with CSF or ECF and was thought to expand gradually due to subsequent internal pressure changes [172]. However, syringomyelia may develop gradually, without an initial incident of spinal cord trauma or hematomyelia. Again, these models are more representative of myelomalacia than of syringomyelia.

1.2.1.6
Secretory Hypothesis

The above-mentioned concepts were based mainly on neuropathological analysis of autopsy cases. Analysis of fluid contained in syrinx cavities led to a number of other hypotheses; these hypotheses were thought to explain the origin of the fluid and the pathways by which this fluid gained access to the central canal or spinal cord parenchyma. The similarity between syrinx fluid and CSF was the basis for Blaylock [19], Durward et al. [46], Rice-Edwards [137], and Wiedemeyer et al. [167] to postulate that ependymal cells produced and secreted CSF, accumulating in the central canal and causing a syrinx if the central canal was obstructed. Some animal studies suggested CSF production of the spinal cord and CSF flow inside the central canal [106]. However, the central canal progressively occludes with age in most people. Syringomyelia would be one of the most common neurological diseases of man if this concept was valid.

1.2.1.7
Transudation Hypothesis

Transudation may play a major role in cyst formation in patients with cystic neoplasms and with some cysts associated with intramedullary tumors [58, 88, 97, 168, 172, 175]. Holmes [80] reported in 1915 that posttraumatic syringomyelia only developed in patients who had an additional intramedullary neoplastic process. However, even in cases associated with intramedullary tumors, this mechanism alone cannot explain why cervical intramedullary tumors are associated with syringomyelia more often than with thoracic or conus tumors of the same histology [142].

1.2.1.8
Hydrodynamic Hypothesis

If CSF is not produced inside the spinal cord, how does it get there? The hydrodynamic theory was first described by Gull in 1862 [68]. He presented a case with progressive muscle atrophy over a period of 13 months where the patient died shortly after admission to the hospital. Unfortunately, only the spinal cord was discussed in the autopsy description. Enormous dilatation of the cervicothoracic cord due to the cyst being lined by ependymal cells led Gull to the assumption that this was an example of accumulation of CSF in the central canal; he termed it "hydromyelus." Lichtenstein [95] took up this idea and proposed in 1942 that a cavity may form in the spinal cord as a result of hydrocephalus and obstruction of all foraminae of the fourth ventricle. Gardner, published in 1959 [60], was the third author to explain the association between syringomyelia and Chiari malformation in this manner, after reviewing 17 cases operated for Chiari I malformation in 1950 [59]. He studied the embryological development of the central nervous system and understood syringomyelia as a dilatation of the central canal due to increased intracranial pressure, which caused CSF to enter the central canal via the obex. The foraminae of Luschka and Magendie open in the fifth month of gestation. If they stay occluded beyond that time, hydrocephalus develops which causes CSF to enter the central canal and to exit at the filum terminale into the SAS. The driving force was thought to be the water hammer effect of the choroid plexus. Gardner observed that the central canal in man progressively occludes with age. A patent central canal was interpreted as a dysraphic defect required for the development of syringomyelia. He preferred the term hydromyelia, to emphasize association with hydrocephalus, and postulated that each syrinx required at least an intermittent hydrocephalus, either prenatally or postnatally. This pathophysiological concept is similar to Chiari's ideas on the development of subtypes of Chiari malformation. He hypothesized that even the malformation itself was caused by prenatal hydrocephalus [29, 30].

The hydrodynamic theory subsequently gained a lot of acceptance. Gardner introduced a surgical method for the treatment of syringomyelia associated with Chiari malformation, which turned out to be quite successful. He performed a medial suboccipital craniectomy, opened the fourth ventricle, closed the obex with a piece of muscle, and performed a duraplasty [60].

An animal model could be established according to this hypothesis. Becker et al. in 1972 [14], Eisenberg in 1974 [47], Hall et al. in several papers since 1975 [70, 71, 72, 73], and Hochwald in 1985 [78] described hydromyelia in cats after injection of kaolin into the cisterna magna. This produced occlusive hydrocephalus with obstruction of all fourth-ventricle outlets and a central canal dilatation, as per Gardner' hypothesis, within a few days. Becker et al. [14] demonstrated that hydromyelia did not develop if the obex was occluded. Furthermore, ligation of the filum terminale and occlusion of the obex in control animals did not cause any dilatation of the central canal. They concluded that hydromyelia in cats after kaolin injection into the cisterna magna was caused by CSF from the fourth ventricle, which had been forced into the central canal via the obex, and that there was no CSF production in the central canal itself. Hall et al. [70] pointed out in their study that ischemia did not play a role in the development of hydromyelia in this animal model. This conclusion was drawn from histological comparison to specimens with spinal cord necrosis. In further experiments, Hall et al. demonstrated flow of CSF into the central canal with radioactive isotopes after injection into the ventricle [71]. Several other investigators described a similar caudal flow of CSF in the central canal of hydrocephalic animals [32, 43, 71, 90, 114]. Hochwald [78] emphasized the increased water content in the posterior white matter in these animals. Likewise, Chakrabortty et al. [27] found histological evidence of white-matter edema in this area, with dilated Virchow-Robin spaces in the subependymal part of the spinal cord. Donauer et al. published a number of papers describing the morphology of the central canal in this animal model [22, 42, 51, 133]. Finally, Babapour et al. [9] demonstrated that prenatal hydrocephalus induced by 6-AN causes obstruction of the foraminae of Luschka and Magendie and hydromyelia, once cranial mechanisms of compensation are exhausted.

However, a number of drawbacks were successively discovered which made this theory inapplicable for the majority of syringomyelia cases. A patent connection between the fourth ventricle and central canal via the obex could not be demonstrated in the majority of syringomyelia patients nor did they have evidence or a history of hydrocephalus [172]. In their paper on the different stages of hydrocephalus, Oi et al. [120] presented a number of children with hydrocephalus and hydromyelia. Adult patients with this constellation rarely are observed. Although the central canal remains patent in a number of mammal species [32], it usually obliterates with age in man, suggesting that the canal plays a less significant role in man than in other species [86, 109, 113, 116].

The surgical procedure introduced by Gardner worked just as well when the obex was not closed with muscle. Pressure gradients measured experimentally by Hall et al. [73] demonstrated a intracranial pressure lower than pressures inside the syrinx cavity, even in hydrocephalic animals. They were unable to lower the pressure inside the hydromyelic cavity by shunting the ventricle and postulated a ball-valve mechanism to explain dilatation of the central canal [73]. Similar observations were made by Dohrmann [41] and Yamada et al. [180]. They even observed hemorrhages in the upper cervical cord after shunting, which they interpreted as venous infarctions. These experimental findings were consistent with clinical experience. Ventriculoperitoneal shunts did not improve neurological symptoms in patients with syringomyelia, even if a connection between the fourth ventricle and dilated central canal was present. Benini and Krayenbühl [15] had suggested ventriculoatrial shunts as a treatment for syringomyelia. In a initial series of 22 patients in 1974, 13 improved, 2 stabilized, and 7 deteriorated during the period of observation [89]. Later, Foster and Hudgson [54] recognized this method but, convinced that it did not address malformations at the craniocervical junction, recommended it for patients with severe arachnoiditis at the foramen magnum. For patients with hydrocephalus and syringomyelia, Williams instructed to treat the hydrocephalus first before operating on the foramen magnum [176]. Milhorat et al. [107] confirmed this view in a recent report.

However, unlike Gardner's theory, recent observations describe a cranial flow of CSF in the central canal of the spinal cord, as per Hall's pressure measurements. After trauma, for instance, blood and necrotic material are transported in a cranial direction in the central canal [69, 106, 108, 163, 178]. Milhorat et al. [106] concluded that the central canal acts like a sink and is of major importance to drain potentially toxic substances away from the area of spinal cord injury.

1.2.1.9
Pressure Dissociation Hypothesis

Williams modified Gardner's ideas as he realized that hydrocephalus could not be made responsible for hydromyelia in each case [168]. He emphasized the importance of CSF flow obstructions to development of syringomyelia, which to this day is his fundamental contribution to our understanding of syringomyelia. Williams performed simultaneous pressure recordings in the SAS intracranially and in the spinal canal in both experimental [171] and clinical settings [169]. According to his concept, partial CSF flow obstructions at the craniocervical junction and elsewhere led to a pressure dissociation; with sudden increases of subarachnoid pressure associated with coughing, sneezing, or Valsalva maneuvers, he was able to demonstrate an intracranial pressure increase which persisted even after the spinal subarachnoid pressure had returned to normal. He suggested a ball-valve mechanism, such as CSF passing the area of obstruction during these maneuvers but being unable to reverse flow after spinal pressure normalization. The intracranial pressure is then normalized, due to CSF flow via the obex into the central canal. This view was supported by clinical descriptions of patients who sometimes experienced quite severe exacerbations of their symptoms with such maneuvers [17].

With this concept, hydrocephalus was not required to explain syringomyelia, but a patent connection was still mandatory between the fourth ventricle and the central canal. Neuropathological studies, however, were unable to demonstrate such a patent connection in the majority of cases. Only for children with hydrocephalus and hydromyelia could patency of this pathway be regularly demonstrated.

Oldfield et al. further modified the pressure dissociation theory [121] in 1994 by emphasizing the importance of a rapid downward motion during systole of cerebellar tonsils in patients with Chiari I malformation. This sudden increase of spinal subarachnoid pressure was thought to cause CSF flow into the spinal cord. Actions such as coughing, etc., would cause a similar reaction.

1.2.1.10
Transmedullary Hypothesis

Ball and Dayan [10] described another hypothesis based on observations after intrathecal injections of water-soluble contrast media. After some time, contrast accumulated in the syrinx [8, 21, 44, 85, 147]. Detailed studies were done to find out whether contrast had entered the cord via the fourth ventricle and obex or with transparenchymal flow. The latter appeared to be the mechanism. Ball and Dayan [10] explained this effect by proclaiming flow of contrast along extracellular pathways (so-called Virchow-Robin spaces) into the cord provided a block of CSF flow, causing a sufficient increase of subarachnoid pressure.

Pressure recordings in the SAS and syrinx cavities, however, proved higher pressure in the syrinx than in the surrounding SAS [36, 48], also calling into question Oldfield' theory [121] mentioned above.

1.2.1.11
Edema Hypothesis

Tannenberg [152] in 1924 and Liber and Lisa [94] in 1937 considered syringomyelia to be the endstage of spinal cord edema. They thought edema fluid accumulated in the cord due to blockage of Virchow-Robin spaces [94] or the central canal [152]. Aboulker [2], Yamada et al. [180], and Taylor and Byrnes [160] further elaborated on these ideas and emphasized the additional importance of venous obstruction which, together with a block of CSF flow, was considered to cause spinal cord edema and later formation of a syringomyelic cavity [2]. Thus, Aboulker combined the transmedullary [10] and edema hypotheses [94, 152]. However, as for Ball and Dayan' hypothesis, Aboulker' theory requires a positive pressure gradient between the SAS and syrinx, whereas measurements suggest a gradient in the opposite direction [36, 48].

References

1. Abbe R, Coley WB (1892) Syringomyelia: operation, exploration of the cord, withdrawal of fluid. J Nerv Ment Dis 19:512–520
2. Aboulker J (1979) La syringomyélie et les liquides intra-rachidiens. Neurochirurgie 25[Suppl]:1–144
3. Adelstein LJ (1938) Surgical treatment of syringomyelia. Am J Surg 40:384–395
4. Alajouanine T, Hornet T, Thurel R, Andre R (1935) Le feutrage arachnoidien postérieur dans la syringomyélie (sa place dans la pathologie des leptomeninges). Rev Neurol (Paris) 64:91–98
5. Allen AR (1911) Surgery of experimental lesion of spinal cord equivalent to crush injury of fracture dislocation of spinal column. A preliminary report. JAMA 57:878–880
6. Allen AR (1914) Remarks of the histopathological changes in the spinal cord due to impact. An experimental study. J Nerv Ment Dis 41:141–147
7. Assenmacher DR, Ducker TB (1971) Experimental traumatic paraplegia. The vascular and pathological changes seen in reversible and irreversible spinal cord lesions. J Bone Joint Surg Am 53:671–680
8. Aubin ML, Vignaud J, Jardin C, Bar D (1981) Computed tomography in 75 clinical cases of syringomyelia. Am J Neuroradiol 2:199–204
9. Babapour B (1999) Experimentelle hydrozephale Hydromyelie. Morphologische und mikroanatomische Veränderungen bei der 6-AN-induzierten hydrozephalen Hydromyelie der Ratte (medical dissertation). Hannover Medical School, Hannover
10. Ball MJ, Dayan AD (1972) Pathogenesis of syringomyelia. Lancet 2:799–801
11. Barbaro NM, Wilson CB, Gutin PH, Edwards MS (1984) Surgical treatment of syringomyelia. Favorable results with syringoperitoneal shunting. J Neurosurg 61:531–538
12. Barnett HJM (1973) Syringomyelia associated with spinal arachnoiditis. In: Barnett HJM, Foster JB, Hudgson P (eds) Syringomyelia. Major problems in neurology. (vol 1) Saunders, London, pp 220–244
13. Bastian HC (1867) On a case of concussion-lesion with extensive secondary degeneration of the spinal cord. Proc R Med Chir Soc London 50:499
14. Becker DP, Wilson JA, Watson GW (1972) The spinal cord central canal: response to experimental hydrocephalus and canal occlusion. J Neurosurg 36:416–424
15. Benini A, Krayenbühl H (1969) Ein neuer chirurgischer Weg zur Behandlung der Hydro- und Syringomyelie: embryologische Grundlage und erste Ergebnisse. Schweiz Med Wochenschr 99:1137–1142
16. Bernstein EP, Horwitt S (1913) Syringomyelia with pathological findings. Med Record 84:698–701

17. Bertrand G (1973) Dynamic factors in the evolution of syringomyelia and syringobulbia. Clin Neurosurg 20:322–333
18. Bielschowsky M, Unger E (1920) Syringomyelie mit Teratom- und extramedullärer Blastombildung: zur Kenntnis der Pathogenese der Syringomyelie. Jahrb Psychiatr Neurol 25:173
19. Blaylock RL (1981) Hydrosyringomyelia of the conus medullaris associated with a thoracic meningeoma. J Neurosurg 54:833–835
20. Boman K, Iivanainen M (1967) Prognosis of syringomyelia. Acta Neurol Scand 43:61–68
21. Bonafe A, Manelfe C, Espagno J, Guirand B, Rascol A (1980) Evaluation of syringomyelia with metrizamide computed tomography myelography. J Comput Assist Tomogr 4:797–802
22. Booz K, Faulhauer K, Donauer E, Nieland F (1979) Morphologische Veränderungen am Zentralkanal der Katze nach Kaolin-Injektion in die Zisterna Magna. Z Mikrosk Anat Forsch 93:643–661
23. Borysowicz J (1967) Results of a treatment of syringomyelia with nitrogen mustard. Pol Med J 6:728–732
24. Bremer FW (1926) Klinische Untersuchungen zur Ätiologie der Syringomyelie, der "Status dysraphicus". Dtsch Z Nervenheilk 95:1–103
25. Brunner JC (1700) Hydrocephalo, sire hydrope capitis. In: Bonneti T (ed) Sepulchretum, Miscellaneous Natural Curios III. (Dec Ann I 1688, 2nd edn, Lib I) Cramer and Perachon, Geneva, p 394
26. Camus J, Roussy G (1914) Cavités médullaires et méningites cervicales: étude expérimentale. Rev Neurol (Paris) 22:213–225
27. Chakrabortty S, Tamaki N, Ehara K, Ide C (1994) Experimental syringomyelia in the rabbit: an ultrastructural study of the spinal cord tissue. Neurosurgery 35:1112–1120
28. Charcot JM, Joffroy A (1869) Deux cas d'atrophie musculaire progressive avec lésions de la substance grise et des faisceaux anterolateraux de la moelle épinière. Arch Physiol 2[Ser 1]:354–367
29. Chiari H (1891) Veränderungen des Kleinhirns infolge von Hydrocephalie des Grosshirns. Dtsch Med Wochenschr 17:1172–1175
30. Chiari H (1896) Über Veränderungen des Kleinhirns, des Pons und der Medulla oblongata infolge von congenitaler Hydrocephalie des Grosshirns. Denkschr Akad Wiss Wien 63:71–116
31. Cho KH, Iwasaki Y, Imamura H, Hida K, Abe H (1994) Experimental model of posttraumatic syringomyelia: the role of adhesive arachnoiditis. J Neurosurg 80:133–139
32. Cifuentes M, Rodriguez S, Perez J, Grondona JM, Rodriguez EM, Fernandez-Llebrez P (1994) Decreased cerebrospinal fluid flow through the central canal of the spinal cord of rats immunologically deprived of Reissner' fibre. Exp Brain Res 98:431–440
33. Cleland J (1883) Contribution to the study of spina bifida, encephalocele, and anencephalus. J Anat Physiol 17:257–291
34. Cohen WA, Young W, DeCrescito V, Horii S, Kricheff II (1985) Posttraumatic syrinx formation: experimental study. AJNR Am J Neuroradiol 6:823–827
35. Czerny LJ, Heinismann JI (1930) Beiträge zur Pathologie und Röntgentherapie der Syringomyelie. Z Neurol Psych 125:573–614
36. Davis CH, Symon L (1989) Mechanisms and treatment in post-traumatic syringomyelia. Br J Neurosurg 3:669–674
37. DeLaPaz RL, Brady TJ, Buonanno FS, New PF, Kistler JP, McGinnis BD, Pykett IL, Taveras JM (1983) Nuclear magnetic resonance (NMR) imaging of Arnold-Chiari type I malformation with hydromyelia. J Comput Assist Tomogr 7:126–129
38. Delherm L, Morel-Kahn M (1930) Treatment of syringomyelia by roentgentherapy. Am J Surg 9:302–314
39. Di Chiro G, Schellinger D (1976) Computed tomography after lumbar intrathecal introduction of metrizamide. Radiology 120:101–104
40. Di Chiro G, Axelbaum SP, Schellinger D, Twigg HL, Ledley RS (1975) Computerized axial tomography in syringomyelia. N Engl J Med 292:13–16
41. Dohrmann GJ (1972) Cervical spinal cord in experimental hydrocephalus. J Neurosurg 37:538–542
42. Donauer E (1989) Syringomyelie. Klinische und experimentelle Studien. Med Habil Univ Homburg, Germany
43. Donauer E, Wussow W, Rascher K, Piepgras U (1986) Radiologic studies in cerebrospinal fluid pathways in experimental hydrocephalus-hydrosyringomyelia. Acta Radiol Suppl 369:251–253
44. Dubois PJ, Drayer BP, Sage M, Osborne D, Heinz ER (1981) Intramedullary penetrance of metrizamide in the dog spinal cord. AJNR Am J Neuroradiol 2:313–317
45. Ducker TB, Kindt GW, Kempe LG (1971) Pathological findings in acute experimental spinal cord trauma. J Neurosurg 35:700–708
46. Durward QJ, Rice GP, Ball MJ, Gilbert JJ, Kaufmann JCE (1982) Selective spinal cordectomy: clinicopathological correlation. J Neurosurg 56:359–367
47. Eisenberg HM, McLennan JE, Welch K (1974) Ventricular perfusion in cats with kaolin-induced hydrocephalus. J Neurosurg 41:20–28
48. Ellertson AB, Greitz T (1970) The distending force in the production of communicating syringomyelia. Lancet 1:1234
49. Elsberg CA (1916) Diagnosis and treatment of surgical diseases of the spinal cord and its membranes. Saunders, Philadelphia
50. Estienne C (1546) La dissection des parties du corps humain divisée en trois livres, book 3. Simon de Collines, Paris
51. Faulhauer K, Donauer E (1985) Experimental hydrocephalus and hydrosyringomyelia in the cat. Radiological findings. Acta Neurochir (Wien) 74:72–80
52. Fehlings MG, Tator CH, Linden RD (1989) The relationship among the severity of spinal cord injury, motor and somatosensory evoked potentials and spinal cord blood flow. Electroencephalogr Clin Neurophysiol 74:241–259
53. Ferry DJ, Hardman JM, Earle KM (1969) Syringomyelia and intramedullary neoplasms. Med Ann Distr Columbia 38:363–365
54. Foster JB, Hudgson P (1973) The surgical treatment of communicating syringomyelia. In: Barnett HJM, Foster JB, Hudgson P (eds) Syringomyelia. Major problems in neurology, vol 1. Saunders, London, pp 64–78

55. Frazier CH (1930) Shall syringomyelia be added to the lesions appropriate for surgical intervention? JAMA 95:1911–1912

56. Frazier CH, Rowe SN (1936) The surgical treatment of syringomyelia. Ann Surg 103:481–497

57. Freeman LW, Wright TW (1953) Experimental observations of concussion and contusion of the spinal cord. Ann Surg 137:433–443

58. Gardner WJ (1965) Hydrodynamic mechanism of syringomyelia: its relationship to myelocele. J Neurol Neurosurg Psychiatry 28:247–259

59. Gardner WJ, Goodall RJ (1950) The surgical treatment of Arnold-Chiari malformation in adults: an explanation of its mechanism and importance of encephalography in diagnosis. J Neurosurg 7:199–206

60. Gardner WJ, Angel J (1959) The mechanism of syringomyelia and its surgical correction. Clin Neurosurg 6:131–140

61. Gardner WJ, Bell HS, Poolos PN, Dohn DF, Steinberg M (1977) Terminal ventriculostomy for syringomyelia. J Neurosurg 46:609–617

62. Giese E, Ossinskaja W (1932) Weitere Beobachtungen über die Röntgentherapie der Syringomyelie. Strahlentherapie 43:739–748

63. Greenwald CH, Eugenio M, Hughes CR, Gardner WJ (1958) The importance of the air shadow of the cisterna magna in encephalographic diagnosis. Radiology 71:695

64. Griffiths IR (1975) Vasogenic edema following acute and chronic spinal cord compression in the dog. J Neurosurg 42:155–165

65. Griffiths IR, Pitts LH, Crawford RA, Trench JG (1978) Spinal cord compression and blood flow. I. The effect of raised cerebrospinal fluid pressure on spinal cord blood flow. Neurology 28:1145–1151

66. Griffiths IR, Trench JG, Crawford RA (1979) Spinal cord blood flow and conduction during experimental cord compression in normotensive and hypertensive dogs. J Neurosurg 50:353–360

67. Grinker RR (1934) Neurology. Charles C. Thomas, Springfield, Illinois, p 914

68. Gull W (1862) Case of progressive atrophy of the muscles of the hands: enlargement of the ventricle of the cord in the cervical region, with atrophy of the gray matter (hydromyelus). Guys Hosp Report 8[Ser 3]:244–250

69. Hackney DB, Asato R, Joseph PM, Carolin MJ, McGrath JT, Grossman RI, Kassab EA, DeSimone D (1986) Hemorrhage and edema in acute spinal cord compression: demonstration by MR imaging. Radiology 161:387–390

70. Hall PV, Muller J, Campbell RL (1975) Experimental hydrosyringomyelia, ischaemic myelopathy, and syringomyelia. J Neurosurg 43:464–470

71. Hall PV, Kalsbeck JE, Wellman HN, Campbell RL, Lewis S (1976) Radioisotope evaluation of experimental hydrosyringomyelia. J Neurosurg 45:181–187

72. Hall P, Godersky J, Muller J, Campbell R, Kalsbeck J (1977) A study of experimental syringomyelia by scanning electron microscopy. Neurosurgery 1:41–47

73. Hall P, Turner M, Aichinger S, Bendick P, Campbell R (1980) Experimental syringomyelia: the relationship between intraventricular and intrasyrinx pressures. J Neurosurg 52:812–817

74. Hallopeau H (1869) Contribution a l'étude de la sclérose diffuse péri-épendymaire. C R Soc Biol 21:169–205

75. Hassin GB (1920) A contribution to the histopathology and histogenesis of syringomyelia. Arch Neurol Psychiatry 3:130–146

76. Henneberg R, Koch M (1923) Zur Pathogenese der Syringomyelie und über Haematomyelie bei Syringomyelie. Monatschr Psychiatr Neurol 54:117–140

77. Hinsdale G (1897) Syringomyelia. International Medical Magazine Company, Philadelphia

78. Hochwald GM (1985) Animal models of hydrocephalus: recent developments. Proc Soc Exp Biol Med 178:1–11

79. Hoffman GS, Ellsworth CA, Wells EE, Frank WA, Mackie RW (1983) Spinal arachnoiditis: what is the clinical spectrum? II. Arachnoiditis induced by Pantopaque/autologous blood in dogs, a possible model for human disease. Spine 8:541–551

80. Holmes G (1915) The Goulstonian Lectures on spinal injuries of warfare. I. The pathology of acute spinal injury. Br Med J 2:769–774

81. Holmes G, Kennedy RF (1909) Two anomalous cases of syringomyelia. Proc R Soc Med 2:1–7

82. Jensen F, Reske-Jensen E (1977) Post-traumatic syringomyelia. Scand J Rehabil Med 9:35–43

83. Jirasek A (1927) Endomyelographie bei Syringomyelie. Zentralbl Chir 54:2447–2452

84. Joffroy A, Achard C (1887) De la myelite cavitaire (observations; reflexions; pathogenie des cavites). Arch Physiol 10[Ser 3, Suppl]:435–472

85. Kan S, Fox AJ, Vinuela F, Barnett HJM, Peerless SJ (1983) Delayed CT metrizamide enhancement of syringomyelia secondary to tumor. AJNR Am J Neuroradiol 4:73–78

86. Kasantikul V, Netsky MG, James AE (1979) Relation of age and cerebral ventricle size to central canal in man. Morphological analysis. J Neurosurg 51:85–93

87. Kirgis HD, Echols DH (1949) Syringo-encephalomyelia. Discussion of related syndromes and pathologic processes, with a report of a case. J Neurosurg 6:368–375

88. Kiwitt JCW, Lanksch WR, Fritsch H, Luis E, Stork W, Roosen N, Schirmer M, Bock W, Marguth F (1988) Magnetic resonance tomography of solid spinal cord tumors with extensive secondary syringomyelia. Adv Neurosurg 16:211–215

89. Krayenbühl H (1974) Evaluation of the different surgical approaches in the treatment of syringomyelia. Clin Neurol Neurosurg 77:110–128

90. Kuwamura K, McLone D, Raimondi AJ (1978) The central (spinal) canal in congenital murine hydrocephalus: morphological and physiological aspects. Child's Brain 4:216–234

91. Laha RK, Malik HG, Langille RA (1975) Post-traumatic syringomyelia. Surg Neurol 4:519–522

92. Lesoin F, Petit H, Thomas CE III, Viaud C, Baleriaux D, Jomin M (1986) Use of the syringoperitoneal shunt in the treatment of syringomyelia. Surg Neurol 25:131–136

93. L'Hermitte J, Boveri P (1912) Sur un cas de cavité médullaire consécutive à une compression bulbaire chez l'homme et étude expérimentale des cavités spinales produites par la compression. Rev Neurol (Paris) 20:385–393

94. Liber AF, Lisa JR (1937) Rosenthal fibres in non-neoplastic syringomyelia: a note on the pathogenesis of syringomyelia. J Nerv Ment Dis 86:549–558

95. Lichtenstein BW (1942) Distant neuroanatomic complications of spina bifida (spinal dysraphism). Hydrocephalus, Arnold-Chiari malformation, stenosis of aquaeduct of Sylvius, etc.; pathogenesis and pathology. Arch Neurol Psychiatry 47:195–214

96. Lichtenstein BW (1943) Cervical syringomyelia and syringomyelia-like states associated with Arnold-Chiari deformity and platybasia. Arch Neurol Psychiatry 49:881–894

97. Lohle PN, Wurzer HAL, Hoogland PH, Seelen PJ, Go KG (1994) The pathogenesis of syringomyelia in spinal cord ependymoma. Clin Neurol Neurosurg 96:323–326

98. Love JG, Olafson RA (1966) Syringomyelia: a look at surgical therapy. J Neurosurg 24:714–718

99. Markow DA, Gorjelik R, Liwschitz S (1932) Über die Röntgentherapie der spinalen Gliose. Strahlentherapie 45:349–354

100. Martinez-Arizala A, Mora J, Green B, Hayashi N (1990) Dorsal spinal venous occlusion model in the rat: preliminary observations. Soc Neurosci Abstr 16:992

101. McConnell AA, Parker HI (1938) A deformity of the hind-brain associated with internal hydrocephalus. Its relation to the Arnold-Chiari malformation. Brain 61:415–429

102. McGrath JT (1965) Spinal dysraphism in the dog with comments on syringomyelia. Pathol Vet 2[Suppl]:1–36

103. McLaurin RL, Bailey OT, Schurr PH, Ingraham FD (1954) Myelomalacia and multiple cavitations of spinal cord secondary to adhesive arachnoiditis. Arch Pathol 57:138–146

104. McVeigh JF (1923) Experimental cord crushes: with special reference to the mechanical factors involved and subsequent changes in the areas of the cord affected. Arch Surg 7:573–600

105. Means ED, Anderson DR, Waters TR, Kalaf L (1981) Effects of methylprednisolone in compressive trauma to the feline spinal cord. J Neurosurg 55:200–208

106. Milhorat TH, Adler DE, Heger IM, Miller JI, Hollenberg-Sher JR (1991) Histopathology of experimental hematomyelia. J Neurosurg 75:911–915

107. Milhorat TH, Johnson WD, Miller JI, Bergland RM, Hollenberg-Sher J (1992) Surgical treatment of syringomyelia based on magnetic resonance imaging criteria. Neurosurgery 31:231–245

108. Milhorat TH, Nobandegani F, Miller JI, Rao C (1993) Noncommunicating syringomyelia following occlusion of central canal in rats. Experimental model and histological findings. J Neurosurg 78:274–279

109. Milhorat TH, Kotzen RM, Anzil AP (1994) Stenosis of central canal of spinal cord in man: incidence and pathological findings in 232 autopsy cases. J Neurosurg 80:716–722

110. Mixter WJ (1936) Discussion of Frazier CH, Rowe SN. The surgical treatment of syringomyelia. Ann Surg 103:497

111. Morgagni GB (Alexander B, translator) (1769) The seats and causes of disease (letter XII, article 9). Millar and Cadel, London, p 370

112. Mucenieks P (1933) Über die operative Therapie der Syringomyelie. Dtsch Z Chir 240:346–361

113. Murthy VS, Deshpande DH (1980) The central canal of the filum terminale in communicating hydrocephalus. J Neurosurg 53:528–532

114. Nakamura S, Camins MB, Hochwald GM (1983) Pressure-absorption responses to the infusion of fluid into the spinal cord central canal of kaolin-hydrocephalic cats. J Neurosurg 58:198–203

115. Netsky MG (1953) Syringomyelia: a clinicopathologic study. Arch Neurol Psychiatry 70:741–777

116. Newman PK, Terenty TR, Foster JB (1981) Some observations on the pathogenesis of syringomyelia. J Neurol Neurosurg Psychiatry 44:964–969

117. Noble LJ, Wrathall WD (1985) Spinal cord contusion in the rat. Morphometric analyses of alterations in the cord. Exp Neurol 88:135–149

118. Noble LJ, Wrathall JR (1989) Correlative analysis of lesion development and functional status after graded spinal cord contusive injuries in the rat. Exp Neurol 103:34–40

119. Norman D, Mills CM, Brant-Zawadski M, Yeates A, Crooks LE, Kaufman L (1983) Magnetic resonance imaging of the spinal cord and canal: potentials and limitations. AJNR Am J Neuroradiol 141:1147–1152

120. Oi S, Kudo H, Yamada H, Kim S, Hamano S, Urui S, Matsumoto S (1991) Hydromyelic hydrocephalus. Correlation of hydromyelia with various stages of hydrocephalus in postshunt isolated compartments. J Neurosurg 74:371–379

121. Oldfield EH, Muraszko K, Shawker TH, Patronas NJ (1994) Pathophysiology of syringomyelia associated with Chiari I malformation of the cerebellar tonsils. Implications for diagnosis and treatment. J Neurosurg 80:3–15

122. Ollivier D'Angers CP (1827) De le moelle épinière et de ses maladies, 2nd edn. Chez Crevot, Paris

123. Oppel WA (1929) Erfahrungen mit der operativen Behandlung der Syringomyelie nach Pousepp. Arch Klin Chir 155:416–434

124. Ostertag B (1925) Zur Frage der dysraphischen Störungen des Rückenmarks und der von ihnen abzuleitenden Geschwulstbildungen. Arch Psychiatr Nervenkr 75:89–143

125. Ostertag B (1930) Weitere Untersuchung über die vererbbare Syringomyelie beim Kaninchen. Zentralbl Ges Neurol Psychiatr 57:426

126. Padovani R, Cavallo M, Gaist G (1989) Surgical treatment of syringomyelia: favorable results with syringosubarachnoid shunting. Surg Neurol 32:173–180

127. Peiper H (1931) Die operative Behandlung der Syringomyelie. Nervenarzt 4:436–453

128. Penfield W, Coburn DF (1938) Arnold-Chiari malformation and its operative treatment. Arch Neurol Psychiatry 40:328–336

129. Philippon J, Sangla S, Lara-Morales J, Gazengel J, Rivierez M, Horn YE (1988) Treatment of syringomyelia by syringo-peritoneal shunt. Acta Neurochir Suppl (Wien) 43:32–34

130. Phillips TW, Kindt GW (1981) Syringoperitoneal shunt for syringomyelia: a preliminary report. Surg Neurol 16:462–466

131. Portal A (1804) Cours d'anatomie médicale, vol 4. Boudouin, Paris

132. Pousepp L (1926) Traitement opératoire dans deux cas de syringomyélie avec amélioration notable. Rev Neurol (Paris) 43:1171–1179

133. Rascher K, Booz KH, Donauer E, Nacimento AC (1987) Structural alterations in the spinal cord during progressive communicating syringomyelia. An experimental study in the cat. Acta Neuropathol (Berl) 72:248–255

134. Raymond F (1905) La syringomyélie. Rev Gen Clin Therapeut 19:817–818

135. Retif J (1964) Syringomyélie et phacomatose. Acta Neurol Belg 64:832–851

136. Rhoton AL Jr (1976) Microsurgery of Arnold-Chiari malformation in adults with and without hydromyelia. J Neurosurg 45:473–483

137. Rice-Edwards JM (1977) A pathological study of syringomyelia. J Neurol Neurosurg Psychiatry 40:198

138. Rivlin AS, Tator CH (1978) Effect of duration of acute spinal cord compression in a new acute injury model in the rat. Surg Neurol 10:39–43

139. Rossier AB, Foo D, Shillito J, Dyro FM (1985) Posttraumatic syringomyelia: incidence, clinical presentation, electrophysiological studies, syrinx protein and results of conservative and operative treatment. Brain 108:439–461

140. Russel DS, Donald C (1935) Mechanism of internal hydrocephalus in spina bifida. Brain 58:203–215

141. Sahatchieff S (1912) Le traitement de la syringomyélie par rayons X. Bulletin Officiel de la Société Française d'Electrothérapie et de la Radiologie Médicale, Paris, p 233

142. Samii M, Klekamp J (1994) Surgical results for 100 intramedullary tumors in relation to accompanying syringomyelia. Neurosurgery 35:865–873

143. Schaeffer H (1932) Le traitment opératoire de la syringomyélie. Presse Med 40:379–383

144. Schlesinger H (1895) Die Syringomyelie. Franz Deuticke, Leipzig, Wien

145. Schmaus H (1890) Commotio spinalis. In: Lubarsch O, Ostertag R (eds) Ergebnisse der allgemeinen Pathologie und pathologischen Anatomie des Menschen und der Tiere. Bergmann, Wiesbaden, pp 674–713

146. Schwarz E (1897) Präparate von einem Falle syphilitischer Myelomeningitis mit Höhlenbildung im Rückenmarke und besonderer degenerativen Veränderungen der Neuroglia. Wien Klin Wochenschr 7:177–178

147. Seibert CE, Dreisbach JN, Swanson WB, Edgar RE, Williams P, Hahn H (1981) Progressive posttraumatic cystic myelopathy: neuroradiologic evaluation. AJR Am J Roentgenol 136:1161–1166

148. Sicard J, Forestier J (1921) Méthode radiographique d'exploration de la cavité épidurale par le lipiodol. Rev Neurol (Paris) 36:1264–1266

149. Simon T (1875) Beiträge zur Pathologie und pathologischen Anatomie des Central-Nervensystems. Arch Psychiatr 5:108–163

150. Spiller WG (1908) The association of syringomyelia with tabes dorsalis. J Med Res 18:149–158

151. Tamaki K, Lubin AJ (1938) Pathogenesis of syringomyelia: case illustrating the process of cavity formation from embryonic cell rests. Arch Neurol Psychiatry 40:748–761

152. Tannenberg J (1924) Über die Pathogenese der Syringomyelie, zugleich ein Beitrag zum Vorkommen von Capillarhaemangiomen im Rueckenmark. Z Neurol 92:119–174

153. Tarlov IM, Klinger H (1954) Spinal cord compression studies. Time limits for recovery after acute compression in dogs. Arch Neurol Psychiatry 71:271–290

154. Tarlov IM, Klinger H, Vitale S (1953) Spinal cord compression studies. Experimental techniques to produce acute and gradual compression. Arch Neurol Psychiatry 70:813–819

155. Tatara N (1992) [Experimental syringomyelia in rabbits and rats after localized spinal arachnoiditis.] No To Shinkei 44:1115–1125

156. Tator CH (1991) Review of experimental spinal cord injury with emphasis on the local and systemic circulatory effects. Neurochirurgie 37:291–302

157. Tator CH, Deecke L (1973) Value of normothermic perfusion, hypothermic perfusion and durotomy in the treatment of experimental acute spinal cord trauma. J Neurosurg 39:52–64

158. Tator CH, Meguro K, Rowed DW (1982) Favorable results with syringosubarachnoid shunts for treatment of syringomyelia. J Neurosurg 56:517–523

159. Tauber ES, Langworthy OR (1935) A study of syringomyelia and the formation of cavities in the spinal cord. J Nerv Ment Dis 81:245–264

160. Taylor AR, Byrnes DP (1974) Foramen magnum and high cervical cord compression. Brain 97:473–480

161. Taylor J, Greenfield JG, Martin JP (1922) Two cases of syringomyelia and syringobulbia, observed clinically over many years, and examined pathologically. Brain 45:323–356

162. Van Houweninge Graftdijk CJ (1932) Over hydrocephalus. Eduard Ijdo, Leyden

163. Vaquero J, Ramiro MJ, Oya S, Cabezudo JM (1981) Ependymal reaction after experimental spinal cord injury. Acta Neurochir (Wien) 55:295–302

164. Wagner FC Jr, Stewart WB (1981) Effect of trauma dose on spinal cord edema. J Neurosurg 54:802–806

165. Wagner FC Jr, Van Gilder JC, Dohrmann GJ (1977) The development of intramedullary cavitation following spinal cord injury. An experimental pathological study. Paraplegia 14:245–250

166. Wedeen VJ, Rosen BR, Chesler D, Brady TJ (1985) MR velocity imaging by phase display. J Comput Assist Tomogr 9:530–536

167. Wiedemayer H, Nau HE, Raukut F, Gerhard L, Reinhard V, Grote W (1990) Pathogenesis and operative treatment of syringomyelia. Adv Neurosurg 18:119–125

168. Williams B (1970) Current concepts of syringomyelia. Br J Hosp Med 4:331–342

169. Williams B (1976) Cerebrospinal fluid pressure changes in response to coughing. Brain 99:331–346

170. Williams B (1978) A critical appraisal of posterior fossa surgery for communicating syringomyelia. Brain 101:223–250

171. Williams B (1980) Experimental communicating syringomyelia in dogs after cisternal kaolin injection. II. Pressure studies. J Neurol Sci 48:109–122

172. Williams B (1980) On the pathogenesis of syringomyelia: a review. J R Soc Med 73:798–806

173. Williams B (1981) Simultaneous cerebral and spinal fluid pressure recordings. I. Technique, physiology, and normal results. Acta Neurochir (Wien) 58:167–185

174. Williams B (1981) Simultaneous cerebral and spinal fluid pressure recordings. II. Cerebrospinal dissociation with lesions at the foramen magnum. Acta Neurochir (Wien) 59:123–142

175. Williams B (1986) Progress in syringomyelia. Neurol Res 8:130–145

176. Williams B (1990) Syringomyelia. Neurosurg Clin N Am 1:653–685

177. Williams B, Page N (1987) Surgical treatment of syringomyelia with syringopleural shunting. Br J Neurosurg 1:63–80

178. Wilson CB, Bertan V, Norrell HA, Hukuda S (1969) Experimental cervical myelopathy. II. Acute ischemic myelopathy. Arch Neurol 21:571–589

179. Wisoff JH, Epstein F (1989) Management of hydromyelia. Neurosurgery 25:562–571

180. Yamada H, Yokota A, Haratake J, Horie A (1996) Morphological study of experimental syringomyelia with kaolin-induced hydrocephalus in a canine model. J Neurosurg 84:999–1005

181. Yeates A, Brant-Zawadski M, Norman D, Kaufman L, Crooks LE, Newton TH (1983) Nuclear magnetic resonance imaging of syringomyelia. AJNR Am J Neuroradiol 4:234–237

182. Yezierski RP, Santana M, Park SH, Madsen PW (1993) Neuronal degeneration and spinal cavitation following intraspinal injections of quisqualic acid in the rat. J Neurotrauma 10:445–456

2 The Pathophysiology of Syringomyelia

We have analyzed more than 500 patients with syringomyelia who were treated within the past 20 years. Either at the craniocervical junction or in the spinal canal, an associated pathology could be found in each patient. Each associated pathology was in close anatomical relation to the syrinx cavity and caused CSF flow obstruction and/or spinal cord tethering to some degree. The best long-term results for treatment of syringomyelia were obtained with successful treatment of the associated pathology.

These observations alone call into question whether a syrinx may develop in its own right or – to put it in other words – whether an idiopathic syrinx exists. A pathophysiological hypothesis of syringomyelia has to analyze the associated pathologies and incorporate studies on CSF circulation, spinal cord mobility, fluid movements in the SAS and central nervous system, and effects of the vascular and respiratory systems.

Harbitz and Lossius already emphasized in 1929 [43] the importance of CSF flow disturbances in patients with syringomyelia. However, they were unable to incorporate this observation into a pathophysiological concept. To do this, a number of questions need to be answered:

1. How is the flow of fluid in the SAS regulated?
2. How is the flow of fluid in spinal cord tissue regulated?
3. How are fluid movements in subarachnoid and extracellular space interrelated?
4. How do arterial and venous pressure changes influence CSF and ECF flow?
5. How does movement of the spinal cord change tissue pressures therein?

2.1
Anatomical Background

Numerous studies have shown that extracellular space (ECS) and SAS are two parts of a single fluid compartment [5, 11, 13, 14, 16, 48, 49, 55, 63, 67, 77, 79, 82, 91, 95, 101, 108, 109, 110]. The only anatomical barriers between them are the pia mater on the surface of the central nervous system and the ependyma cells of ventricles or central canal.

The ependyma allows a slow passage of substances between ECS and SAS and is part of a metabolic system which eliminates toxic waste products from CSF and ECF [5, 19]. Free fluid passage across the ependymal layer does not exist under physiological conditions. In the central canal of man, fluid moves from the spinal canal toward the cranial cavity. Guillain proposed in 1899 [39] that fluid flow from the central canal into the ventricle system was an important part of the lymphatic system of the central nervous system. Figure 2.1 demonstrates the extraordinarily rare observation of such fluid transport in the central canal. In the patient of the figure, a dermoid cyst at level L3 to L5 was successively drained into the central canal, which expanded over several months due to this fatty fluid and formed a syrinx up to the level of C2.

At the surface of the brain and spinal cord, the situation is different. Pia mater cells are connected by desmosomes and so-called gap junctions [1, 9, 47, 56, 108]. Electron microscopic studies were able to demonstrate fenestrations in the pia mater of the spinal canal, predominantly at the root entry zones [13, 55, 63]. In this way, free communication exists between SAS and perivascular spaces (i.e., Virchow-Robins spaces) of the ECS [1, 13, 20, 47, 48, 53, 55, 56, 63, 70, 95, 113].

The cells of the arachnoid, unlike the pia mater, are connected by so-called tight junctions, so that this layer is not fluid permeable [60, 108]. The accumulation of water-soluble contrast media in the parenchyma of the central nervous system after intrathecal injection can be explained on this anatomical basis [2, 23, 26, 34, 49, 50, 108, 113]. The pia mater functions as a barrier only for cells or substances of high molecular weight [47, 113]. Perivascular spaces can be found throughout the central nervous system, reaching from the surface to the ependymal layer in close relationship to capillaries, arterioles, and venules [20]. Further analysis of perivascular spaces revealed that they contained a complex array of collagen fibers and free cells which may differentiate to macrophages. During inflammatory reactions, these cells can alter their shape in such a way that they may penetrate through the pia mater fenestrations and move into the SAS [63]. Therefore, pia mater fenestrations are important for transfer of fluid between SAS and ECS

[113] and for immunological reactions of the central nervous system [30, 63]. Additional studies have demonstrated further connection of the SAS to the extracranial lymphatic system [7, 8, 31], similar to the ideas originally suggested by Guillain in 1899 [39].

2.2
Fluid Movements in the Extracellular and Subarachnoid Spaces

Two forms of fluid movement have to be distinguished: diffusion and bulk flow. Diffusion describes the passage of fluid according to chemical concentration gradients. Bulk flow, however, consists of fluid movement according to pressure gradients. Most studies regarding fluid movements in the ECS concentrate on the genesis and resorption of edema. In this condition, bulk flow plays a predominant role. It could be demonstrated that edema fluid expands along perivascular channels and is cleared toward the SAS [15, 35, 37, 38, 44, 45, 68, 71, 72, 81, 90, 102]. The expansion of posttraumatic edema in the spinal cord, for instance, is guided by bulk flow [100]. Arachnoid scarring in the spinal canal alters CSF flow and changes subarachnoid and intraparenchymal pressures so that interstitial edema of the spinal cord may develop due to aggravation of ECF flow [54]. Lowering the arterial blood pressure slows down bulk flow in the ECS and, thus, the resorption of edema fluid [61].

Whether or not bulk flow occurs under physiological conditions is a matter of debate [17, 40, 54, 62, 71, 83]. During cardiac systole, blood enters the brain and spinal cord, resulting in a volume increase of these organs. This volume effect has consequences for CSF and ECF flow. In SAS, the arachnoidal cisterns are compressed, so that CSF is pushed out of the cisterns into the SAS. In ECS, perivascular spaces along arterioles are likewise compressed, whereas those along venules dilate [87].

During cardiac diastole, blood returns to the heart with a consequent decrease of brain and spinal cord volumes. Basal cisterns dilate, which causes CSF flow into the cisterns, and perivascular channels along arterioles expand while those along venules become compressed [87].

These volume changes in perivascular spaces may induce fluid movements in the ECS, i.e., bulk flow. It has been proposed that, during systole, ECF flows toward and into the SAS; whereas, during diastole, CSF enters the parenchyma and ECF is directed towards the ependyma [5, 30, 79, 95]. Additionally, pressure in the SAS is governed by arterial pressure during systole and by venous pressure during diastole [42]. By ligating the aorta to block arterial flow, no pulsations in Virchow-Robin spaces [61, 79] or subarachnoid cisterns occur [87]. Hence, flow of CSF and ECF ceases, except for flow phenomena according to respiratory

pressure changes mediated to the spinal SAS along the epidural venous plexus [33, 52, 59, 74, 88, 104, 106, 107].

In the spinal canal, CSF flow velocities decrease toward the lumbar region; the highest velocities are observed in the cervical and thoracic canal [24, 28, 36, 76, 85, 92, 93]. Rennels et al. [80] could demonstrate faster flow of horseradish peroxidase (HRP) from the SAS into the ECS of the spinal cord if the marker was injected into the cisterna magna versus injection into the lumbar SAS. In other words, flow of HRP across the pia mater into the ECS was faster in areas of higher CSF flow velocities. This finding would be in accordance with the assumption that CSF and ECF flow are related to each other [46, 54, 96]. Pressure changes in the SAS are mediated to dura mater, epidural space on one side, and spinal cord on the other side – and vice versa [25]. Therefore, alterations of CSF flow will have a direct impact on ECF flow [54, 96].

The pressure in the SAS also has an impact on microcirculation and vice versa. Bower et al. [6] could show that lowering CSF pressure by aspiration of CSF significantly improves microcirculation of the spinal cord in dogs after ligation of the thoracic aorta, presumably by lowering the perfusion pressure in the cord along with the subarachnoid pressure. On the venous side Cassar-Pullicino et al. [10] were able to demonstrate, in cases of spinal trauma, reverse flow in the paravertebral venous plexus. This elevated venous pressure interferes with spinal cord venous drainage and causes an elevation of pressure in the SAS. This may cause an increase of ECF in the spinal cord, diluting potentially toxic material, but may also be one mechanism of edema formation in patients after spinal cord trauma. Necrotic material, blood products, and other substances are then transported in the central canal in cranial direction, as shown in animal experiments [65] and neuroradiological studies in man [41].

2.3
Tethered Cord and Extracellular Space

Effects of tethering on the spinal cord have only been investigated in two aspects: metabolism and microcirculation [21, 22, 75, 111]. Fuse et al. demonstrated that axonal transport of HRP is not altered in animals with a tethered cord [32]. The influence of spinal cord movements on fluid transport in the ECS have not yet been studied.

However, patients with syringomyelia report quite often that they can provoke symptoms by exerting certain movements of their neck or head [97]. Tachibana et al. [98] demonstrated in dogs that intramedullary pressure increased with neck flexion and decreased with retroflexion or extension. After transsection of nerve roots and dentate ligaments, neck movements no longer changed the intramedullary pressure.

In man, the most extensive spinal cord movements can be observed in the cervical area. A 1.8–2.8 cm range of movement has been measured [73]. The interplay of spinal cord movements, CSF flow, and ECF flow may be altered significantly by spinal cord tethering. Patients may experience pathological intramedullary pressure changes when exerting certain neck movements, if mobility of the cervical cord is restricted as suggested by animal experiments [54]. This may explain why a syrinx can occur in a patient with a tethered cord but without associated disturbances of CSF flow [51, 70, 86].

2.4
Pathophysiological Concept

Syringomyelia is a collection of ECF in the spinal cord and is associated with an increase of ECF volume and aggravated bulk flow in the ECS (Fig. 2.1). Depending on local flow resistances, ECF may accumulate predominantly in the central canal or in the spinal cord ECS itself. The following mechanisms may be responsible:

▶ Aggravation of ECF flow exceeding ECS capacities
- Due to obstruction of CSF flow
- Due to altered spinal cord movements associated with a tethered cord
- Due to altered spinal cord microcirculation
▶ Obstruction of ECF flow toward SAS
- Due to higher viscosity of ECF
- Due to obstruction of perivascular spaces
- Due to altered spinal cord microcirculation

With obstruction of CSF flow, all forces promoting CSF flow are still acting on the SAS [107] and are mediated toward the ECS. With increased flow resistance in the SAS, fluid movements are aggravated in the ECS; i.e., ECF flow and volume increase because, in contrast to the SAS, flow resistances are not elevated in the ECS [54]. Li and Chui [57] showed that water-soluble contrast injected into the SAS accumulates faster in the spinal cord than in the controls, as is consistent with an increase of ECF flow in patients with syringomyelia. Observation of profound fluid movement in the syrinx itself is in accordance with this concept [4, 29, 52, 92, 94, 99] and may resemble the effect, which Williams [105] named "slosh".

If ECF cannot be cleared sufficiently into the SAS [3, 12, 103], perivascular channels dilate [12, 54, 66, 78, 89], ECF volume increases, and a syrinx develops. Exchange between CSF and ECF may be further interrupted due to arachnoid adhesions [58] obstructing the pia mater fenestrations. This concept also explains the results of subarachnoid and syrinx pressure recordings. Pressure is higher inside the syrinx than in the surrounding SAS [18, 27]. Neuropathological studies show that approxi-

mately 22–37% of the syringomyelic cavities had perforated the pia mater to establish free communication with the SAS [67], adding further evidence that syrinx pressures exceed subarachnoid pressures. Similarly, intramedullary pressures are higher than in the SAS adjacent to the level of arachnoid scarring, where interstitial edema develops [54]. In patients with a tethered cord, spine movements may cause altered intramedullary pressures [98]; thus, pressure gradients and fluid flow in the SAS and ECS may be altered.

The relationship to spinal cord blood flow was analyzed by Young et al. [112] who demonstrated reduced spinal cord blood flow prior to shunting of the syrinx. This finding could indicate a reduced perfusion pressure due to the syrinx. Once the syrinx was opened and collapsed with insertion of the drain, blood flow improved.

Alterations of spinal cord microcirculation could form the basis of syringomyelia associated with vascular anomalies such as hemangioblastomas. Small tumor nodules may cause significant cystic cavitations in the spinal cord, due to aggravated ECF flow combined with a disruption of the blood–brain barrier so that exudate may accumulate in the ECS. The high viscosity of the exudate prohibits an easy clearance towards the SAS and favors the development of an intramedullary cyst.

The major pathophysiological mechanism in patients with intramedullary tumors, however, may be obstruction of ECF flow pathways. The incidence of syringomyelia is higher in tumors which compress and displace spinal cord tissue, i.e., ependymomas, angioblastomas, etc., than in infiltrating neoplasms, such as astrocytomas. Furthermore, the incidence of syringomyelia increases according to the spinal level – i.e., the cervical area with the highest CSF and, presumably, the highest ECF flow velocities is the predominantly affected area [84]. Obstruction of Virchow-Robin spaces, changes of ECF flow in highly vascularized tumors, and changes of ECF viscosity due to higher protein content may act synergistically and ultimately lead to formation of a syrinx.

If we understand syringomyelia as a state of chronic interstitial edema, where ECF is trapped in the spinal cord due to CSF flow obstruction, spinal cord tethering, or an intramedullary tumor, then we can explain all of the experimental and clinical observations mentioned in the historical and pathophysiological overviews presented so far. The following chapters of this book will provide treatment strategies for patients with syringomyelia based on this pathophysiological concept.

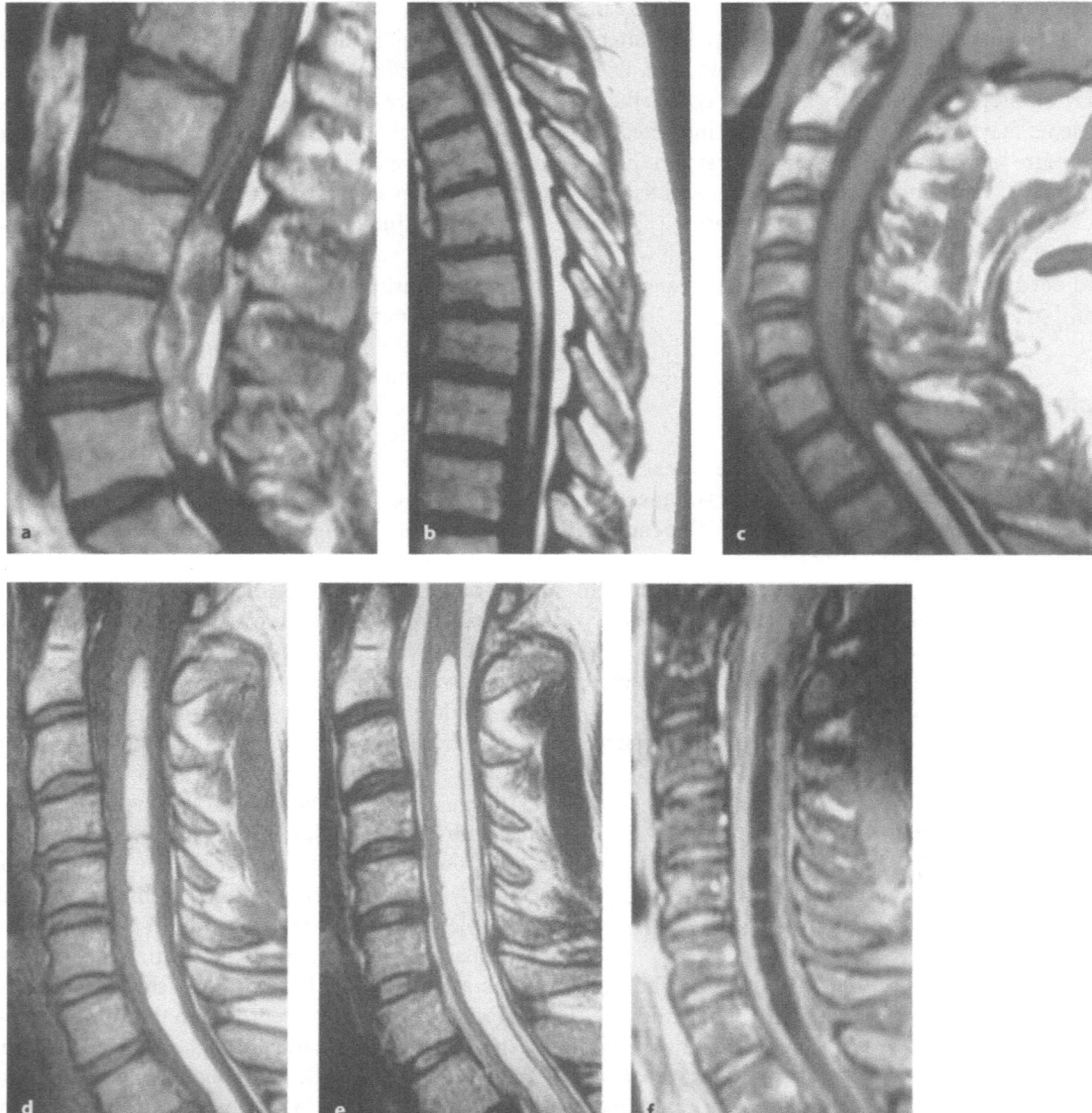

Fig. 2.1 a–f. This 33-year-old man presented with slight back pain and minor sensorimotor deficits of his lower limbs. (a) The MRI shows a large dermoid cyst from the levels of L3 to L5. At that time, a scan of the thoracic spine demonstrated distension of the central canal area by a substance that resembled fat in terms of its signal properties. (b) This phenomenon could be observed up to the level of Th1 (c). The scan was repeated 6 months later. Now a large cyst could be seen up to the level of C2 (d–f). T1- (d), T2- (e), and T2-weighted images under fat suppression (f) all demonstrated signal properties suggestive of fat. Therefore, it was concluded that the dermoid cyst had ruptured into the central canal so that the fluid was successively drained in cranial direction. The unphysiologically high viscosity of this fluid might have been responsible for the sustained dilatation of the central canal, resulting in syringomyelia

2.5
Disorders Associated with Syringomyelia

Idiopathic syringomyelia does not exist. Therefore, successful management of patients with syringomyelia requires, foremost, identification and appropriate management of the underlying disorder. If this can be achieved, syringomyelia no longer poses a threatening clinical problem because, at least, further progression of neurological symptoms will be prevented. Outcome and prognosis of patients with syringomyelia are determined primarily by the disease process which has caused the syrinx. In other words, it is not the syringomyelia but the causative pathology that primarily needs treatment. Table 2.1 gives an overview of the pathologies which may be associated with syringomyelia.

Apart from clinical analysis, modern imaging techniques such as MRI and phase-contrast cine MRI offer the opportunity to diagnose syringomyelia easily; these methods can also follow, neuroradiologically, how a syrinx develops and how different treatment modalities influence the extent and caliber of a syrinx. However, additional imaging modalities, such as myelography or CT, may still be required to identify the underlying disorder. With careful review of neuroradiological studies of the entire spinal axis, the underlying disorder usually becomes obvious. MRI studies should always demonstrate the entire syrinx as the underlying cause may be located at either end. These should always include a study with gadolinium to search for an intramedullary tumor.

However, sometimes standard techniques do not disclose the underlying pathology. What should be done in such a patient? If syringomyelia develops due to CSF flow obstruction, spinal cord tethering, or a neoplastic process, we may draw two important conclusions in our search for the underlying pathology in a patient presenting with a syrinx.

1. Clinically, the first neurological symptoms to appear will most likely be related to the disorder that causes the syrinx, rather than the syrinx itself. In other words, a carefully taken case history provides important information for identification of the underlying disorder. The first symptoms noted by the patient usually point to the anatomical region where the disorder will be found.
2. Radiologically, a syrinx expands directionally away from the underlying pathology. Classically, the upper or lower part of the syrinx will be in close anatomical contact to this pathology. Serial MRI studies taken over months or years, even, may disclose the spinal level of the underlying disorder by depicting changes of syrinx diameter and extension. The diameter of the syrinx is usually largest at

Table 2.1

1. Syringomyelia in association with diseases at the craniocervical junction

   Malformations

      Chiari malformation

      Basilar invagination

      Disorders associated with a small volume of the posterior fossa

      Rhombencephalic malformations

   Arachnopathy

      Postmeningitic

      Postsurgical

      Posthemorrhagic

      Posttraumatic

   Tumors of the posterior fossa

   Supratentorial tumors

2. Syringomyelia in association with diseases of the spinal canal

   Malformations

      Spina bifida

      Tethered cord syndrome

      Diastematomyelia

   Tumors

      Intramedullary

      Extramedullary

      Extradural

   Arachnopathy

      Posttraumatic

      Postmeningitic

      Postsurgical

      Posthemorrhagic

   Degenerative diseases of the spine

      Disc Disease

      Scoliosis

      Kyphosis

the level closest to the pathology and the syrinx will progress to further spinal levels at the opposite end; i.e., if the syrinx progresses caudally, the underlying pathology will be found at the cranial pole of the syrinx and vice versa.

With these assumptions in mind, it can usually be decided quite easily whether a syrinx has developed due to pathology at the craniocervical junction or elsewhere in the spinal canal. The following chapters will deal with each of the disease processes shown in Table 2.1 and will present guidelines toward their diagnosis, prognosis, surgical indications, treatment modalities, and clinical outcomes.

References

1. Alcolado R, Weller RO, Parrish EP, Garrod D (1988) The cranial arachnoid and pia mater in man: anatomical and ultrastructural observations. Neuropathol Appl Neurobiol 14:1–17
2. Aubin ML, Vignaud J, Jardin C, Bar D (1981) Computed tomography in 75 clinical cases of syringomyelia. AJNR Am J Neuroradiol 2:199–204
3. Avrahami E, Tadmor R, Cohn DF (1989) Magnetic resonance imaging in patients with progressive myelopathy following spinal surgery. J Neurol Neurosurg Psychiatry 52:176–181
4. Barkovich AJ, Sherman JL, Citrin CM, Wippold FJ II (1987) MR of postoperative syringomyelia. AJNR Am J Neuroradiol 8:319–327
5. Borison HL, Borison R, McCarthy LE (1980) Brain stem penetration by horseradish peroxidase from the cerebrospinal fluid spaces in the cat. Exp Neurol 69:271–289
6. Bower TC, Murray MJ, Gloviczki P, Yaksh TL, Hollier LH, Pairolero PC (1989) Effects of thoracic aortic occlusion and cerebrospinal fluid drainage on regional spinal cord blood flow in dogs: correlation with neurologic outcome. J Vasc Surg 9:135–144
7. Bradbury MWB, Cserr HF, Westrop RJ (1981) Drainage of cerebral interstitial fluid into deep cervical lymph of the rabbit. Am J Physiol 240:F329–F336
8. Brierley JB (1950) The penetration of particulate matter from the cerebrospinal fluid into the spinal ganglia, peripheral nerves, and perivascular spaces of the central nervous system. J Neurol Neurosurg Psychiatry 13:203–215
9. Brightman MW, Reese TS (1969) Junctions between intimately apposed cell membranes in the vertebrate brain. J Cell Biol 40:648–677
10. Cassar-Pullicino VN, Colhoun E, McLelland M, McCall IW, El Masry W (1995) Hemodynamic alterations in the paravertebral venous plexus after spinal injury. Radiology 97:659–663
11. Castro ME, Portnoy HD, Maesaka J (1991) Elevated cortical venous pressure in hydrocephalus. Neurosurgery 29:232–238
12. Chakrabortty S, Tamaki N, Ehara K, Ide C (1994) Experimental syringomyelia in the rabbit: an ultrastructural study of the spinal cord tissue. Neurosurgery 35:1112–1120
13. Cloyd MW, Low FN (1974) Scanning electron microscopy of the subarachnoid space in the dog. I. Spinal cord levels. J Comp Neurol 153:325–368
14. Cserr HF (1971) Physiology of the choroid plexus. Physiol Rev 51:273–311
15. Cserr HF, Ostrach LH (1974) Bulk flow of interstitial fluid following intracranial injection of Blue Dextran 2000. Exp Neurol 45:50–60
16. Cserr HF, Cooper DN, Milhorat TH (1977) Flow of cerebral interstitial fluid as indicated by the removal of extracellular markers from rat caudate nucleus. In: Bito LZ, Davson H, Fenstermacher JD (eds)The ocular and cerebrospinal fluids. Exp Eye Res [Suppl 25]:461–473
17. Cserr HF, Cooper DN, Suri PK, Patlak CS (1981) Efflux of radiolabeled polyethylene glycols and albumin from rat brain. Am J Physiol 240:F319–F328
18. Davis CH, Symon L (1989) Mechanisms and treatment in post-traumatic syringomyelia. Br J Neurosurg 3:669–674
19. Del Bigio MR (1995) The ependyma: a protective barrier between brain and cerebrospinal fluid. Glia 14:1–13
20. Desaga U, Leonhardt H (1976) Bindegewebe in perivaskulären Räumen subependymaler Kapillaren des Rückenmarks beim Kaninchen. Z Mikrosk Anat Forsch 90:801–815
21. Dolan EJ, Transfeld EE, Tator CH, Simmons EH, Hughes KF (1980) The effect of spinal distraction on regional spinal cord blood flow in cats. J Neurosurg 53:756–764
22. Donaldson I, Gibson R (1982) Spinal cord atrophy associated with arachnoiditis as demonstrated by computed tomography. Neuroradiology 24:101–105
23. Drayer RP, Rosenbaum AE (1977) Metrizamide brain penetrance. Acta Radiol Suppl 555:280–293
24. Du Boulay G (1966) Pulsatile movements in the CSF pathways. Br J Radiol 39:255–262
25. Du Boulay GH, O'Connell JEA, Cume J, Bostik T, Verity P (1972) Further investigations on pulsatile movements of the cerebrospinal fluid pathways. Acta Radiol 13:496–523
26. Dubois PJ, Drayer BP, Sage M, Osborne D, Heinz ER (1981) Intramedullary penetrance of metrizamide in the dog spinal cord. AJNR Am J Neuroradiol 2:313–317
27. Ellertson AB, Greitz T (1970) The distending force in the production of communicating syringomyelia. Lancet 1:1234
28. Enzmann DR, Pelc NJ (1991) Normal flow patterns with phase-contrast cine MRI imaging. Radiology 178:467–474
29. Enzmann DR, O'Donehue J, Rubin JB, Shuer L, Cogen P, Silverberg G (1987) CSF pulsations within nonneoplastic spinal cord cysts. AJR Am J Roentgenol 149:149–157
30. Esiri MM, Gay D (1990) Immunological and neuropathological significance of the Virchow-Robin space. J Neurol Sci 100:3–8
31. Foldi M (1977) Pre-lymphatic drainage of the brain. Am Heart J 93:121–124
32. Fuse T, Patrickson JW, Yamada S (1989) Axonal transport of horseradish peroxidase in the experimental tethered spinal cord. Pediatr Neurosci 15:296–301
33. Gillilan LA (1970) Veins of the spinal cord. Anatomic details, suggested clinical applications. Neurology 20:860–868
34. Golman K (1973) Distribution and retention of 121I-labeled metrizamide after intravenous and suboccipital injections in rabbit, rat and cat. Acta Radiol Suppl 335:300–311

35. Green BA, Wagner FC Jr (1973) Evolution of edema in the acutely injured spinal cord: a fluorescence microscopic study. Surg Neurol 1:98–101

36. Greitz D (1993) Cerebrospinal fluid circulation and associated intracranial dynamics. A radiologic investigation using MR imaging and radionuclide cisternography. Acta Radiol Suppl 386:1–23

37. Griffiths IR (1975) Vasogenic edema following acute and chronic spinal cord compression in the dog. J Neurosurg 42:155–165

38. Griffiths IR, Miller R (1974) Vascular permeability to protein and vasogenic oedema in experimental concussive injuries to the canine spinal cord. J Neurol Sci 22:291–304

39. Guillain G (1899) La circulation de la lymphe dans la moelle épinière. Rev Neurol (Paris) 7:796–859

40. Guyton AC, Coleman TG (1968) Regulation of the interstitial fluid volume and pressure. Ann N Y Acad Sci 150:537–547

41. Hackney DB, Asato R, Joseph PM, Carolin MJ, McGrath JT, Grossman RI, Kassab EA, DeSimone D (1986) Hemorrhage and edema in acute spinal cord compression: demonstration by MR imaging. Radiology 161:387–390

42. Hamer J, Alberti E, Hoyer S, Wiedemann K (1977) Influence of systemic and cerebral vascular factors on the cerebrospinal fluid pressure waves. J Neurosurg 46:36–45

43. Harbitz F, Lossius E (1929) Extramedullary tumor. Arachnoiditis fibrosa cystica et ossificans. Gliosis of the medulla. Acta Psychiatr Neurol 4:51–64

44. Hattori H, Kimura M, Takahashi M, Hashimoto S (1990) Morphological estimation of brain extracellular fluid dynamics in cold-induced edema from the aspect of cerebrospinal fluid–extracellular fluid communication. Acta Pathol Jpn 40:314–321

45. Hossmann KA, Bothe HW, Bodsch W, Paschen W (1983) Pathophysiological aspects of blood–brain barrier disturbances in experimental brain tumors and brain abscesses. Acta Neuropathol Suppl (Berl) 8:89–102

46. Hurth M, Parker F (1999) Histoire, controverses et pathogénie. Neurochirurgie 45[Suppl 1]:138–157

47. Hutchings M, Weller RO (1986) Anatomical relationships of the pia mater to cerebral blood vessels in man. J Neurosurg 65:316–325

48. Iida F (1966) Elektronenmikroskopische Untersuchungen am oberflächlichen Anteil des Gehirns bei Hund und Katze. Arch Histol Jpn 27:267–285

49. Ikata T, Masaki K, Kashiwaguchi S (1988) Clinical and experimental studies on permeability of tracers in normal spinal cord and syringomyelia. Spine 13:737–741

50. Isherwood I, Fawcitt RA, Forbes WSC, Nettle JRL, Pullan BR (1977) Computer tomography of the spinal canal using metrizamide. Acta Radiol Suppl 355:299–305

51. Iskandar BJ, Oakes WJ, McLaughlin C, Osumi AK, Tien RD (1994) Terminal syringohydromyelia and occult spinal dysraphism. J Neurosurg 81:513–519

52. Itabashi T (1990) Quantitative analysis of cervical CSF and syrinx fluid pulsations. Nippon Saikingaku Gakkai Zasshi 64:523–533

53. Jones EG (1970) On the mode of entry of blood vessels into the cerebral cortex. J Anat 106:507–520

54. Klekamp J, Völkel K, Bartels CJ, Samii M (2001) Disturbances of cerebrospinal fluid flow attributable to arachnoid scarring cause interstitial edema of the cat spinal cord. Neurosurgery 48:174–186

55. Krahn V (1982) The pia mater at the site of entry of blood vessels into the central nervous system. Anat Embryol 164:257–263

56. Krisch B, Leonhardt H, Oksche A (1984) Compartments and perivascular arrangement of the meninges covering the cerebral cortex of the rat. Cell Tissue Res 238:459–474

57. Li KC, Chui MC (1987) Conventional and CT metrizamide myelography in Arnold-Chiari malformation and syringomyelia. AJNR Am J Neuroradiol 8:11–17

58. Liber AF, Lisa JR (1937) Rosenthal fibres in non-neoplastic syringomyelia: a note on the pathogenesis of syringomyelia. J Nerv Ment Dis 86:549–558

59. Lockey P, Poots G, Williams B (1975) Theoretical aspects of the attenuation of pressure pulses within the CSF pathways. Med Biol Eng 14:861–869

60. Lopes CAS, Mair WGP (1974) Ultrastructure of the arachnoid membrane in man. Acta Neuropathol (Berl) 28:167–173

61. Maas AIR (1977) Cerebrospinal fluid enzymes in acute brain injury. I. Dynamics of changes in CSF enzyme activity after acute experimental brain injury. J Neurol Neurosurg Psychiatry 40:655–665

62. Martakas F, Stechele S, Keller F (1978) Microcirculation within the cerebral extracellular space. In: Cervos-Navarro J, Ferszt R (eds) Advances in neurology, vol 20. Raven Press, New York, pp 125–131

63. Merchant RE, Low FN (1979) Scanning electron microscopy of the subarachnoid space in the dog: evidence for a non-hematogenous origin of subarachnoid macrophages. Am J Anat 156:183–206

64. Milhorat TH (1975) The third circulation revisited. J Neurosurg 42:628–645

65. Milhorat TH, Adler DE, Heger IM, Miller JI, Hollenberg-Sher JR (1991) Histopathology of experimental hematomyelia. J Neurosurg 75:911–915

66. Milhorat TH, Nobandegani F, Miller JI, Rao C (1993) Noncommunicating syringomyelia following occlusion of central canal in rats. Experimental model and histological findings. J Neurosurg 78:274–279

67. Milhorat TH, Capocelli AL, Anzil AP, Kotzen RM, Milhorat RH (1995) Pathological basis of spinal cord cavitation in syringomyelia: analysis of 105 autopsy cases. J Neurosurg 82:802–812

68. Nemecek S, Petr R, Suba P, Rozsival V, Melka O (1977) Longitudinal extension of oedema in experimental spinal cord injury – evidence for two types of posttraumatic oedema. Acta Neurochir (Wien) 37:7–16

69. Nicholas DS, Weller RO (1988) The fine anatomy of the human spinal meninges: a light and scanning electron microscopy study. J Neurosurg 69:276–282

70. O'Neill OR, Roman-Goldstein S, Piatt JH Jr (1994) Sacral agenesis associated with spinal cord syrinx. Pediatr Neurosurg 20:217–220

71. Ohata K, Marmarou A (1992) Clearance of brain edema and macromolecules through the cortical extracellular space. J Neurosurg 77:387–396

72. Ohata K, Marmarou A, Povlishock JT (1990) An immunocytochemical study of protein clearance in brain infusion edema. Acta Neuropathol (Berl) 81:162–177

73. Ommaya AK (1968) Mechanical properties of tissues of the nervous system. J Biomech 1:127–138

74. Ponssen H, Van den Bos G (1971) Influence of the circulation on the CSF pressure waves. J Neurol Neurosurg Psychiatry 34:108

75. Purtzer TJ, Yamada S, Tani S (1985) Metabolic and histologic studies of chronic model of tethered cord. Surg Forum 36:612–614

76. Quencer RM, Post MJD, Hinks RS (1990) Cine MRI in the evaluation of normal and abnormal CSF flow: intracranial and intraspinal studies. Neuroradiology 32:371–391

77. Rapoport SI (1976) Sites and functions of the blood–brain barrier. In: Rapoport SI (ed) Blood–brain barrier in physiology and medicine. Raven Press, New York, pp 43–86

78. Reddy KKV, Del Bigio MR, Sutherland GR (1989) Ultrastructure of the human posttraumatic syrinx. J Neurosurg 71:239–243

79. Rennels ML, Gregory TF, Blaumanis OR, Fujimoto K, Grady PA (1985) Evidence for a paravascular fluid circulation in the mammalian central nervous system, provided by the rapid distribution of tracer protein throughout the brain from the subarachnoid space. Brain Res 326:47–63

80. Rennels ML, Blaumanis OR, Grady PA (1990) Rapid solute transport throughout the brain via paravascular fluid pathways. Adv Neurol 52:431–439

81. Reulen HJ, Graham R, Spatz M, Klatzo I (1977) Role of pressure gradients and bulk flow in dynamics of vasogenic brain edema. J Neurosurg 46:24–35

82. Reulen HJ, Tsuyumu M, Tack A, Fenske AR, Prioleau GR (1978) Clearance of edema fluid into cerebrospinal fluid. J Neurosurg 48:754–764

83. Rosenberg GA, Kyner WT, Strada E (1980) Bulk flow of brain interstitial fluid under normal and hyperosmolar conditions. Am J Physiol 238:F42–F49

84. Samii M, Klekamp J (1994) Surgical results for 100 intramedullary tumors in relation to accompanying syringomyelia. Neurosurgery 35:865–873

85. Schellinger D, Le Bihan D, Rajan SS, Cammarata CA, Patronas NJ, Deveikis JP, Levy LM (1992) MR of slow CSF flow in the spine. AJNR Am J Neuroradiol 13:1393–1403

86. Schlesinger AE, Naidich TP, Quencer RM (1986) Concurrent hydromyelia and diastematomyelia. AJNR Am J Neuroradiol 7:473–477

87. Schroth G (1991) Physiologie und Pathologie der intrakraniellen Liquordynamik. Jahrbuch der Radiologie, pp 287–290

88. Schroth G, Klose U (1992) Cerebrospinal fluid flow. II. Physiology of respiration-related pulsations. Neuroradiology 35:10–15

89. Schuster P (1915) Beitrag zur Kenntnis der Anatomie und Klinik der Meningitis serosa spinalis circumscripta. Monatschr Psychiatr Neurol 37:341–373

90. Shapiro K, Shulman K, Marmarou A, Poll W (1977) Tissue pressure gradients in spinal cord injury. Surg Neurol 7:275–279

91. Shapiro WR (1988) Cerebrospinal fluid circulation and the blood–brain barrier. Ann N Y Acad Sci 531:9–14

92. Sherman JL, Barkovich AJ, Citrin CM (1986) The MR appearance of syringomyelia: new observations. AJNR Am J Neuroradiol 7:985–995

93. Sherman JL, Citrin CM, Bowen BJ, Gangarosa RE (1986) MR demonstration of cerebrospinal fluid flow by obstructive lesions. AJNR Am J Neuroradiol 7:571–579

94. Sherman JL, Barkovich AJ, Citrin CM (1987) The MR appearance of syringomyelia: new observations. AJR Am J Roentgenol 148:381–391

95. Stoodley MA, Jones NR, Brown CJ (1996) Evidence for rapid fluid flow from the subarachnoid space into the spinal cord central canal in the rat. Brain Res 707:155–164

96. Stoodley MA, Gutschmidt B, Jones NR (1999) Cerebrospinal fluid flow in an animal model of noncommunicating syringomyelia. Neurosurgery 44:1065–1076

97. Tachibana S, Iida H, Yada K (1992) Significance of positive Queckenstedt test in patients with syringomyelia associated with Arnold-Chiari malformation. J Neurosurg 76:67–71

98. Tachibana S, Kitahara Y, Iida H, Yada K (1994) Spinal cord intramedullary pressure. A probable factor in syrinx growth. Spine 19:2174–2178

99. Tobimatsu Y, Nihei R, Kimura T, Suyama T, Kimura H, Tobimatsu H, Shirakawa T (1995) A quantitative analysis of cerebrospinal fluid flow in post-traumatic syringomyelia. Paraplegia 33:203–207

100. Wagner FC Jr, Stewart WB (1981) Effect of trauma dose on spinal cord edema. J Neurosurg 54:802–806

101. Wagner HJ, Pilgrim C, Brandl J (1974) Penetration and removal of horseradish peroxidase injected into the cerebrospinal fluid: role of cerebral perivascular spaces, endothelium and microglia. Acta Neuropathol (Berl) 27:299–315

102. Weller RO, Kida S, Zhang ET (1992) Pathways of fluid drainage from the brain – morphological aspects and immunological significance in rat and man. Brain Pathol 2:277–284

103. Williams B (1972) Pathogenesis of syringomyelia. Lancet 2:969–970

104. Williams B (1976) Cerebrospinal fluid pressure changes in response to coughing. Brain 99:331–346

105. Williams B (1980) On the pathogenesis of syringomyelia: a review. J R Soc Med 73:798–806

106. Williams B (1981) Simultaneous cerebral and spinal fluid pressure recordings. I. Technique, physiology, and normal results. Acta Neurochir (Wien) 58:167–185

107. Williams B (1981) Simultaneous cerebral and spinal fluid pressure recordings. II. Cerebrospinal dissociation with lesions at the foramen magnum. Acta Neurochir (Wien) 59:123–142

108. Winkler SS, Sackett JF (1980) Explanation of metrizamide brain penetration: a review. J Comput Assist Tomogr 4:191–193

109. Woollam DHM, Millen JW (1958) Observations on the production and circulation of the cerebrospinal fluid. In: Wolstenholm GE, O'Connor CM (eds) Ciba Foundation Symposium on the cerebrospinal fluid. Little and Brown, Boston, pp 124–146

110. Wright PM, Nogueira GJ, Levin E (1971) Role of pia mater in the transfer of substances in and out of the cerebrospinal fluid. Exp Brain Res 13:294–305

111. Yamada S, Iacono RP, Andrade RP, Mandybur G, Yamada BS (1995) Pathophysiology of tethered cord syndrome. Neurosurg Clin N Am 6:311–323

112. Young WF, Tuma R, O'Grady T (2000) Intraoperative measurement of spinal cord blood flow in syringomyelia. Clin Neurol Neurosurg 102:119–123

113. Zhang ET, Inman CBE, Weller RO (1990) Interrelationships of the pia mater and the perivascular (Virchow-Robin) spaces in the human cerebrum. J Anat 170:111–123

3 Syringomyelia Associated with Diseases at the Craniocervical Junction

Diseases at the craniocervical junction that lead to syringomyelia interfere with CSF circulation and physiological movements of the cerebellum and brainstem. Clinical presentation typically starts with symptoms related to compression of the brainstem and cervical cord at the foramen magnum. Clinical signs of the syringomyelia develop at a second stage. The most common, by far, pathology at the craniocervical junction associated with syringomyelia is Chiari I malformation.

3.1
Chiari Malformations

In his two monographs, published in 1891 [54] and 1896 [55], Chiari described four types of anomalies at the craniocervical junction. Types I–III are characterized by different degrees of caudal displacement of cerebellum and brainstem into the spinal canal; whereas, type IV consists of cerebellar hypoplasia.

The most common Chiari malformation – and the one most often associated with syringomyelia – is type I (CMI) (Fig. 3.1). Studies have shown that approximately 75–85% of patients with CMI will develop syringomyelia [7, 8, 11]. CMI is characterized by herniation of cerebellar tonsils below the level of the foramen magnum. A herniation of more than 5 mm is considered pathological for adults [3]. Other parts of the central nervous system, such as cerebellar vermis or brainstem, are not displaced in CMI and remain in their normal anatomic position.

In Chiari type II malformation (CMII), cerebellar vermis and brainstem are herniated into the spinal canal (Fig. 3.2). Unlike CMI, the foramen magnum rather than the level of maximum compression is enlarged. Instead, compression of the brainstem occurs in the cervical spine. With downward displacement

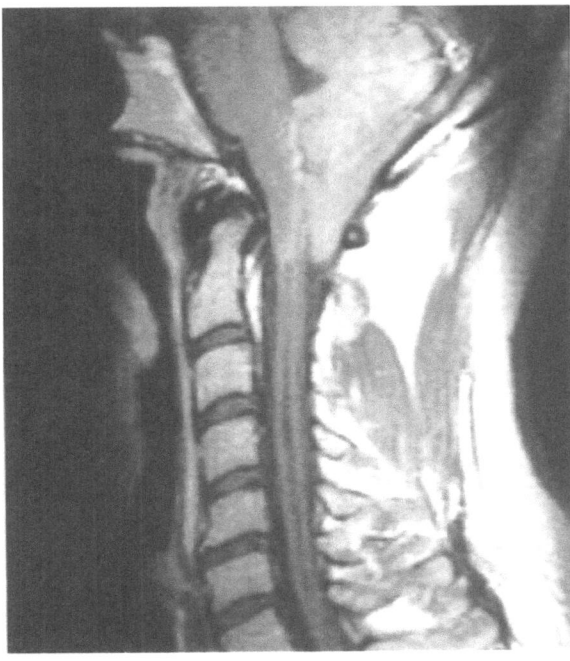

Fig. 3.1. T1-weighted sagittal MRI scan of a 49-year-old woman with typical Chiari I malformation and syringomyelia. The posterior fossa is small and shallow. The tentorium reaches down close to the foramen magnum uand well below the level of the external occipital protuberance. The tonsils extend below C1. The syrinx starts at C3 and extends to the midthoracic cord

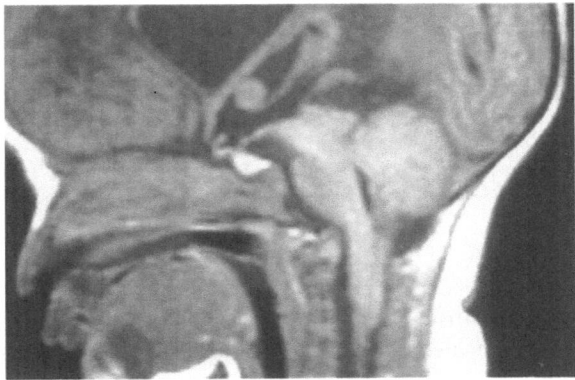

Fig. 3.2. T1-weighted sagittal MRI scan of a 4-month-old girl with Chiari II malformation. The lumbosacral myelomeningocele was closed on the day of birth and a ventriculoperitoneal shunt was placed soon after. Since then the child was repeatedly troubled by pneumonia and apnea attacks. MRI shows descent of the vermis and cerebellar tonsils to the level of C4. Note the insertion of the tentorium just at the posterior margin of the enlarged foramen magnum, indicating the position of the torcula at that level. There appears to be some additional anterior compression due to some degree of basilar invagination. Despite a functioning ventriculoperitoneal shunt, the ventricles are considerably enlarged. As a typical dysplastic feature of Chiari II malformation, a deformity of the midbrain is apparent

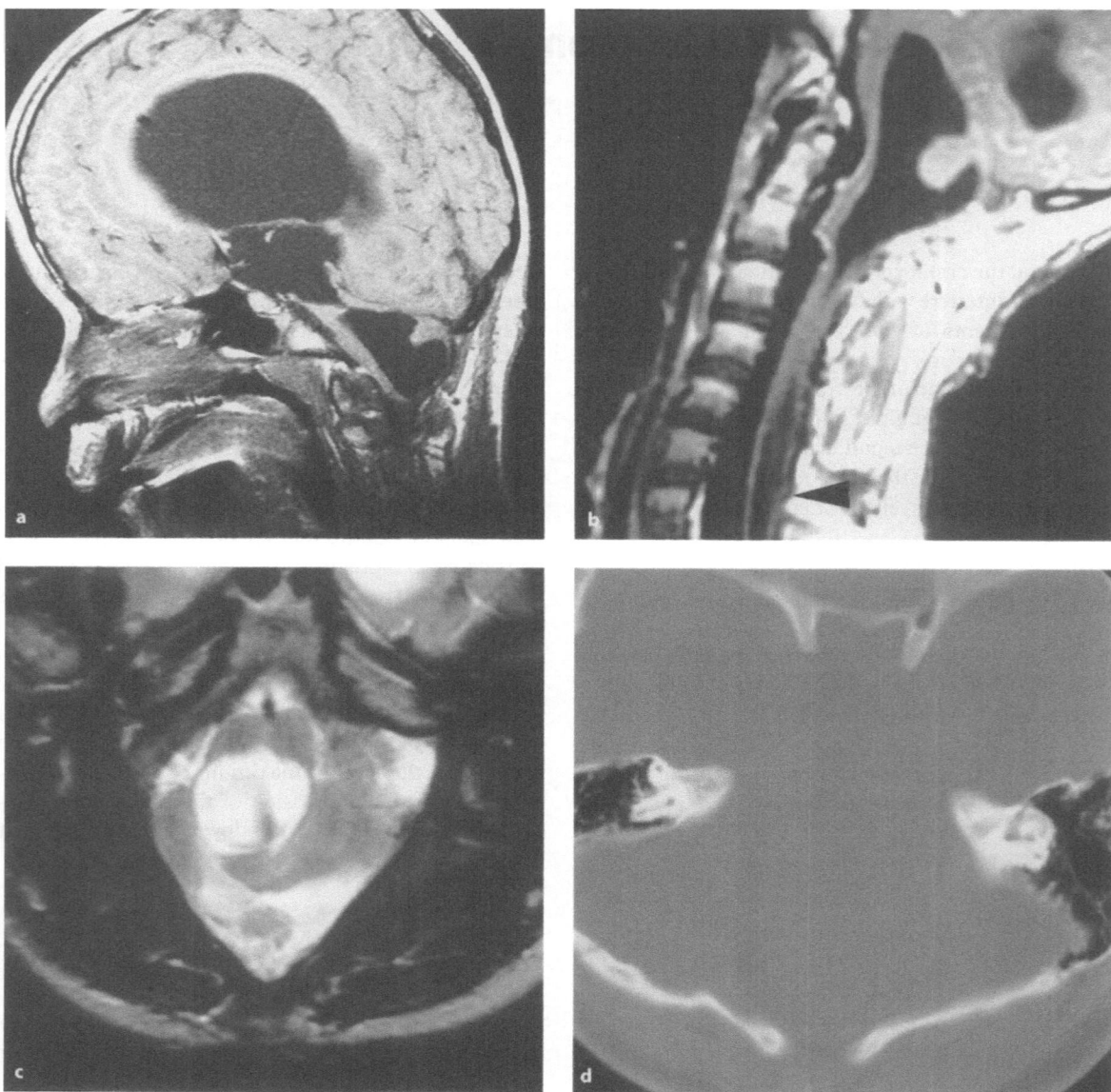

Fig. 3.3 a–d

of the brainstem, the fourth ventricle becomes markedly elongated. The obex may be located as low as the tip of the cerebellar tonsils, which may reach down to the lower cervical segments. Always associated with CMII are hydrocephalus, due to obstruction of foramina of Magendie and Luschka, and lumbar myelomeningocele. Sometimes additional features can be observed, such as a spina bifida of the upper cervical segments, dysplasia of the brainstem (especially midbrain), agenesis of the corpus callosum, hypoplasia of the tentorium, and bony anomalies of petrous bone and clivus [75, 208]. In Chiari type III malformation (CMIII), herniation of the cerebellum is combined with craniocervical meningoen-cephalocele and aplasia of the tentorium [208, 230] (Fig. 3.3). Chiari type IV malformation (CMIV) is characterized by hypoplasia or even aplasia of the cerebellar vermis. This malformation is discussed in the chapter section on rhombencephalic malformations (Sect. 3.2).

Chiari himself suspected that these malformations were caused by congenital hydrocephalus in conjunction with a small posterior fossa. John Cleland, who had described a patient with CMII a few years earlier [59], considered the malformations to be anomalies of the central nervous system itself, rather than secondary effects of congenital or even prenatal hydrocephalus. To date, this controversy is still not completely

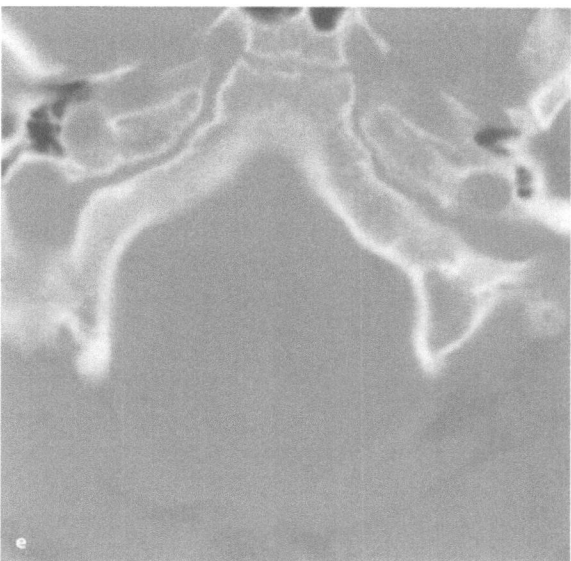

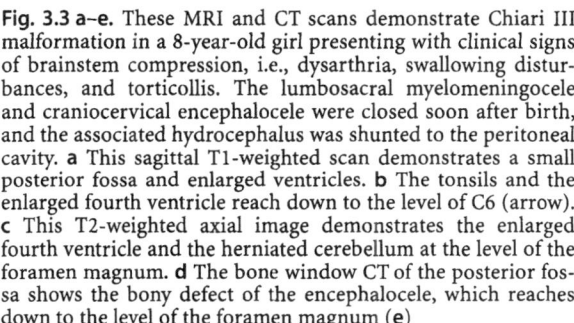

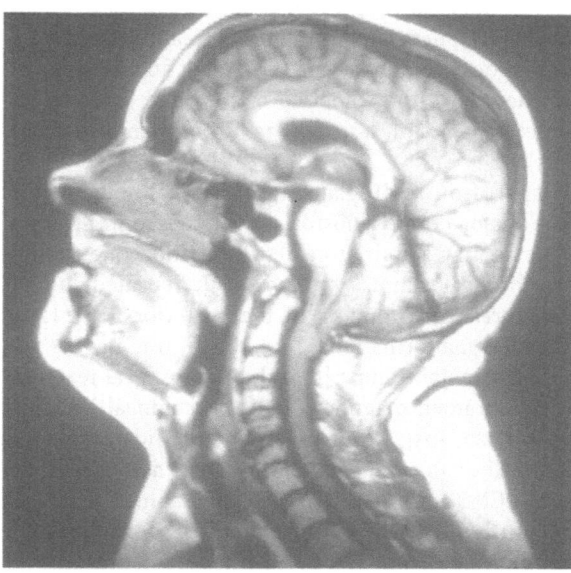

Fig. 3.3 a–e. These MRI and CT scans demonstrate Chiari III malformation in a 8-year-old girl presenting with clinical signs of brainstem compression, i.e., dysarthria, swallowing disturbances, and torticollis. The lumbosacral myelomeningocele and craniocervical encephalocele were closed soon after birth, and the associated hydrocephalus was shunted to the peritoneal cavity. **a** This sagittal T1-weighted scan demonstrates a small posterior fossa and enlarged ventricles. **b** The tonsils and the enlarged fourth ventricle reach down to the level of C6 (arrow). **c** This T2-weighted axial image demonstrates the enlarged fourth ventricle and the herniated cerebellum at the level of the foramen magnum. **d** The bone window CT of the posterior fossa shows the bony defect of the encephalocele, which reaches down to the level of the foramen magnum (**e**)

Fig. 3.4. This T1-weighted sagittal MRI scan of a 62-year-old woman with Chiari I malformation and syringobulbia demonstrates beaking of the cervical cord right below the tip of the tonsils at C2. Please note the hyperlordosis of the cervical spine, lowering compression of the brainstem and spinal cord at the foramen magnum

solved – more than 100 years later. However, there is increasing evidence that at least CMI, if not also CMII, is an anomaly of skull development foremost and not primarily a malformation of the central nervous system [22, 58, 157, 172, 184, 230, 236]. Experimentally, CMI can be produced in animals by interfering with bone growth of the posterior fossa [98, 148, 260, 262]. A small posterior fossa forces the cerebellum and brainstem into the cervical canal. In CMI, the herniation is of a minor degree, so that the fourth ventricle is not completely obstructed and hydrocephalus does not develop in most patients. Sometimes a small hump of the upper cervical cord can be observed below the tonsillar tips, but no further dysplastic changes of the cerebellum or cerebrum take place (Fig. 3.4). In CMII, however, the herniation is of such magnitude that the fourth ventricle becomes completely obstructed and hydrocephalus develops. Whether the dysplastic features of the brain in CMII are secondary events due to brainstem compression and hydrocephalus [156, 213] or are a malformation of the central nervous system in itself [24] is still a controversial issue. There is growing evidence, however, that at least some of the dys-

plastic changes are indeed secondary changes [157]. McLone and Knepper [157] proposed an elegant theory for the series of events that lead to CMII and the other dysplastic changes seen in this patient group. Due to continuous drainage of CSF from the myelomeningocele into the amniotic fluid during gestation, the intracranial pressure is lowered to such a degree that the posterior fossa is underdeveloped and migration deficits of neuroblasts may result. With continuous flow of CSF into the amniotic fluid, the nervous structures of the posterior fossa start to gain volume; therefore, upward and downward herniation of the cerebellum and brain stem may result, causing dysplasia of the tentorium and hydrocephalus due to obstruction of the fourth ventricle and subarachnoid space despite an enlarged foramen magnum.

If this assumption is valid, it should be possible to prevent these central nervous system manifestations or even to reverse them, provided decompression of the displaced structures and treatment of the hydrocephalus are performed early enough. Some reports clearly indicate this. In CMI, it could be shown that decompression of the foramen magnum reverses tonsillar herniation [215, 250] and the medullary buckle frequently seen below the tip of the tonsils. In patients with myelomeningocele, the low percentage of CMII or hydrocephalus during the fetal period versus the almost obligatory combination of myelomeningocele with CMII and hydrocephalus postnatally [31, 219] suggest that CMII and hydrocephalus develop secondarily [21]. Successful intrauterine treatment of myelomeningocele may prevent CMII and further dysplastic changes of the spinal cord [164] and brain in humans [248, 249], as well as experimental animals [165].

Apart from CMI related to congenital bony malformations or craniosynostosis [273], a second group of patients may acquire tonsillar herniation due to lumboperitoneal shunts [57, 239, 263], repeated lumbar punctures [218], tumors of the posterior fossa [130], vascular malformations [92], birth trauma [5, 105, 265], postnatal trauma [5, 114], or meningeal reactions at the foramen magnum due to mechanical irritation [1, 2, 5, 20, 105]. Williams [265] and Hida [105] were the earliest to point out the frequent association between CMI and birth injury. They assumed that, during birth, the cerebellum is pushed down into the foramen magnum due to an increase of intracranial pressure and to deformation of the skull in the birth canal. In cases of birth complications, a meningeal tear may occur, with rupturing of small perforating vessels, and cause arachnoiditis at the foramen magnum. With the passage of time, an arachnoid scar develops and anchors the tonsils in an abnormal position at or below the foramen magnum [266]. With profound arachnoid scarring, hydrocephalus may even develop [264].

3.1.1
Clinical Presentation

In our series, patients with CMI presented at an average age of 40±17 years, with an average clinical history of 75±106 months. Similar figures were published in a multicenter study on 285 patients with CMI in France [5]. Of those with CMII, patients were considerably younger (11±10 years) and demonstrated a much shorter history of 22±52 months. CMI and CMII may cause neurological symptoms by a number of pathomechanisms:

1. Compression of brainstem and cervical cord
2. CSF flow obstruction at the foramen magnum due to tonsillar tissue and arachnoid adhesions causing syringomyelia or syringobulbia
3. Obstruction of the fourth ventricle causing hydrocephalus
4. Tethering of the brainstem or cervical cord by arachnoid adhesions
5. Craniocervical instabilities associated with bony malformations

Each of these pathomechanisms may cause symptoms independently and will determine the clinical course. Theoretically, clinical and diagnostic evalua-

Table 3.1. Growth parameters of the human brain

Brain part	Size at birth (%)	Growth period (months)
Cerebellum	15	18
Cerebrum	29	22
Thalamus	48	17
Basal ganglia	38	22
Cerebral white matter	29	56
Cerebral neocortex	32	165
Hippocampus	27	27
Entire brain	24	20

tion of each individual patient should reveal which pathomechanisms are producing symptoms in order to appropriately plan the surgical strategy. In practice, however, such differential analysis cannot be separately made for all these components.

The second major influence on the clinical course is the age at which neurological symptoms start. Initially, most patients complain about signs of brainstem compression. Depending on the age of the patient, symptoms of brainstem compression may vary in their form, severity, and progression. Children under the age of 2 years become symptomatic with feeding problems, a weak cry, inspiratory stridor, apnea, cyanotic spells, or increased muscle tone. Clinically, they may deteriorate rapidly in this age group, with a significant risk for life-threatening respiratory problems in particular [31, 52, 60, 128, 189, 198, 199, 201, 208, 255, 272]. Between 2 years and 12 years of age, a common problem is the development of scoliosis [273]. Symptoms of coordination difficulties or gait ataxia may also appear but progress much less rapidly than for infants [31, 208, 273]. In youths and adults, common initial manifestations of brainstem compression are occipital headaches, nystagmus, or hypesthesia in the trigeminal distribution [31, 192, 208].

These age-related differences in clinical onset and progression may be related to growth of the cerebellum. In man, the cerebellum is one of the smallest parts of the brain at the time of birth in relation to its final size in adulthood. Only 15% of the adult cerebellum volume is present, versus other parts of the brain which are already about twice as large (Table 3.1) [129, 211]. This rather small cerebellar volume at birth may actually be a safeguard against inadvertent brainstem compression during delivery. The major growth period of the cerebellum extends from birth to approximately 18 months of age. During this short time peri-

Table 3.2. First clinical symptoms for patients with Chiari I and II malformations

First symptom	CMI with syrinx, n=166	CMI without syrinx, n=64	CMII, n=12
Occipital headache	31%	44%	8%
Gait ataxia	12%	23%	8%
Swallowing disturbance	2%	12%	15%
Autonomic dysfunction	–	3%	31%
Sleep apnea	1%	3%	–
Motor weakness	15%	3%	23%
Hypesthesia	19%	9%	–
Dysesthesias	17%	–	8%
Sphincter disturbance	1%	–	–
Hydrocephalus	–	2%	–
Scoliosis	1%	–	8%

CMI, Chiari I malformation; CMII, Chiari II malformation

od, it enlarges to approximately 90% of its adult size [211].

Therefore, the very dramatic clinical course in children under the age of 2 years may be explained by rapid growth of the displaced cerebellar tissue in a compartment that cannot accommodate this volume increase. Incidentally, CMI is one of the few malformations that usually does not cause symptoms in childhood. The overwhelming number of patients – approximately 90% in our series – become symptomatic in adulthood. Given the fact that the cerebellum has already reached most of its adult volume by the age of 2 years, i.e., the anatomical relations responsible for the clinical picture barely change after that time, this slowly progressive course is quite remarkable.

At the start of clinical symptoms, patients in our series reported occipital headaches, gait ataxia, and swallowing dysfunctions with adult onset or dysfunctions of caudal cranial nerves, apnea, and autonomic dysregulations if problems started in infancy [5] (Table 3.2). In CMI, occipital headaches are the first symptom for patients without (44%) and with (31%) accompanying syringomyelia; they are the most common first manifestation. Classically, these occipital headaches can be provoked by Valsalva maneuvers, coughing, sneezing, or anteflexion of the neck. The pain may come instantly, originating in the occipital area and radiating anteriorly [190]. Some patients report a feeling as if the head would burst. The pain may be unilateral and accompanied by autonomic dysfunctions, such as respiratory problems, irregula-

rities of heart rate, etc. These symptoms may be so severe that the patient is rendered suddenly unconscious [234]. Other than this rather typical situation of occipital headache provoked by increases of intracranial pressure, a classical Chiari-type headache does not exist. Distinguishing these from cervicogenic headaches may be very difficult, especially in patients with associated cervical disc problems [190, 228].

Gait ataxia is reported as the first clinical symptom by 15% of patients with CMI (23% without and 12% with syringomyelia, respectively). Swallowing difficulties are much more common in the group without syringomyelia at the beginning of the disease (12% and 2%, respectively), and are a result of brainstem compression at the foramen magnum rather than being related to syringomyelia. However, patients with concurrent CMI and syringomyelia more often report motor weakness (15% and 3%, respectively), sensory disturbances (19% and 9%, respectively), or dysesthesias (17% and 0%, respectively) as the first clinical problem.

Gait problems arise as a consequence of impaired coordination rather than lower extremity weakness. Patients report difficulties with walking in the dark. Others mention a combination of ataxia and occipital headaches while climbing down stairs when they have to look down and bend their neck forward to watch where they are stepping.

In terms of motor weakness, distal hand muscles are usually the first to be affected and are quite often atrophied by the time the patient consults a physician. In most instances, symptoms are observed on only one side at first. Later, the contralateral hand also becomes weaker. Throughout the clinical course, the side affected first usually remains the most affected. Lower extremity weakness is not observed at the start of clinical disease in a patient where the syringomyelia is related to the foramen magnum.

Dysesthesias may be reported as a tingling or burning sensation or as a feeling of tightness. Sometimes patients are able to provoke dysesthesias with the same Valsalva maneuvers used to provoke occipital headaches.

Rare initial presentations of CMI in adults include hydrocephalus, sleep apnea [14, 78, 102, 126, 167, 180, 183, 187], scoliosis, sphincter disturbances, or autonomic dysfunctions [6, 7, 9, 14, 40, 43, 64, 142, 225]. Several authors reported patients who suddenly died due to respiratory or cardiac arrest associated with an undiagnosed or untreated CMI [124, 212]. Alegre et al. [6] published about a 31-year-old patient with acute cardiac arrest after a sudden neck movement. Another author reported about a 13-year-old child with cardiac and respiratory arrest after a minor trauma [146]. Many patients report a stepwise progression of their

Table 3.3. Symptoms of patients with Chiari I and II malformations at the time of operation

Symptom		CMI with syrinx		CMI without syrinx		CMII	
Hypesthesia		91%		44%		88%	
Occipital headache		70%		71%		50%	
Dysesthesias		69%		31%		25%	
Motor weakness		69%		22%		75%	
Gait ataxia	Unable to walk	65%	12%	72%	10%	100%	75%
Sphincter disturbance	Incontinence	38%	6%	22%	7%	88%	75%
Trigeminal hypesthesia		21%		4%		8%	
Swallowing dysfunction		18%		33%		38%	
Vocal cord paralysis		8%		12%		31%	
Facial palsy		–		4%		–	
Palsies CN III, IV and VI		3%		18%		16%	
Nystagmus		6%		43%		8%	
Sleep apnea		2%		6%		–	
Autonomic dysregulation		3%		6%		46%	
Horner's syndrome		5%		–		–	

CMI, Chiari I malformation; CMII, Chiari II malformation

clinical symptoms, often provoked by sudden uncontrolled movements or after an otherwise harmless fall [229]. Instantly severe and life-threatening symptoms or situations, however, are extremely rare in patients with CMI. In CMII, severe autonomic dysfunctions are observed more often, especially if symptoms start to develop in infancy. Medullary dysfunctions are still the leading cause of death in this age group [44]. Nevertheless, it is our opinion that prophylactic surgery of asymptomatic patients with Chiari malformations is not warranted.

By the time the patient seeks an operation, neurological symptoms have changed (Table 3.3). Almost every patient experiences a progression of neurological symptoms with the passage of time, either gradually or stepwise [5, 11, 39, 48, 104, 221]. The speed of neurological deterioration, however, is extremely variable once the patient has passed infancy. We have seen a patient with very slow progression over 50 years still have just minor symptoms and other patients being admitted in a wheelchair within a few years time after the first signs had appeared. To date, the largest study on the natural history of syringomyelia was performed by Hertel et al. [104] who studied 323 patients over a large number of years. They documented a slowly progressive course in 65% of patients, a stepwise progression in 29% of patients, and a rapid deterioration in 6% of patients. Recently, Moriwaka et al. [176] pub-

lished a nationwide epidemiological survey on syringomyelia in Japan. Among 1243 cases of syringomyelia, 684 (51.2%) were associated with CMI. The clinical course was slowly progressive in the great majority of cases (82.5%), but in 202 patients (16.2%) a rather stable course was observed, while spontaneous resolution of symptoms was observed in only 29 patients (2.3%) (Fig. 3.5).

Spontaneous resolution of a syrinx requires spontaneous improvement of CSF flow. In children, skull growth still continues after the cerebellum has reached more than 90% of its final size at the age of 2 years [211]. Therefore, tonsils may regress intracranially in relation to the growing skull [166] to the extent that free CSF passage is established, allowing the syrinx to decrease in size or even to disappear completely.

Of six adult cases, including the one shown in Fig. 3.5, significant improvement of CMI accompanied the resolution of syringomyelia in three patients [186, 193], while CMI remained unchanged in the other three cases. A changed ratio between cerebellar and intracranial volumes cannot explain the disappearance of CSF flow obstruction and syringomyelia in adults. The most likely explanation is spontaneous improvement of CSF circulation at the foramen magnum. Arachnoid pathology may have caused significant CSF flow obstruction in these cases. With the rupture of an

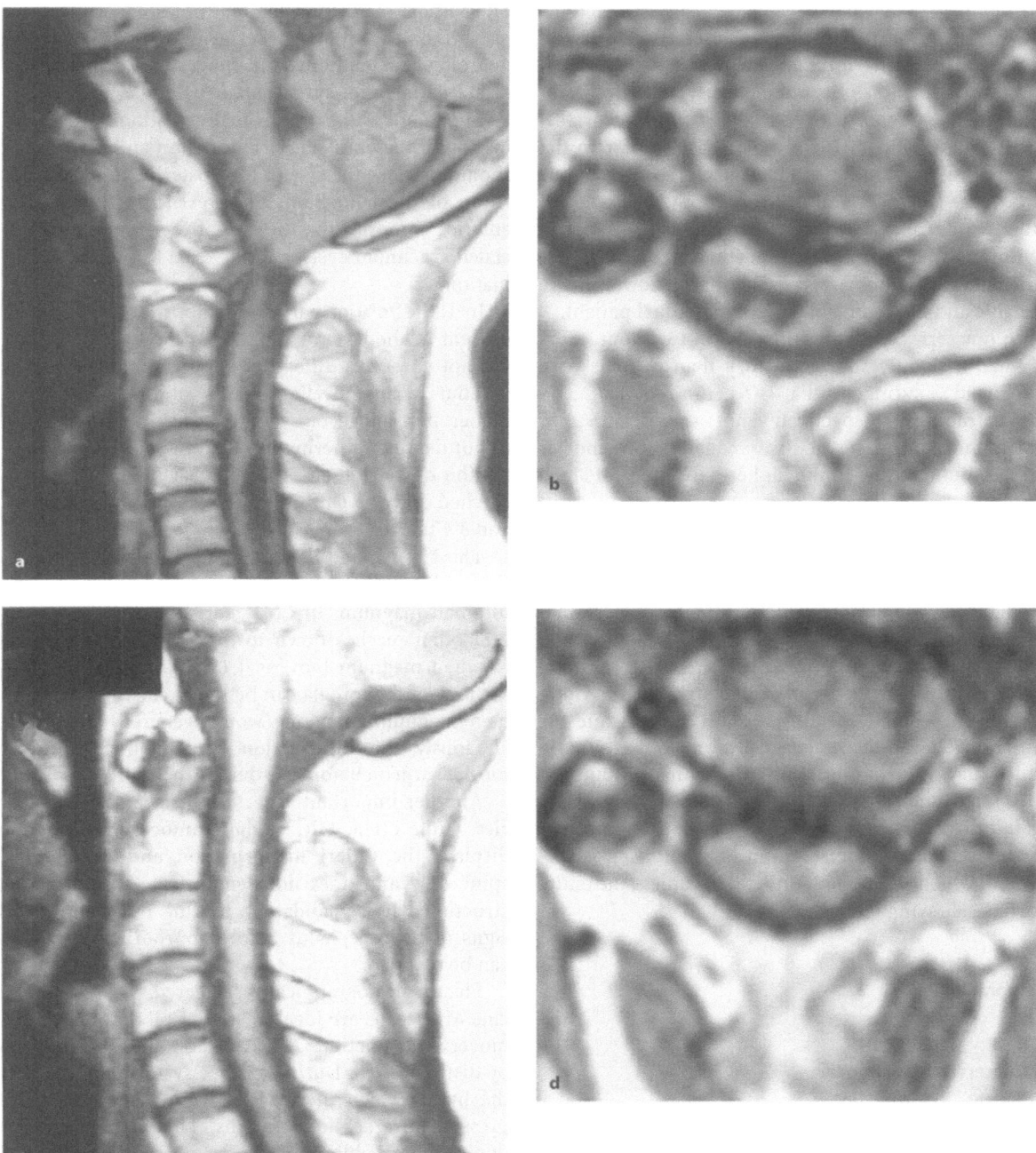

Fig. 3.5 a–d. This 37-year-old female patient presented with a 3-month history of burning type dysesthesias in her right arm. On neurological examination, hypesthesia for light touch, pain, and temperature was found in her right arm and right trigeminal distribution. The remainder of the examination was normal with no long tract signs. The T1-weighted MRI scan demonstrated a classic Chiari I malformation with syringomyelia between C2 and Th2. **a** The sagittal scan shows the obstruction of the cisterna magna by cerebellar tonsils which reach down to C1. There was no hydrocephalus. **b** The axial scan at the level of C5 demonstrates a large syrinx on the right side of the cord. The advantages and risks of surgery were discussed with the patient. Within the next couple of months, symptoms started to regress spontaneously so that surgery was postponed. Later, after 32 months, the patient was asymptomatic and underwent a control MRI showing complete resolution of the Chiari malformation (**c**) and syringomyelia (**d**). The patient did not recall any specific incidents associated with sudden changes of symptoms in these 2 years but reported a gradual disappearance of sensory and dysesthetic symptoms

arachnoid membrane, CSF flow may have improved to such an degree that the cerebellar tonsils retracted intracranially, as can be observed after successful decompression at the foramen magnum [215, 250]. To date, very few cases of spontaneous syringomyelia resolution in patients with CMI have been accurately documented with MRI. Only ten cases similar to the patient presented in Fig. 3.5 have been reported to our knowledge [18, 19, 51, 121, 186, 193, 217, 237, 238, 270]. In other words, once a syrinx has produced neurological symptoms, the clinical situation will almost always deteriorate with time. Degree and pace, however, are variable and unpredictable for an individual patient.

In our series, patients with CMI but without a syrinx had a slightly shorter history than patients with associated syringomyelia (64±100 months and 72±100 months, respectively; not significant). For CMII, the clinical history was considerably shorter (22±52 months) due to the higher percentage of small children.

Again, comparison of symptoms between CMI patients with and without syringomyelia reveals significant differences, even though it remains impossible to predict the presence of syringomyelia by clinical analysis alone in an individual patient (Tables 3.2 and 3.3). Of particular importance are the quite common swallowing disturbances in patients with CMI [199]. We recommend performing a chest X-ray while the patient swallows a contrast agent to rule out aspiration which may occur unnoticed by the patient. A pure inspection of the throat to test gag reflex and sensibility of the throat or movement of vocal cords is not enough. Sometimes, coordination of swallowing is disturbed, which will remain undetected unless the entire act of swallowing is analyzed.

3.1.2
Neuroradiology

3.1.2.1
Craniocervical Junction

CMI is characterized by tonsillar herniation below the foramen magnum. In adults, herniation of more than 5 mm is considered pathologic [3]. Mikulis et al. [166] demonstrated a physiological ascension of the cerebellar tonsils with ongoing age. The postnatal volume increase of the cerebellum causes a physiologic herniation of the tonsils until age 10 years. In adulthood, herniation of up to 5 mm is considered to be within the normal range. In old age, brain atrophy causes ascent of the tonsils, so that values of more than 3 mm are pathologic.

Meadows et al. [158] performed a survey on 22,591 unselected patients undergoing MRI scans for various reasons. Among these, 175 patients (0.77%) demon-strated evidence of CMI; and 14% were asymptomatic. The authors concluded that neuroradiological features of CMI alone may not necessarily be associated with neurological symptoms and suggested to reserve surgical treatment for symptomatic patients.

In patients with a Chiari malformation, MRI examination of the craniocervical junction and entire head should disclose the size of the posterior fossa, the position of the tentorium, the presence or absence of anterior compression, the size of the ventricles, associated arachnoid cysts, and the extent of tonsillar herniation.

In CMI, 70% of patients demonstrated a tonsillar descent to the level of C1, 28% to the level of C2. We did not observe a difference between patients with or without syringomyelia. Some authors observed a higher percentage of syringomyelia in patients with minor degrees of herniation than in patients with herniation of more than 15 mm [152, 235]. In CMII, 15% reached down to C1, 39% to C2, 15% to C3, 23% to C4, and 8% to C6.

The MRI should be studied carefully to determine the position of the tentorium and its relation to the foramen magnum. In CMII, for instance, the tentorium often reaches down to the posterior rim of the foramen magnum [201, 257] (Fig. 3.2). Even in CMI, the area of the torcula can be much closer to the foramen magnum than one would generally anticipate. Obviously, this information is of major importance for the surgeon before the dura is incised!

Another important aspect is the size of the ventricles. Quite often, MRI of the craniocervical junction displays the Chiari malformation and the cervical spine only and does not demonstrate supratentorial structures. It is mandatory to rule out radiological signs of hydrocephalus before appropriate treatment can be planned.

Electrocardiographically triggered, phase-contrast cine MRI scans are ideal to study CSF flow at the craniocervical junction. A CSF systole and diastole can be distinguished. During cardiac systole, blood enters the brain, which increases in volume causing compression of arachnoid cisterns. This volume change, due to arterial blood, starts in the frontal lobes and then progresses posteriorly. Therefore, cisterns and ventricles are compressed in a systematic cascade of events. With cisternal compression, CSF flows out of the cistern so that a complex CSF flow pattern is regulated in this manner [70, 79, 84, 96, 97, 149, 258]. Within the cisterna magna, rapid flow of CSF into the spinal canal is observed during systole [15, 36, 79, 117, 205]. In diastole, brain volume decreases in reverse fashion, cisterns dilate and CSF flows toward cisterns. In the cisterna magna, diastole is characterized by a reverse flow of CSF from the spinal canal back to the cistern. Compared with systole, flow velocities are

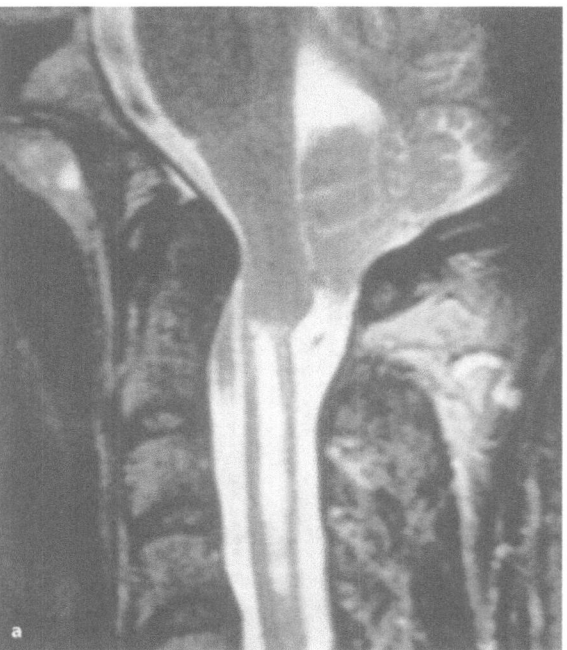

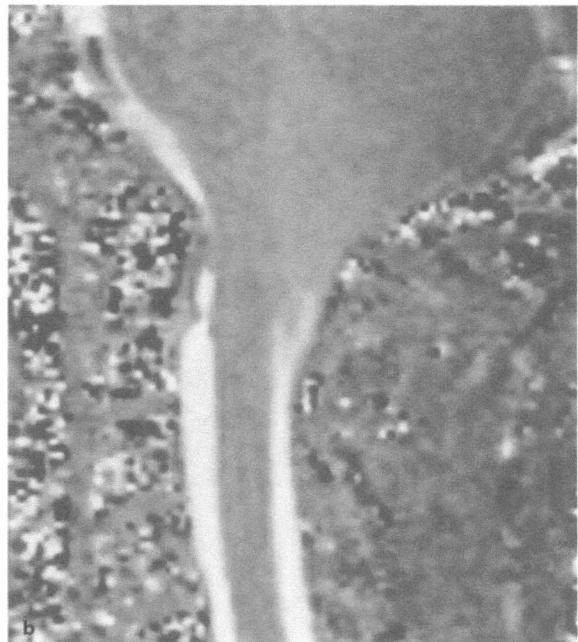

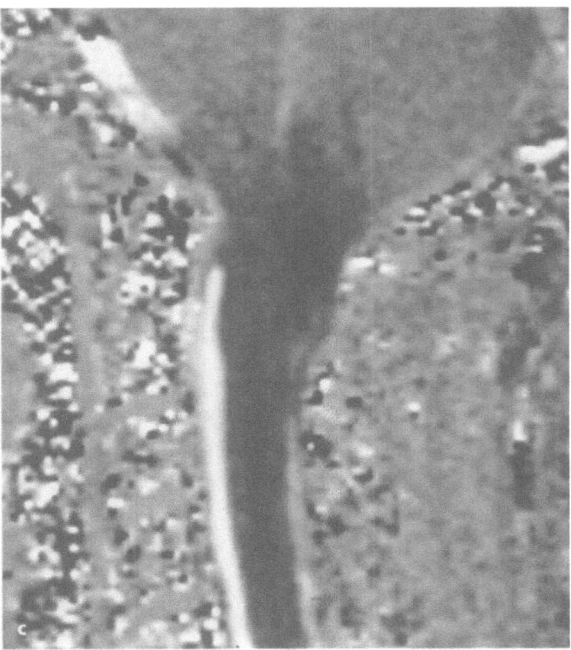

considerably lower in diastole [15, 36, 79, 117, 205]. In this way, pendulous flow of CSF across the foramen magnum is created [70, 73, 117, 136, 144, 222]. A second major influence on CSF flow is respiration. With inspiration, thoracic pressure decreases, while expiration increases it. Epidural veins transmit these pressure changes to the subarachnoid space of the spinal canal. Inspiration favors flow of CSF into the spinal canal, whereas expiration has the opposite effect [71, 224].

Cardiac-gated MRI demonstrated obstruction of CSF flow at the craniocervical junction, due to obliteration of the cisterna magna in all patients who were studied (Fig. 3.6) [15, 36, 41, 42, 73, 117, 134, 269]. We consider this imaging modality to be the method of choice to determine which patients with "borderline" tonsillar herniation may benefit from decompression. Furthermore, it is the ideal method of postoperative control.

During systole, a rapid downward motion of the tonsils [79, 203, 243, 258, 269] and spinal cord [107] was sometimes observable, which can be explained due to volume increase and intracranial CSF flow toward the cisterna magna during systole. When present, an associated syrinx usually started at the level of C1 or C2. Communication between the cyst and fourth ventricle could not be observed in any patient with CMI or CMII on MRI, even though a number of authors reported this phenomenon [95, 117, 135, 197, 223]. Dynamic MRI scanning demonstrated pulsations within the syrinx, indicating profound fluid motion within the syrinx cavity with each cardiac cycle [27, 41,

Fig. 3.6 a–c. a The sagittal T2-weighted MRI scan of this 47-year-old woman shows Chiari I malformation with syringomyelia. The compression of the medulla oblongata at the foramen magnum from posterior by cerebellar tonsils and anterior due to slight basilar invagination is apparent. The systolic (**b**) and diastolic (**c**) phase-contrast cine MRI scans demonstrate normal flow pattern of the anterior and posterior part of the cervical subarachnoid space, but no flow across the foramen magnum, and absent flow signals in the cisterna magna. In diastole, a profound flow signal is apparent in the syrinx

Table 3.4. Bony anomalies in patients with Chiari I malformation

Anomaly	n
Occipital bone – hyperostosis of crista occipitalis	25
Foramen magnum and C1	
Occipitalization of C1	3
Subluxation of C1	4
Spina bifida of C1	1
Aplasia of C1	1
Basilar invagination	8
Cervical spine	
Klippel-Feil C1/C2	2
Klippel-Feil C2/C3	2
Craniocervical instability	3
Total	49 (21%)

42, 73, 80, 154, 205, 227]. Fluid flow inside the syrinx was directed caudally in systole and reverse in diastole. Velocity measurements indicated even faster velocities inside the syrinx than in the subarachnoid space [41, 117].

Apart from a small posterior fossa, it is important to recognize other craniocervical anomalies before surgery (Table 3.4) (Figs. 3.7, 3.8) [4, 5, 17, 28, 37, 56, 63, 66, 77, 81, 125, 133, 138, 140, 155, 163, 173, 196, 220, 223, 232, 252, 253, 259]. Anterior and posterior craniocervical bony anomalies may contribute considerably to clinical symptoms, as well as to constriction of the subarachnoid space, and may need to be addressed surgically. We would like to point out, in particular, that craniocervical instabilities may be associated with CMI or may be induced by posterior bony removal [5, 159, 163]. In our series, three patients with craniocervical instability were detected.

The method of choice to study bony anatomy in Chiari malformations remains the CT with bone window (Fig. 3.7). In CMII, compression occurs in the upper cervical spine so that standard CT, or even a conventional X-ray study of the cervical spine, is sufficient to examine this region for the presence of spina bifida. As this patient group consists predominantly of children, further X-ray examinations are not necessary and can be avoided. With CMI in adults, however, the anatomical situation is more variable; a 3D reconstruction can help to plan the exposure and to provide bony landmarks for better intraoperative orientation if the MRI suggests an abnormality of this kind. Modern techniques allow to reconstruct the bony anatomy

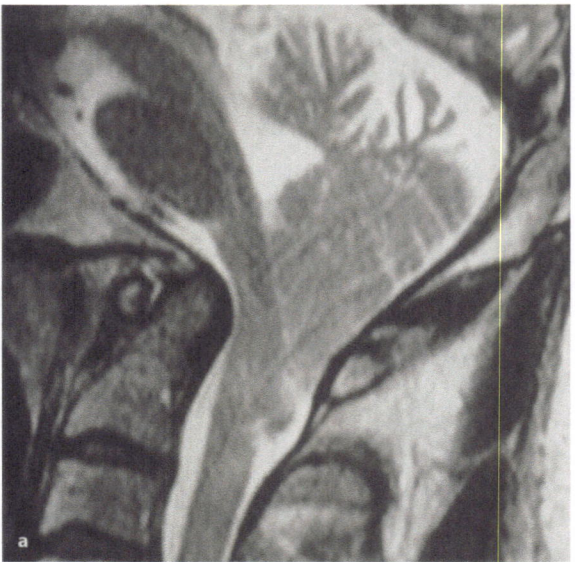

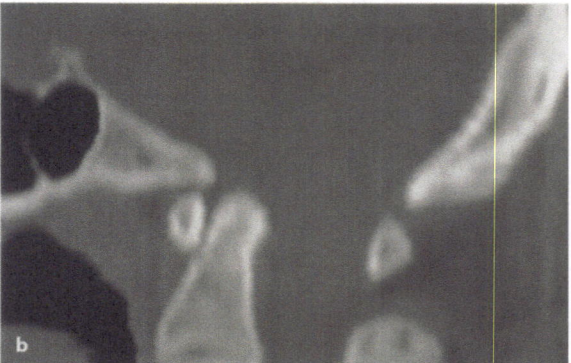

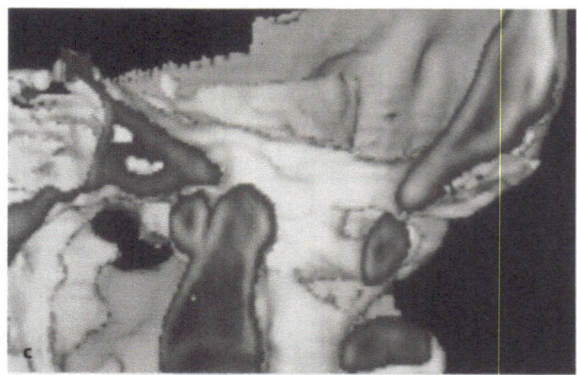

Fig. 3.7 a–c. a The sagittal T2-weighted MRI scan of this 37-year-old patient with swallowing problems, dysarthria, nystagmus, vocal cord palsies, and gait ataxia demonstrate a basilar invagination and Chiari I malformation. The bony anatomy in the sagittal plane can be studied using bone window CT (**b**) or 3D reconstructive techniques (**c**). The management of this patient is discussed in Sect. 3.1.4.4 (Fig. 3.27)

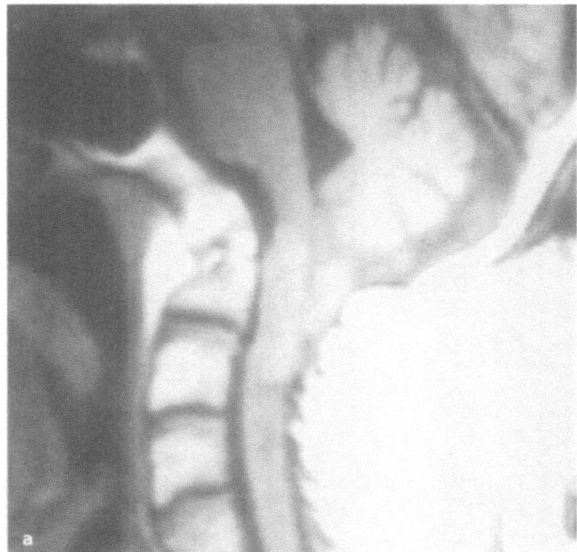

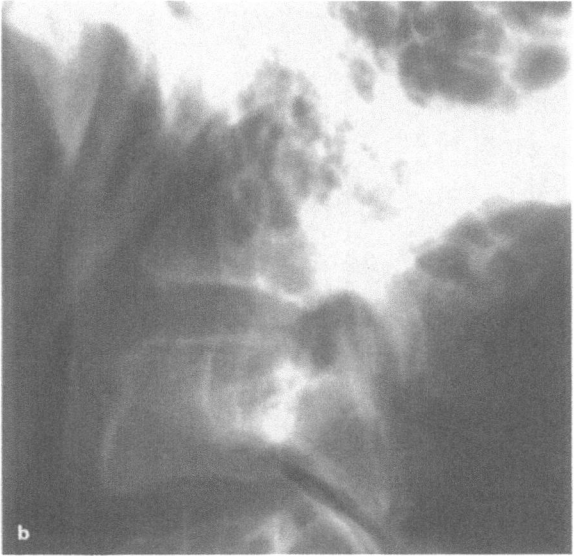

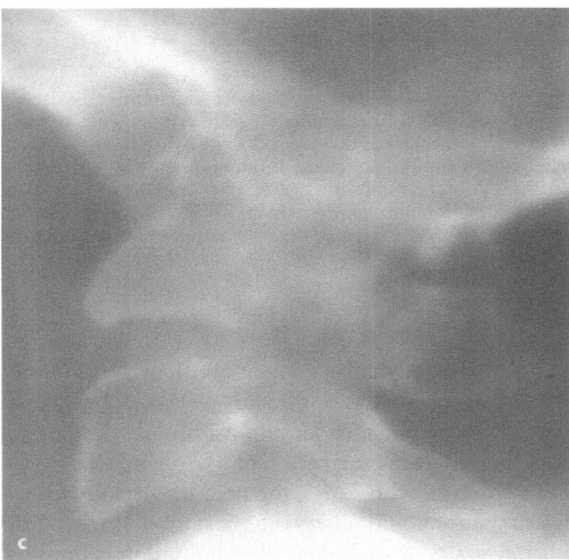

Fig. 3.8 a–c. a The T1-weighted MRI scan of this 46-year-old man with Chiari I malformation demonstrates an abnormality of the anterior foramen magnum region involving clivus, C1, and C2. b Conventional lateral X-ray of the cervical spine already suggests occipitalization of C1. c A lateral tomography provides the best visualization, showing the assimilation of C1 to the clivus and occiput, as well as a bony fusion of the C1/C2 joint

3.1.2.2
Spine and Spinal Cord

Whereas a syrinx was associated with CMI in 73% and with CMII in 54% in our cases (not significant), syringobulbia was more common in patients with CMII than with CMI (23% and 3%, respectively; Chi-square test: $P<0.02$). A correlation between the extent of the syrinx and severity of neurological symptoms could not be detected [95, 223].

In patients with an associated syrinx, the spinal cord should be examined with and without gadolinium to demonstrate the entire extension of the syrinx and to rule out an associated spinal tumor. Two spinal tumors were diagnosed in addition to the craniocervical malformation in our patient series (Fig. 3.9) [143].

In adult patients, the cervical spine should be studied carefully. With a long-standing history of CMI or CMII, hyperlordotic deformity of the cervical spine may develop (Fig. 3.10). This profound retroflexion of the head provides some relief at the foramen magnum. With anteflexion of the head, compression of the cervical cord and brainstem increase, while retroflexion has the opposite effect [178, 240]. This abnormal position of the cervical spine may predispose to degenerative problems. Other abnormalities, such as fusion of the atlas to the occiput (Fig. 3.8), or a Klippel-Feil syndrome (Fig. 3.11), may also provoke degenerative pro-

in every desired plane and to calculate 3D models of the foramen magnum area.

Furthermore, preoperative imaging should consist of plain X-ray films of the cervical spine, including lateral images in ante- and retroflexion. If instability of the craniocervical spine is suspected or additional bony anomalies of the craniocervical junction are present (such as basilar invagination), conventional lateral tomograms with ante- and retroflexion of the neck are recommended. Even though this modality has come somewhat out-of-fashion, it still remains the best way to identify instabilities in this region (Fig. 3.8).

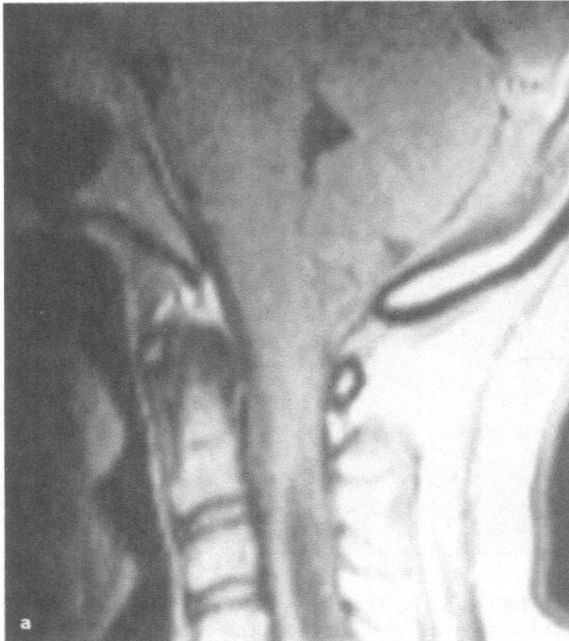

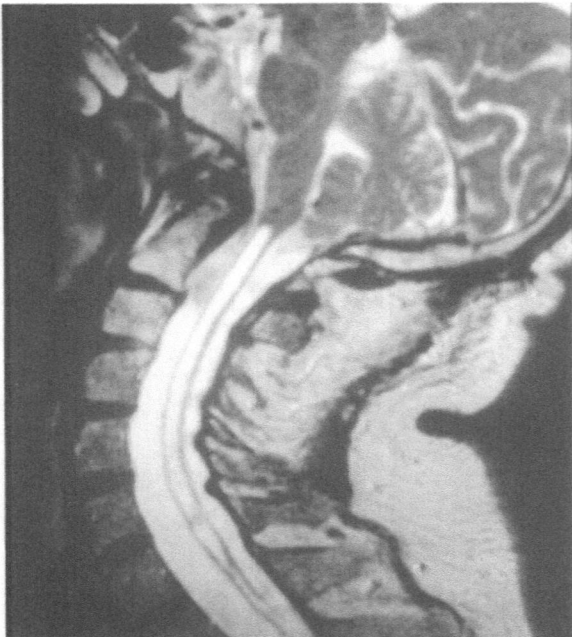

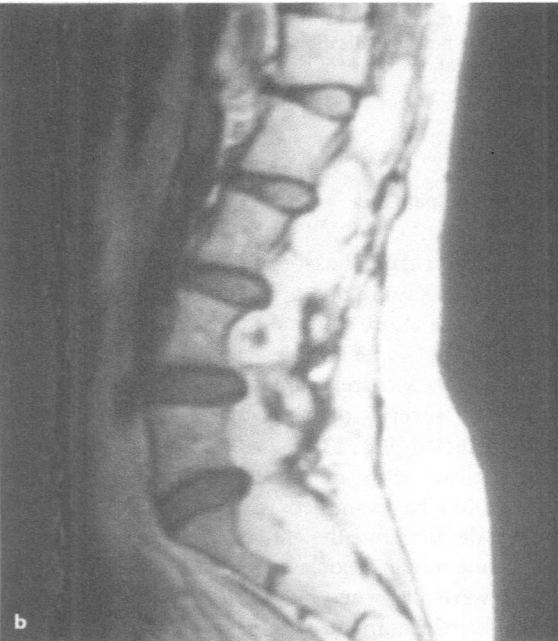

Fig. 3.10. The T2-weighted sagittal MRI scan of this 60-year-old patient with Chiari I malformation and syringomyelia demonstrates hyperlordosis of the cervical spine, which achieves some relief from compression at the foramen magnum. The patient became symptomatic at the age of 18 years and was misdiagnosed to have multiple sclerosis. More than 40 years elapsed until this MRI scan disclosed the true nature of his neurological disease

Fig. 3.9 a, b. The T1-weighted MRI scans with gadolinium of this 35-year-old woman with gait ataxia reveal a classic Chiari I malformation with syringomyelia (**a**) and an extensive ependymoma of the filum terminale, filling the entire spinal canal between sacrum and L1 (**b**)

blems. In a particular patient, radicular symptoms due to degenerative disc diseases or cervical myelopathy may be responsible for clinical progression, rather than the Chiari malformation or syringomyelia.

In children with CMII, the area of myelomeningocele repair should always be examined with MRI whenever a neuroradiological examination is required (Fig. 3.12). Clinical symptoms, as well as a new or reappearing syrinx, may be related to either the foramen magnum pathology or a re-tethered cord [46, 156, 273].

Another problem associated with Chiari malformations and syringomyelia is spinal scoliosis [13, 34, 53, 82, 113, 177, 180, 202, 247, 271, 273]. Overall, approximately 73% of patients with CMI will demonstrate some degree of scoliosis [72]. Scoliosis may be the first manifestation of syringomyelia, especially in childhood (Fig. 3.13). In children, CMI without scoliosis almost does not exist [177, 273]. Therefore, every child with scoliosis should undergo an MRI examination as soon as the slightest neurological sign is detected or orthopedic surgery is considered. If CMI or CMII is detected, it should be treated first in these cases [177], even though it alone may not be sufficient enough to

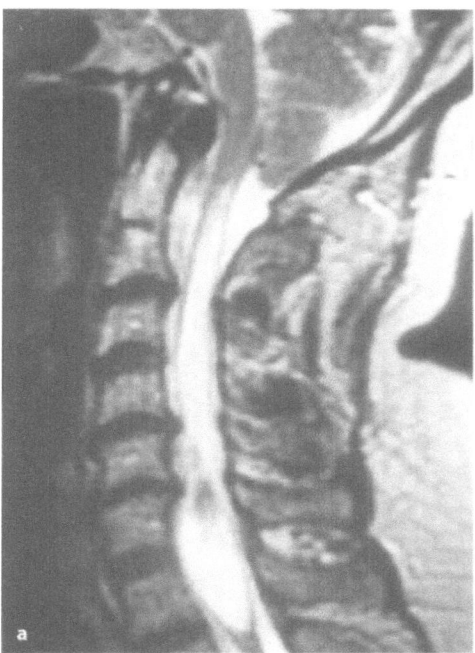

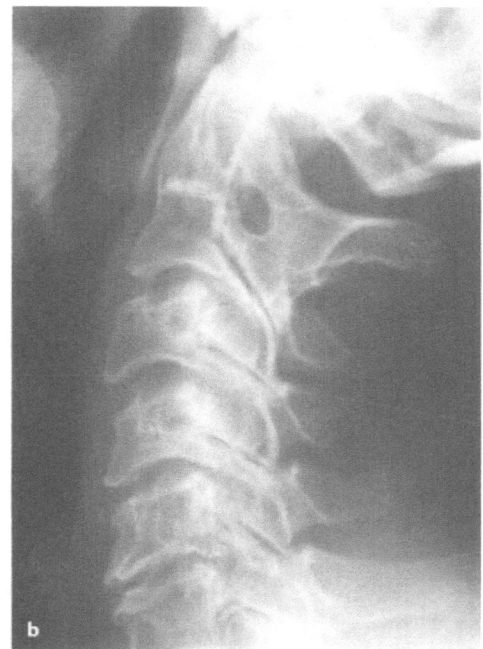

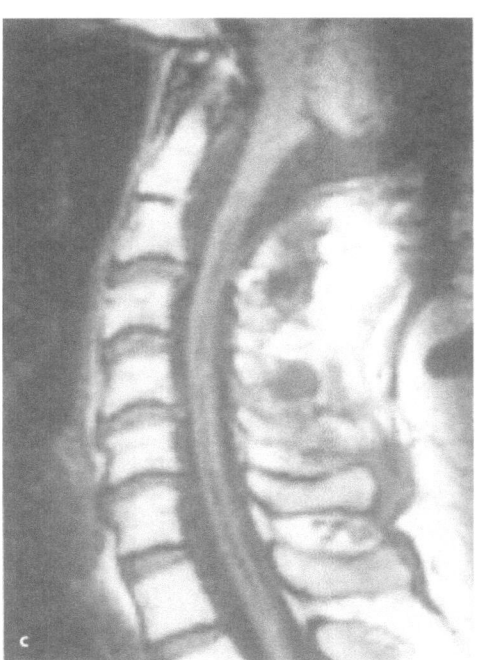

Fig. 3.11 a–c. This 58-year-old woman presented with a long history of occipital and neck pain. She had slight weakness and hypesthesia of her entire right hand and some tingling sensation not representative of a particular nerve root affection. The remainder of the neurological examination was normal. The T2-weighted MRI scan showed CMI with syringomyelia (**a**) and a Klippel-Feil syndrome at C2/3 was detected using conventional X-rays (**b**). Marked degenerative changes of cervical discs are visible at C3/4, C5/6, and C6/7 (**a**). After foramen magnum decompression the syrinx decreased in size and pain, motor weakness, and dysesthesias resolved. One year later, the patient started to complain of neck and shoulder pain on the right side. This can be provoked by turning the head to the right. She experienced some relief with physiotherapy. **c** The T1-weighted MRI scan demonstrates that the foramen magnum is well decompressed and the syrinx collapsed. However, degenerative changes of the cervical spine are unchanged, especially for the segment C3/4 on the right side, which corresponds to the patients' complaints. Even though surgery for C3/4 was discussed with the patient, she choose to continue with conservative treatment. Her status has remained unchanged for 2 years now

3.1.3
Neurophysiology

Neurophysiological findings in Chiari malformations are as variable as their clinical pictures. The relevant investigations are somatosensory-evoked potentials (SSEP) and motor evoked potentials (MEP), by which some information on long tracts may be obtained. Investigations of the cranial nerves and nuclei such as auditory brainstem responses (ABR), blink reflexes, trigeminal evoked responses (TEP), or visually evoked potential (VEP) may be examined if involvement is suspected.

stabilize the scoliosis [82, 273]. Interestingly, a left thoracic curve is seen more often in neurogenic scoliosis than are idiopathic forms [177]. Other features that should alert the physician to perform MRI on a child with scoliosis are rapid progression, pain, and onset before 2 years of age [177].

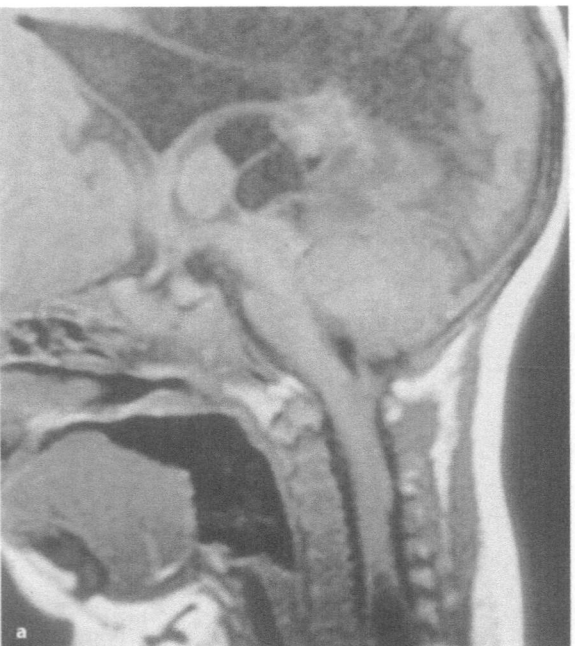

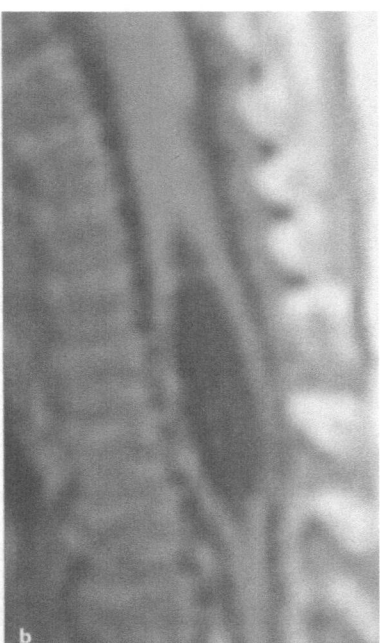

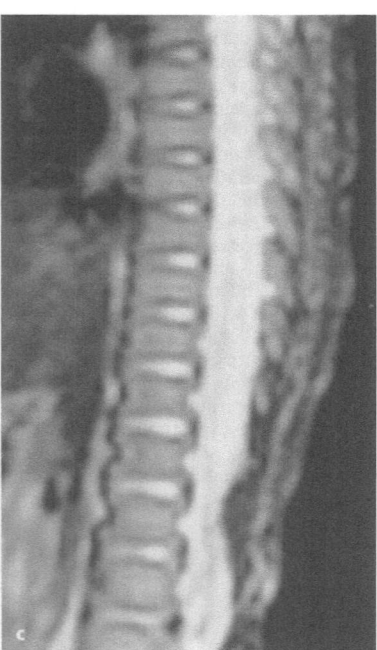

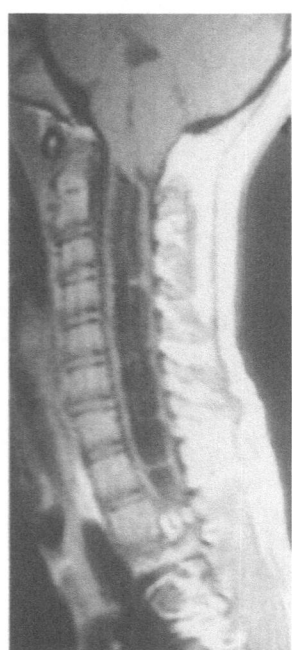

Fig. 3.12 a–c. The T1-weighted MRI scans of this 5-month-old girl demonstrate Chiari II malformation (**a**) with tonsils reaching down to the level of C4 and the upper end of a syrinx at C6. MRI scan of the cervicothoracic spine (**b**) shows the extent of the syrinx between C6 and Th3. The remainder of the spinal examination in T2-weighted images (**c**) shows normal findings down to the level of the myelomeningocele repair. With a history of repeated shunt revisions and meningitis, this syrinx is caused by CSF flow obstruction at the craniocervical junction, rather than re-tethering of the spinal cord

Fig. 3.13. The T1-weighted sagittal MRI scan of this 13-year-old girl with Chiari I malformation and syringomyelia illustrates the problem of imaging the entire syrinx in patients with marked scoliosis. The spinal cord leaves the plane of imaging at the level of Th2. In such instances, each spinal segment has to be studied via a separate axial MRI examination, if the entire syrinx is to be visualized

To date, little is known about typical patterns of presentation and susceptibility to neurosurgical manipulations in patients with CMI. For the diagnosis of syringomyelia, neurophysiological examinations are of minor importance. Median nerve evoked sensory potentials (MSEP) were found to be normal in 5 of 18 patients studied by Forcardas et al. [86]. Pathological findings were interpreted to correlate with proprioceptive deficits. In our own series, approximately 25% of patients exhibited normal SSEP waveforms with normal latencies and amplitudes, while over 50% showed significant deformations but had reproducible waveforms. The extent of SSEP deterioration seems to correlate to some extent with the patient's history and, in particular, the duration of sensory deficits. Some authors tried to identify specific SSEP changes, such as deformation or loss of the cervical and brainstem components [61, 176, 204, 209, 256, 261]. Most authors consider tibial SSEP (TSEP) especially sensitive and superior to MSEP [111, 120, 150, 151, 256, 261] because pathological values are more often detectable.

The major application of SSEP studies is for intraoperative monitoring. All surgical procedures at the craniocervical junction may be potentially harmful for the brainstem, especially in CMI with compression at this level. To increase intraoperative safety, we apply SSEP monitoring routinely during the entire neurosurgical procedure. MSEP and, in some cases, also TSEP are tested at all relevant steps of the procedure:

▶ At the start after induction of anesthesia, i.e., baseline
▶ Positioning of the patient
▶ After 10 minutes post-positioning
▶ Laminectomy of C1
▶ Opening of foramen magnum
▶ Dura opening
▶ Arachnoid opening and dissection
▶ Coagulation of the tonsils
▶ Opening of the fourth ventricle
▶ Insertion of the dural patch
▶ Soft tissue closure
▶ End of the procedure

Three periods are the most interesting during foramen magnum decompression:

▶ The baseline study with the patient on his back in neutral position
▶ The positioning of the patient
▶ During coagulation of the cerebellar tonsils and opening of the fourth ventricle

At the baseline study, absence of SSEP is a very rare finding in CMI. But, in some patients, the SSEP components show such a lack of reproducibility with varying latencies and amplitudes that a reliable baseline cannot be obtained and criteria of preserved SSEP are not fulfilled. This may occur uni- or bilaterally. Bilateral absence is quite unusual but unilateral absence is present in a considerable number of patients. In those cases, the stimulation intensity is increased up to threefold to find out whether at least a few tracts are functioning. With this adjustment, recordings are obtainable in some patients but may remain absent in others.

Severely distorted SSEP are another common phenomenon. Distortions are characterized by an increased latency of the spinal and bulbar (N13, N15) SSEP components, the central (N20, P25) SSEP components, a broadening of the individual components (N15, N20, P25), and a reduced amplitude of individual components.

The presence of a reproducible SSEP is a precondition for any further use as a controlling measure during positioning and surgery. A pathological SSEP at baseline serves as additional proof of craniocervical compression. Neurophysiological findings during positioning, especially during anteflection of the patient's head under general anesthesia, must be recorded without any interruption and continued for at least 10 min after final head fixation. Typical changes during positioning maneuvers are: latency increase of single components, amplitude reduction of individual components, or loss of some or of all components. Figure 3.14 provides an example of MSEP changes during positioning of the patient and their subsequent recovery with correction of the positioning and decompression of the foramen magnum.

In case of SSEP deterioration, the surgeon is immediately informed and a modification of the positioning is suggested to enable a wave recovery. In such an instance, it is advisable to extend the neck and to retroflex the head slightly as this manoeuvre lowers pressure on the brainstem and cervical cord at the foramen magnum.

A latency increase of individual components is carefully looked for, so as to detect indicators of a possible wave disappearance as early as possible. A latency increase of 1 ms is regarded as acceptable, if it stops. If the latency increase continues, a modification of positioning is suggested.

Likewise, amplitude reduction of individual components may indicate an impeding wave loss. An amplitude reduction by a third is regarded as acceptable, if it stops. If it continues, a modification of positioning is recommended.

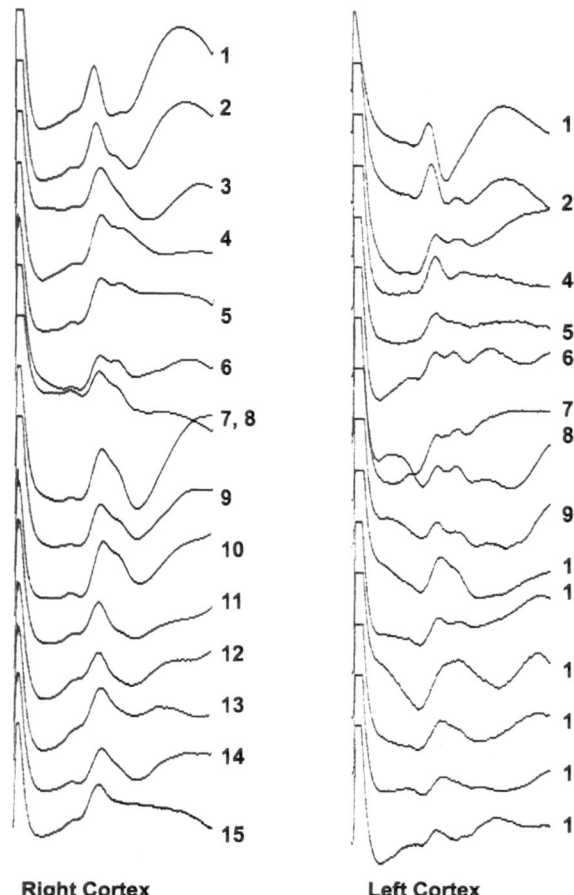

Right Cortex   **Left Cortex**

Fig. 3.14. Overview of intraoperative changes of medianus SSEP recordings in a 40-year-old patient with Chiari I malformation and syringomyelia. Recordings are numbered consecutively for both sides. Recording no.*1* represents the baseline with the patient under general anesthesia. The patient is brought into the semi-sitting position (no. *2*) and the Mayfield clamp is applied (no. *3*). Upon extension and anteflexion of the neck (no. *4*), SSEP starts to deteriorate with prolongation of latencies. Upon fixation of this position (no. *5*), further changes occur with a decrease of amplitudes. The positioning is corrected by applying more extension and less anteflexion (no. *6*). After some time, SSEP recovery is seen (no. *7*) so that surgery was continued. Nos. *8* and *9* show the recordings during bone removal of C1 and occipital bone, respectively. The dura is opened (no. *10*). Upon coagulation of the tonsils and opening of the fourth ventricle (nos. *11, 12*), SSEP latencies improve considerably. The dura patch is inserted (no. *13*) and SSEP improves further during soft tissue closure (no. *14*). Finally, the SSEP recordings made an almost complete recovery during this operation (no. *15*). The patient did not acquire any neurological deficit. Occipital pain and sensory changes improved

A loss of some or all components may occur as a consequence of increasing deterioration of latencies and amplitudes or may occur all of a sudden. Immediate correction of head and neck position are mandatory. Intraoperative recovery of SSEP changes requires early detection of signs of deterioration and immediate modification of an unfavorable position. However, re-

covery of the components – once they have been lost – may take a long time and is not guaranteed. If in doubt, we terminate the operation at this stage and let the patient recover to avoid any risk of severe spinal cord or brainstem compression by continuing the surgery.

Intraoperatively, we sometimes observed transient SSEP deteriorations during coagulation of cerebellar tonsils. However, long-lasting changes were not provoked by this maneuver.

In terms of postoperative clinical function, there is no strict correlation between clinical symptoms and the quality of preserved SSEP [111, 261]. So far, the SSEP of an individual patient is of uncertain significance. Moreover, it is not known precisely which deteriorations are tolerated and whether there are definite or individual limits. Nonetheless, it is known from other SSEP investigations for pathologies at the brainstem and upper cervical cord that SSEP deteriorations are often followed by at least transient deteriorations of neurological function. Furthermore, we know from the postoperative course of patients with CMI that surgical decompression might alleviate occipital pain and signs of brainstem compression, but motor function and coordination are only stabilized in most cases. This aspect indicates the limited tolerance of the medulla and spinal cord to any further trauma and change. Therefore, it is presumed that any neurophysiological deterioration should be prevented during surgery.

Over 75% of patients in our series maintained their level of SSEP quality or regained it – after temporary deterioration – during foramen magnum decompression. A small group of approximately 5% showed improvement of SSEP, while the rest demonstrated some minor intraoperative deteriorations. In the worst cases, a single component became lost, but a more dramatic wave loss did not ever occur. As long as SSEP are preserved, a stable or improved clinical outcome may be assumed. Improvement of SSEP were especially observed during bony decompression, such as removal of the atlas or opening of the foramen magnum.

MEP recordings showed good correlation to preoperative motor deficits in these patients [61]. However, no correlation existed to postoperative outcome [111]. Even in patients with successful decompression, no improvement of MEPs could be demonstrated.

Mori et al. [174] found pathological values for auditory evoked potentials (AEP) in 12 of 16 patients with CMI. As with other types of neurophysiological examinations, no correlation could be found between AEP changes and clinical prognosis in CMI. For infants with CMII, however, several studies suggest good correlation between AEP changes and neurological symptoms related to brainstem compression [108, 241].

Electromyographic (EMG) examinations were able to demonstrate fibrillations, a reduced number of motor units, and chronic changes, but no specific findings [256].

3.1.4
Surgical Management

Surgery should be indicated for adult patients with a Chiari malformation as soon as neurological symptoms are present. If in doubt, cardiac-gated cine MRI may help to identify patients with CSF flow obstruction at the foramen magnum. In children older than 2 years of age, a period of observation may be warranted. If the anatomical situation improves with time, surgery may not be required. However, in infants with CMII, surgery should be considered as soon as symptoms are detected, despite a functioning ventricular shunt. The craniocervical malformation is the most common cause of death in untreated children with CMII [44]. The following surgical strategy should be followed step by step:

1. Treatment of hydrocephalus – if present
2. Decompression of the foramen magnum and cervical canal
3. Stabilization of the craniocervical junction – if instability is present

3.1.4.1
Hydrocephalus and Chiari Malformation

Patients who present clinical signs of hydrocephalus should first be treated for the hydrocephalus [17, 49, 264, 266]. Basically, two possibilities exist: (1) shunting of the ventricle to either the peritoneal cavity or right atrium and (2) third ventriculostomy.

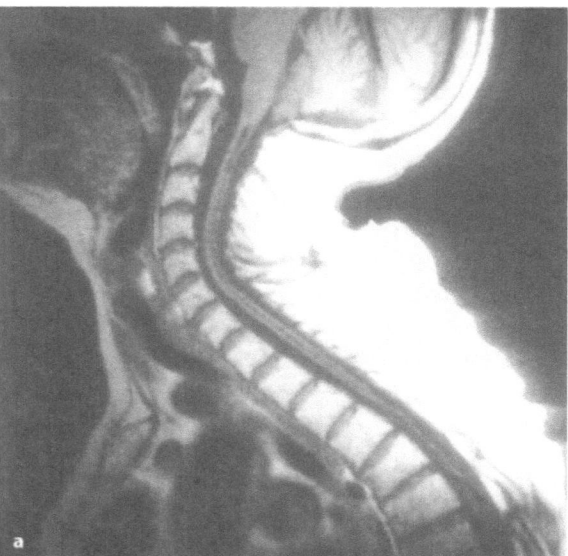

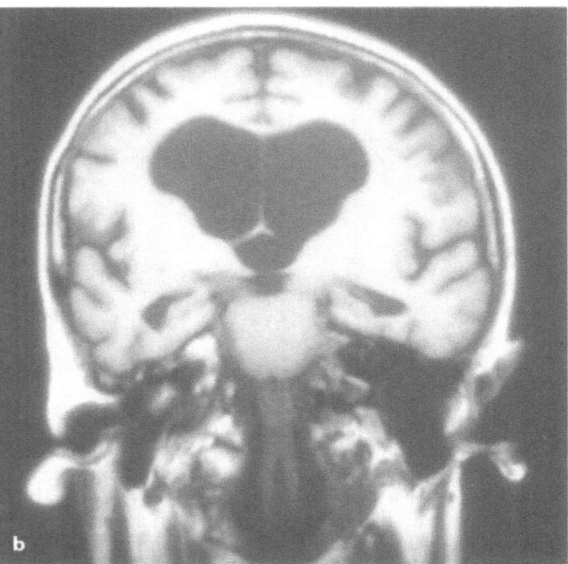

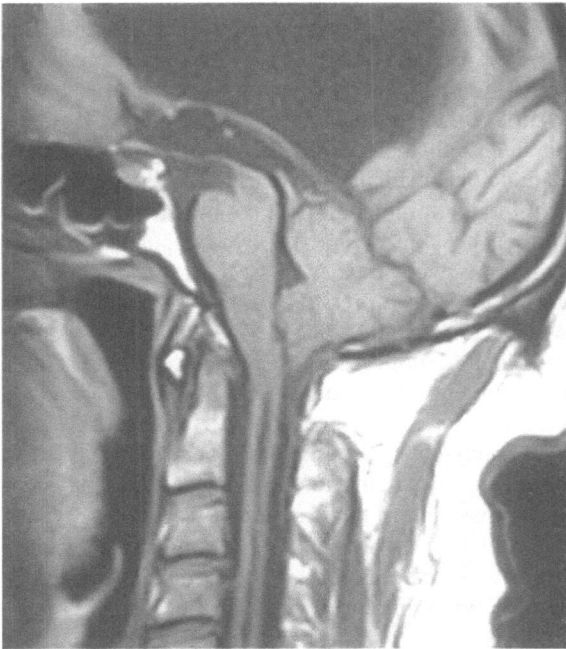

Fig. 3.15. The sagittal T1-weighted MRI scan of this 63-year-old man revealed a Chiari I malformation, syringomyelia, and marked ventricular dilation. The patient complained about slight headache provoked by exertion but revealed no other neurological symptoms. An ophthalmological examination was normal with no evidence of papilledema. In the absence of relevant neurological symptoms, the decision was made to follow this patient clinically and to postpone surgical therapy until symptoms appear

Fig. 3.16 a, b. This 69-year-old woman was admitted with a 4-year history of progressive gait ataxia and hypesthesia in her left leg. For the past 3 months she had experienced bladder incontinence and an organic psychosyndrome. On sagittal (**a**) and coronal (**b**) sections in MRI, hydrocephalus, Chiari I malformation, and syringomyelia were diagnosed. The cervical cord appeared atrophic with a small syrinx cavity. The patient underwent ventriculoperitoneal shunting and demonstrated improvements of gait and bladder function postoperatively

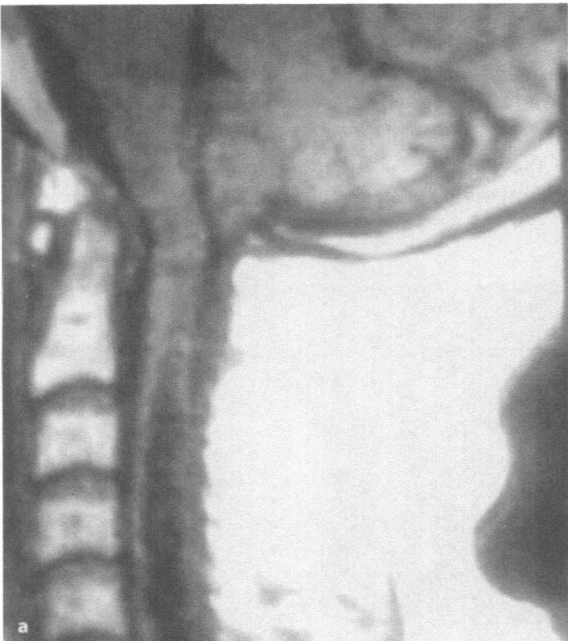

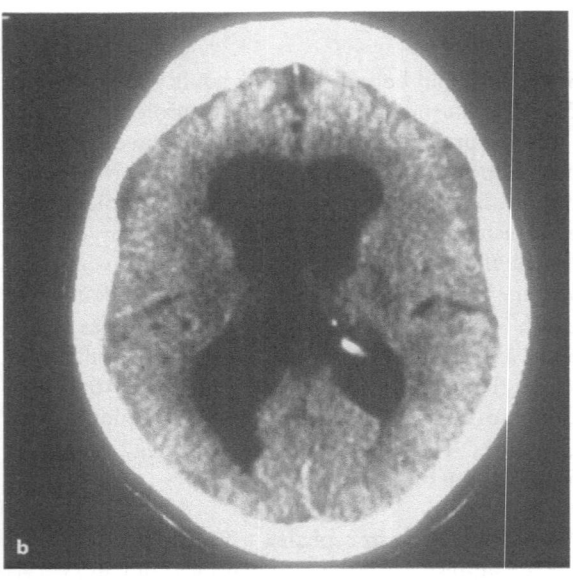

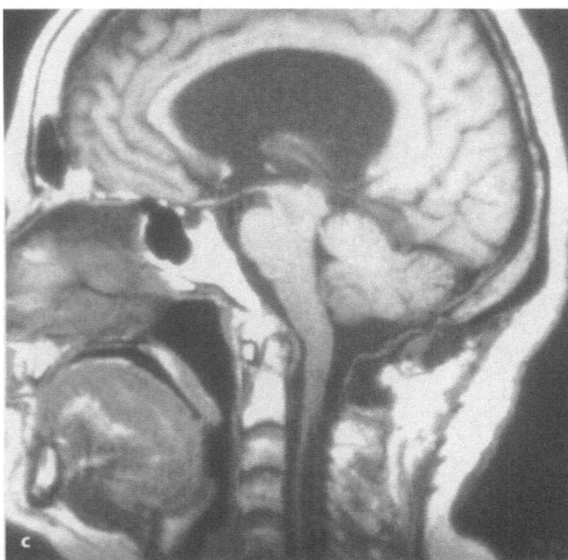

Fig. 3.17 a–c. a The sagittal T1-weighted MRI scan of this year 61-year-old woman with a 2-year history of occipital headaches demonstrates Chiari I malformation with syringomyelia. The size of the ventricles cannot be examined on this scan. **b** CT reveals a marked dilation of the supratentorial ventricles. The patient underwent foramen magnum decompression. **c** The postoperative MRI scan after 1 week shows good decompression of the foramen magnum, collapse of the syrinx, and unchanged ventricle sizes. A small subfascial CSF collection resolved spontaneously. The patient improved postoperatively and is doing well 6 years later

Dilated ventricles were present in 8% of patients with CMI and syringomyelia, 13% of those with CMI but without syringomyelia, and 92% of patients with CMII in our series (Figs. 3.15, 3.16, 3.17). In CMI, two patients demonstrated clinical signs of hydrocephalus and, in both cases, a ventriculoperitoneal shunt was inserted primarily. Postoperatively, only clinical signs related to the hydrocephalus improved. The size of the syrinx remained unchanged in both cases. However, neither of them required further surgical treatment. Radiological evidence of ventricular dilation was present in an additional 21 CMI patients. These, however, showed no clinical signs of hydrocephalus and their symptoms were related to CMI or the syrinx only. Therefore, decompression of the foramen magnum was performed. Just one of these patients required ventriculoperitoneal shunting as a second subsequent procedure because clinical signs of hydrocephalus developed after decompression. All others showed no hydrocephalic symptoms postoperatively. In CMII, however, all patients underwent ventriculoperitoneal shunt insertion as the first line of treatment, if ventricular dilation was evident on MRI and clinical signs of brainstem compression or hydrocephalus were present. If symptoms progressed further, decompression of the brainstem was performed as the second step.

From our experience, we would conclude that hydrocephalus should be treated first in patients with CMII and in those with CMI who present clinical signs related to it (Fig. 3.16). With successful treatment of the hydrocephalus chances are favorable that no further intervention may be necessary [47, 273]. In patients with CMI and ventricular dilation but without clinical signs of hydrocephalus, no shunt seems to be

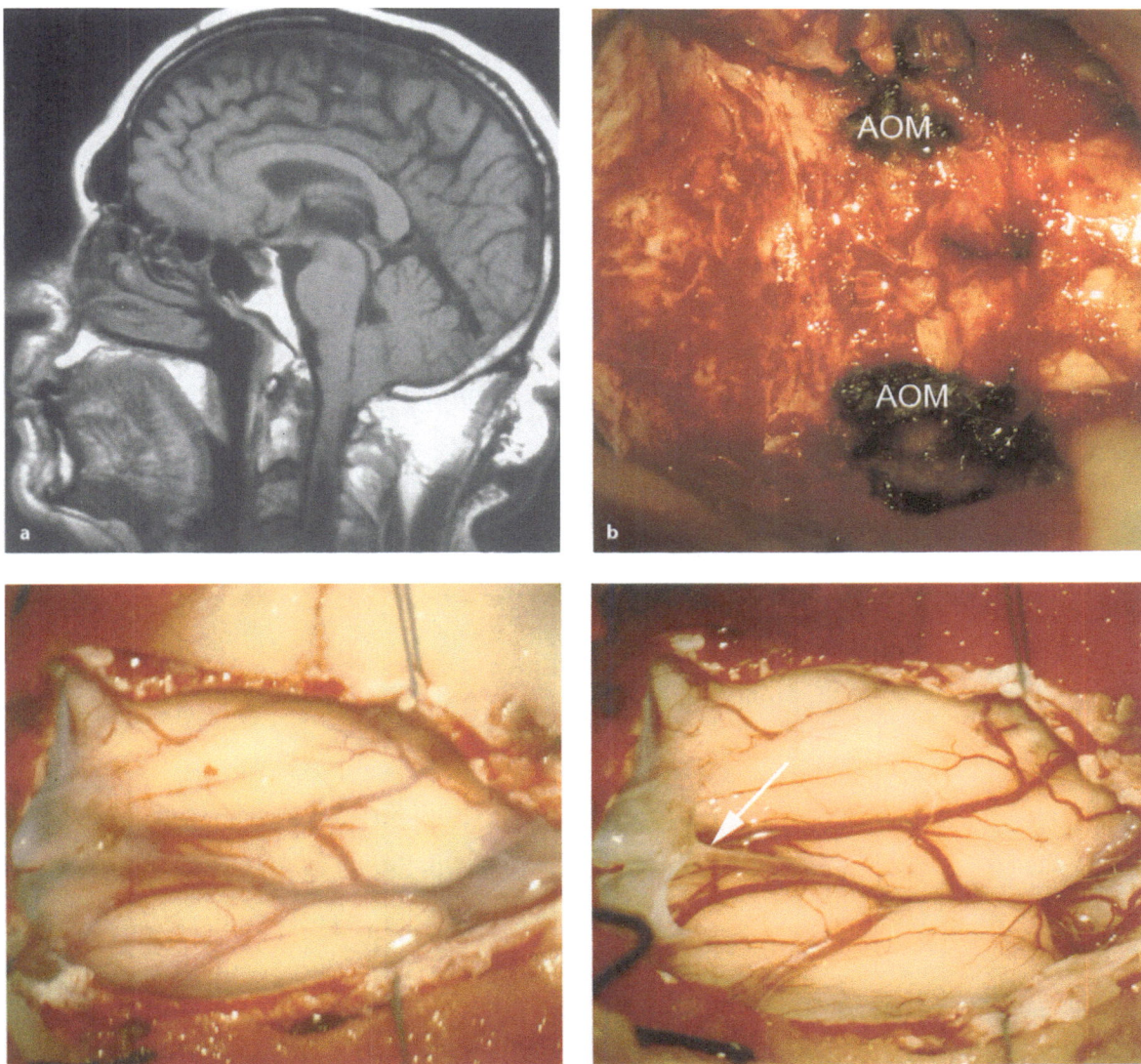

Fig. 3.18 a–j. a The T1-weighted sagittal MRI scan of this 67-year-old man with occipital headaches, marked swallowing problems, and gait ataxia shows typical Chiari I malformation with syringomyelia. Apart from a small posterior fossa, no other anatomical anomalies of the craniocervical junction are noticeable. **b** This intraoperative picture reveals the situation before dura opening. The atlantooccipital membrane (AOM) has been coagulated and dissected laterally and marks the level of the foramen magnum. Please note the extent of the craniectomy, which does not exceed the width of the spinal canal. **c** After opening of the dura in Y-shaped fashion, retention sutures have been applied. The arachnoid is still intact and translucent. The right PICA can just be seen at the tip of the right tonsil at the level of C1. **d** This picture shows the situation after arachnoid opening. The *arrow* marks a small perforating artery extending into the arachnoidal layer (continued on p. 47)

required and foramen magnum decompression alone is sufficient (Fig. 3.17). If in doubt, an external ventricular drain can be inserted to monitor the situation after decompression.

In several scientific meetings, reports have started to appear concerning ventriculostomies for patients with CMI. Successful procedures were even able to reverse the tonsillar herniation, due to the change of CSF circulation caused by this procedure. However, long-term studies need to be performed before a recommendation of this strategy can be given.

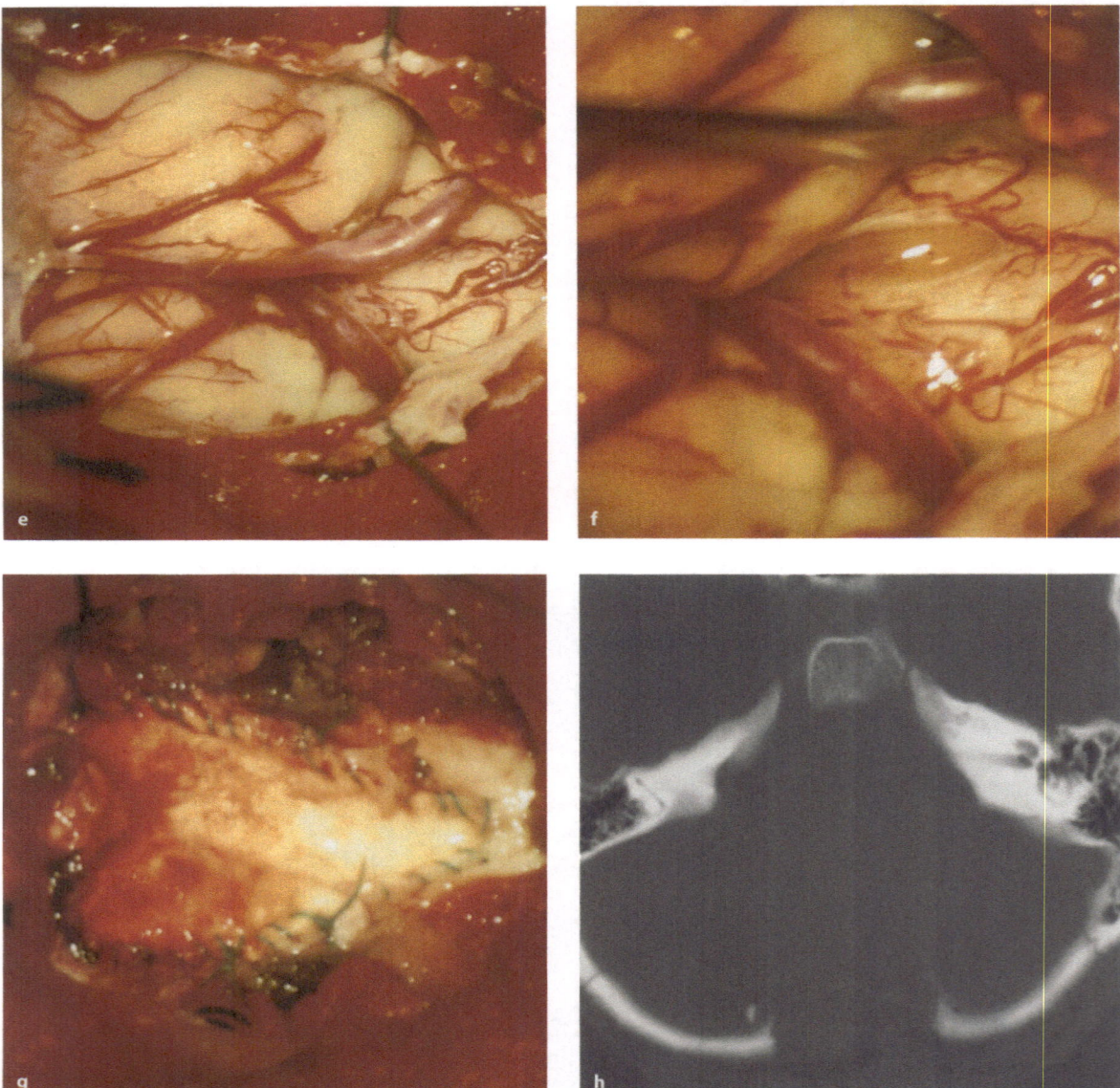

3.1.4.2
Decompression for Chiari I Malformation

Patients should be operated on in the prone position. This position offers a perfect access to the craniocervical junction and avoids risks of the semi-sitting position such as air embolism. The semi-sitting position, which was routinely used until 1995, is now reserved for patients in whom severe arachnoid scarring is suspected in order to use continuous irrigation during microsurgical dissection of the arachnoid. During positioning, we recommend monitoring of evoked sensory potentials (SSEP) to prevent any undue compression of the brainstem. Flexion of the neck in particular may cause significant compression at the foramen magnum

(Fig. 3.14). After a midline incision, detachment of the neck muscles from the occipital bone and the arches of C1, and – depending on the extent of tonsillar herniation – further cervical laminae, then a small laminectomy of the exposed arches and a craniectomy is performed, which includes the foramen magnum. Figure 3.18 demonstrates the individual surgical steps. The width of the craniectomy is adjusted to the width of the upper cervical dural sac and should not exceed 3 cm. Likewise, the upper extension of the craniectomy is tailored to create a cisterna magna and to visualize the foramen of Magendie. Therefore, it is not necessary to expose the transverse sinus and the longitudinal extent of the craniectomy can be limited to approximately 3 cm as well. The occipital bone can be quite thickened.

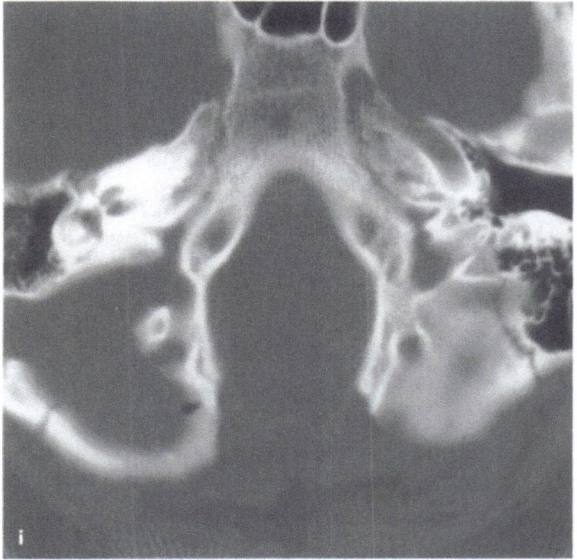

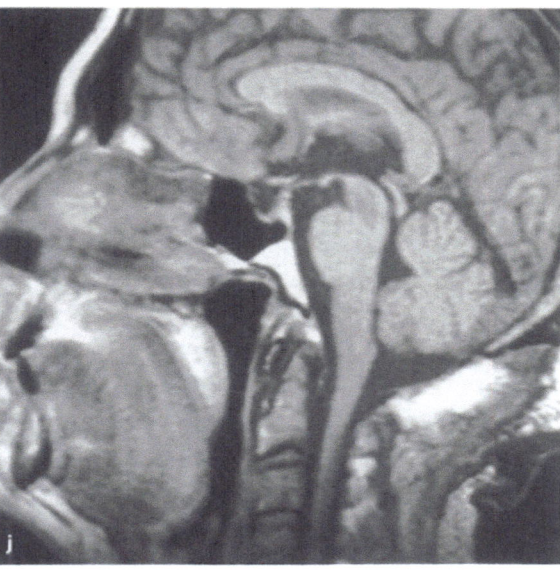

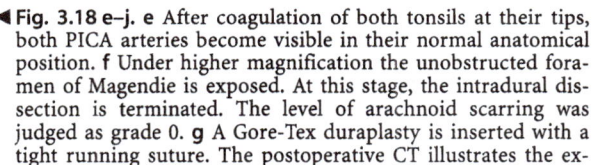

◀ **Fig. 3.18 e–j. e** After coagulation of both tonsils at their tips, both PICA arteries become visible in their normal anatomical position. **f** Under higher magnification the unobstructed foramen of Magendie is exposed. At this stage, the intradural dissection is terminated. The level of arachnoid scarring was judged as grade 0. **g** A Gore-Tex duraplasty is inserted with a tight running suture. The postoperative CT illustrates the ex-

tent of the bony removal (**h, i**). **j** The postoperative sagittal T1-weighted MRI scan after 3 months demonstrates decompression of brain stem and spinal cord at the foramen magnum, a normally sized cisterna magna, and a complete disappearance of the syrinx. The preoperative symptoms had resolved almost completely at this time

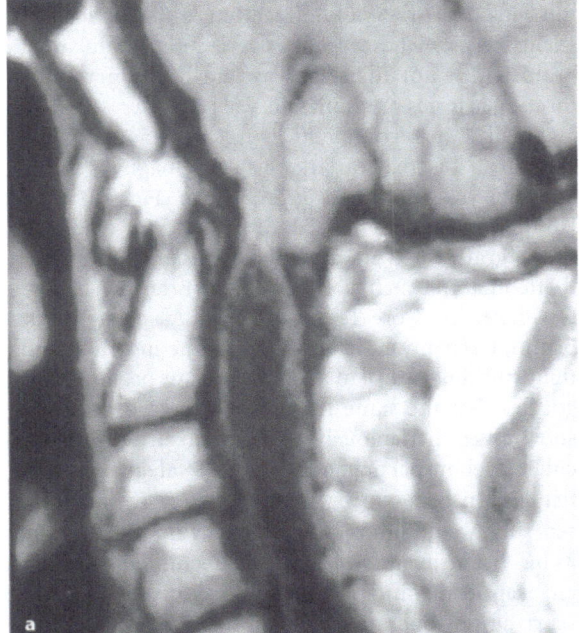

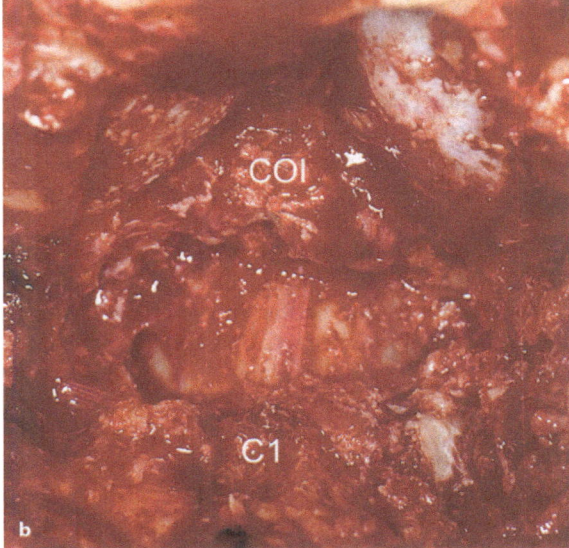

Fig. 3.19 a, b. a The sagittal T1-weighted MRI scan of this 56-year-old man with Chiari I malformation and syringomyelia shows a marked thickening and elevation of the occipital bone at the foramen magnum, causing a bony stenosis. This patient was operated on in semi-sitting position. **b** Intraoperatively, the space of the cisterna magna is completely occupied by this occipital bone, representing a hyperostosis of the crista occipitalis interna (COI). The former level of C1 is marked for better orientation

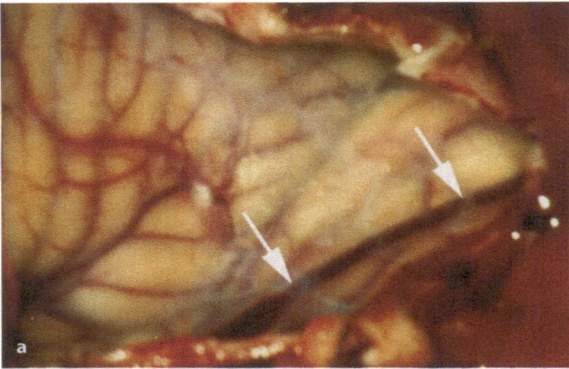
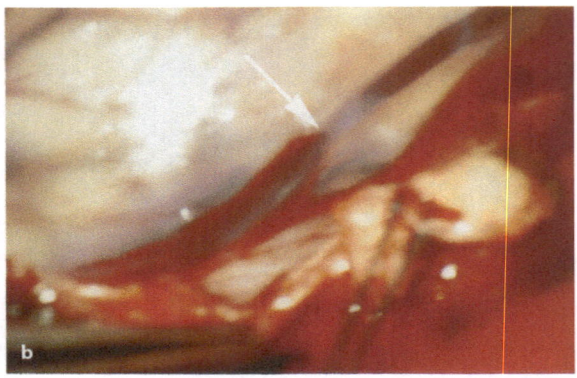

Fig. 3.20 a, b. a This intraoperative view after dura opening in a patient with CMI shows a large bridging vein extending from the spinal cord to the suboccipital sinus, running over the left tonsillar surface (*arrows*). **b** Under higher magnification the area of arachnoidal penetration (*arrow*) can be demonstrated

Particularly in the midline, the crista occipitalis interna can be so enlarged that the entire space of the cisterna magna is completely taken up by bone (Fig. 3.19).

Once bone removal is complete, pulsations of the dura are usually not observed. A thickened part of the atlantooccipital membrane may constrict the dura at the level of the foramen magnum and usually contains a vein. This constricting dural band needs to be transected and should be mobilized off the dura a few mm from both sides to facilitate dura closure at the end of the procedure (Fig. 3.18c).

The dura is incised in a Y-shape. Upon opening of the dura, venous sinuses may be encountered. The suboccipital sinus may persist in the midline in the dura of the posterior fossa. An oblique occipital sinus may be located at the foramen magnum encircling the spinal cord at this level. If present, these have to either be closed by suturing or the dura incision has to be altered to avoid their injury. Upon opening the dura, one has to watch out for bridging veins from the cervical cord, brainstem, or cerebellum, which may enter these sinuses to avoid their rupture (Fig. 3.20).

After dura opening, the arachnoid should be inspected carefully for evidence of scarring (Fig. 3.21b–d) and underlying bridging veins or perforating arteries which may be attached to it (Fig. 3.22d). We strongly recommend avoiding blunt dissection of the arachnoid, as this may injure such vessels, and emphasize to use sharp dissection instead. To establish adequate CSF flow, the arachnoid is dissected in the midline first. The cerebellar tonsils are gently spread apart with two microdissectors. Neuropathological studies [35] have shown that herniated tonsils consist of atrophic, ischemic, and nonfunctioning tissue. Therefore, coagulation and shrinkage of this tissue during surgery does not carry a risk in terms of postoperative neurological deficits, provided unusual variants of the posterior inferior cerebellar artery (PICA) are respected (Fig. 3.23). Coagulation of the tonsils at their tips and medial surface sometimes provides a tremendous amount of space for the cisterna magna and easy access to the foramen of Magendie (Fig. 3.24) [100]. In patients with large cerebellar tonsils, these may be reduced with subpial suction [28, 29]. Once a free outflow from the fourth ventricle has been achieved (Fig. 3.21), arachnoid adhesions may be transected toward the cerebellopontine cisterns or spinal canal (Fig. 3.22). Dissection remains close to the midline for this purpose. Arachnoid dissection should concentrate exclusively on these points. Dissection lateral of the brainstem is not advised so as to avoid injury to perforating arteries or cranial nerves [268].

Finally, we recommend using a spacious artificial dura graft to create a large cisterna magna which we consider essential for this procedure (Figs. 3.18, 3.22) [196]. To minimize the risk of postoperative adhesion of the graft, we avoid autologeous tissue and use synthetic material such as Neuropatch (Braun Melsungen, Germany) or Gore-Tex (Gore and Associates, Putzbrunn, Germany). The graft should be inserted with a tight running suture to avoid fistulas or pseudomeningoceles. For the same reason, we recommend closing soft tissues meticulously. A good closure of the muscular layer in particular is the best safeguard against fistulas. In order to prevent postoperative arachnoid scarring, we do not recommend leaving the dura open as has been suggested [267]. This technique may cause an aseptic meningitis and, thus, provoke arachnoid scarring postoperatively, presumably due to contamination of the subarachnoid space with proteinaceous material from the musculature and breakdown products of blood.

In our series, 190 decompressions of the foramen magnum were done as the primary surgical procedure, while an additional 6 patients underwent this operation after a previous shunt of an associated syr-

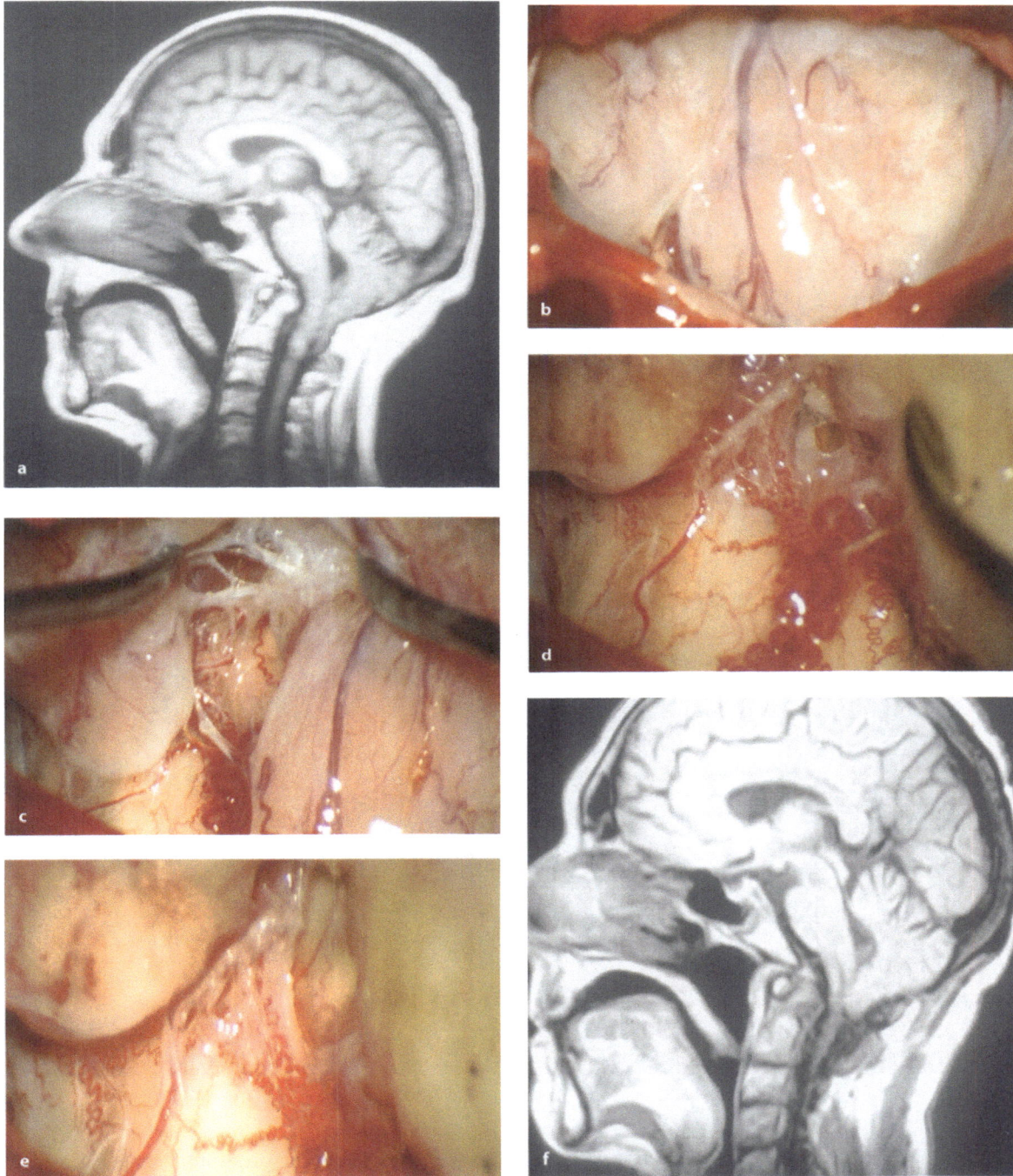

Fig. 3.21 a–f. a The T1-weighted sagittal MRI scan of this 66-year-old woman with swallowing problems and vocal cord paralysis illustrates Chiari I malformation and syringomyelia in connection with basilar invagination. The patient had just recovered from aspiration pneumonia. No instability was present. The decision was made to decompress the foramen magnum posteriorly. b After dura opening in the semi-sitting position, the cerebellar tonsils are seen to be covered by thickened arachnoid. c After arachnoid opening and dissection, the tonsils are held apart with two microdissectors, revealing dense ar-achnoid adhesions between tonsils and brain stem. d Under higher magnification, and after some further dissection, the almost complete occlusion of the foramen of Magendie can be seen. The arachnoid scarring was categorized as grade 1. e This photograph shows the final situation after opening of the foramen. A duraplasty was inserted and the patient recovered with marked improvement of swallowing over a period of 4 weeks. f The postoperative MRI scan demonstrates a decompression of the foramen magnum and ascent of the tonsils

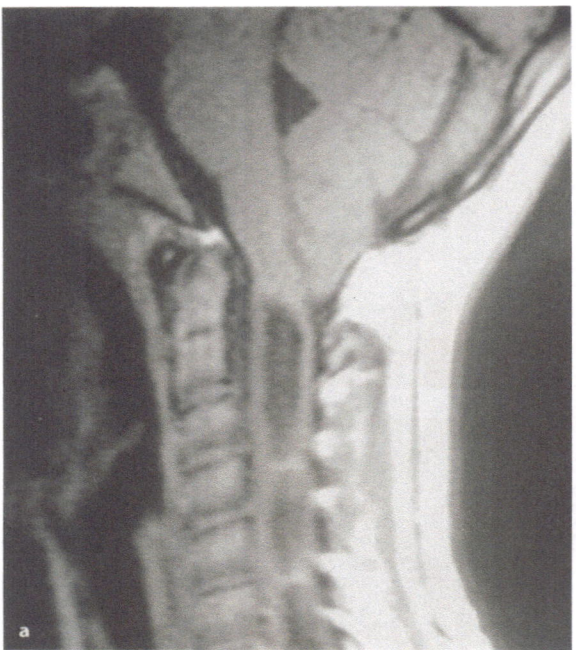

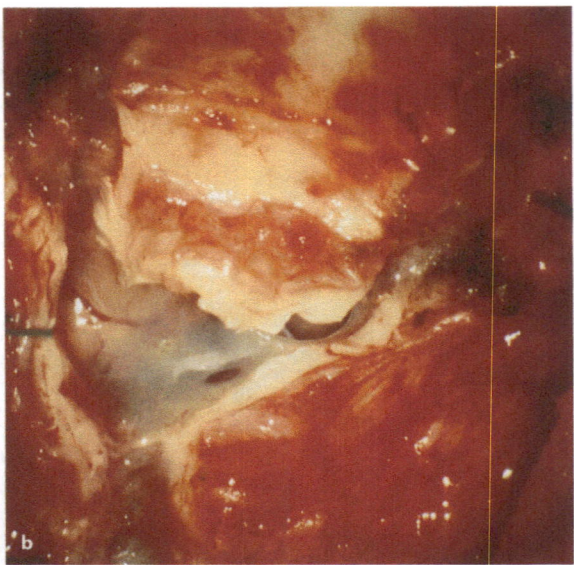

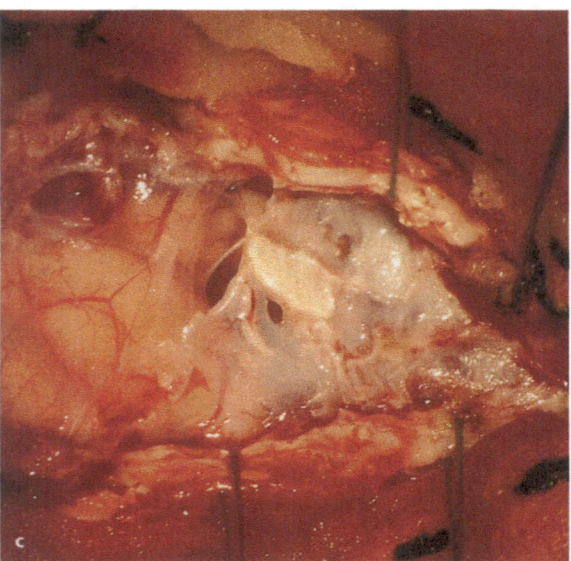

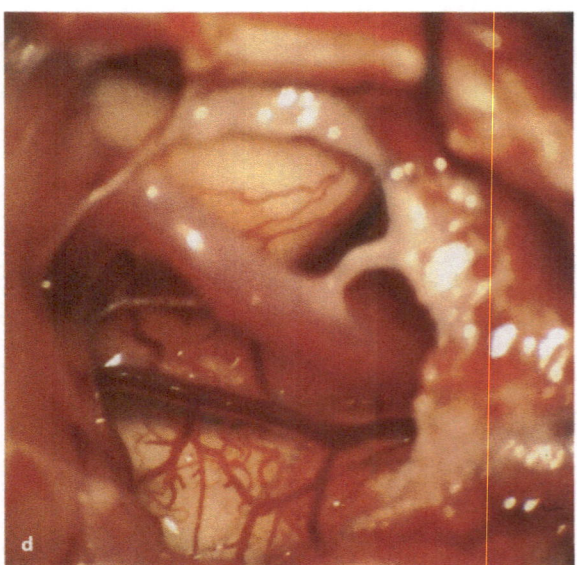

Fig. 3.22 a–h. a The T1-weighted sagittal MRI scan of this 13-year-old girl demonstrates classic Chiari I malformation with syringomyelia. **b** At dura opening, marked arachnoid thickening is apparent. **c** After careful dissection to separate arachnoid and dura, retention sutures could finally be applied to the dura, revealing thick arachnoid scarring, particularly in the area of the cisterna magna. **d** Under higher magnification, a small arterial branch of the right PICA terminating in the arachnoid scar is visible (continued on next page)

inx. Of these, 140 decompressions were performed according to the surgical protocol just presented. In 21 patients the arachnoid was not opened after dural opening, because no arachnoid pathology was apparent and the surgeon considered decompression of the brainstem and CSF flow to be adequate. In 115 instances, an artificial graft material was used, whereas autologous material was employed for the remainder. The remaining 55 decompressions included maneuvers such as obex plugging or extensive craniectomy. These techniques have been abandoned due to unfavorable clinical results.

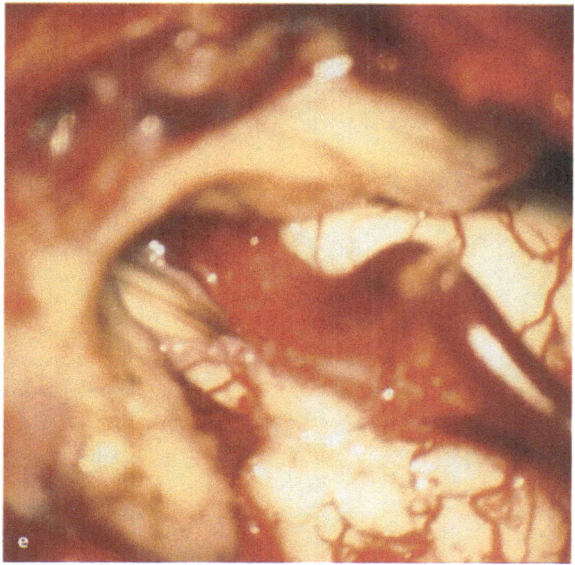

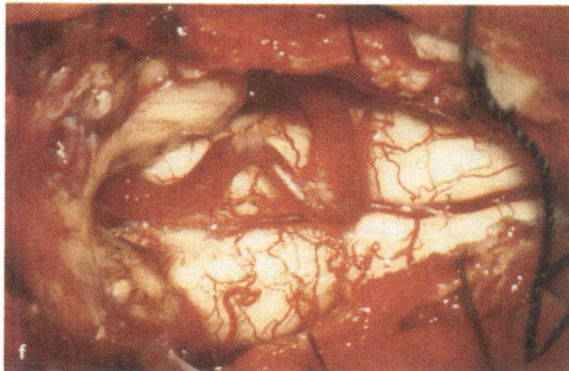

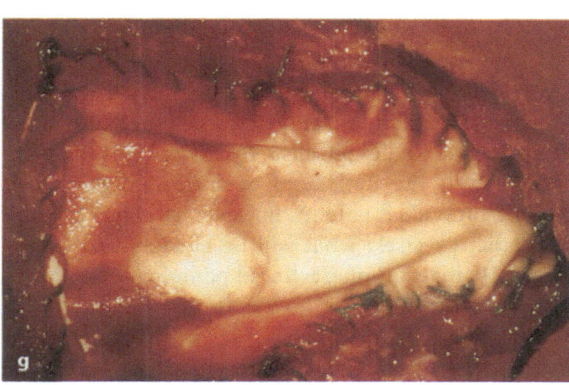

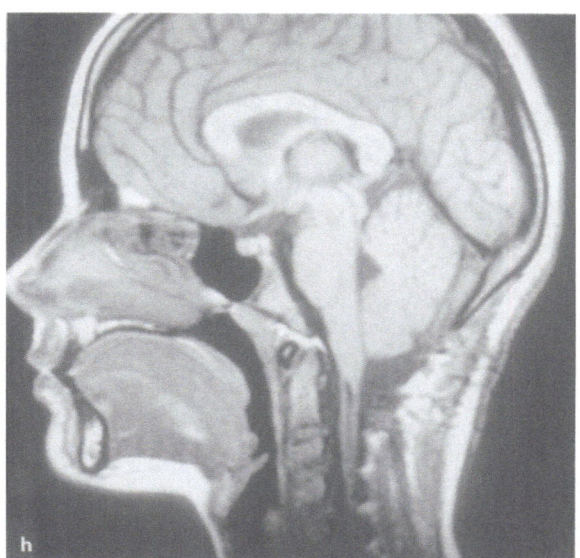

Fig. 3.22 e–h. e After coagulation and transsection of this artery, the tonsils are coagulated medially, so that the foramen of Magendie can be inspected. **f** This picture shows the final view before the duraplasty was inserted. Despite this severe arachnoid pathology (grade 2), all CSF pathways could be opened. **g** The Gore-Tex duraplasty is in place. **h** The postoperative MRI scan after 10 days demonstrates good decompression and collapse of the syrinx

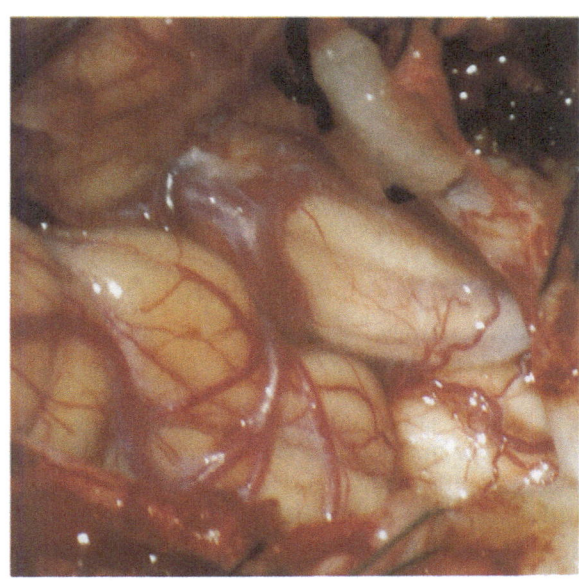

Fig. 3.23. This intraoperative photograph of a patient with Chiari I malformation shows an anatomical variant of the right PICA, which runs over the right tonsil toward the fourth ventricle

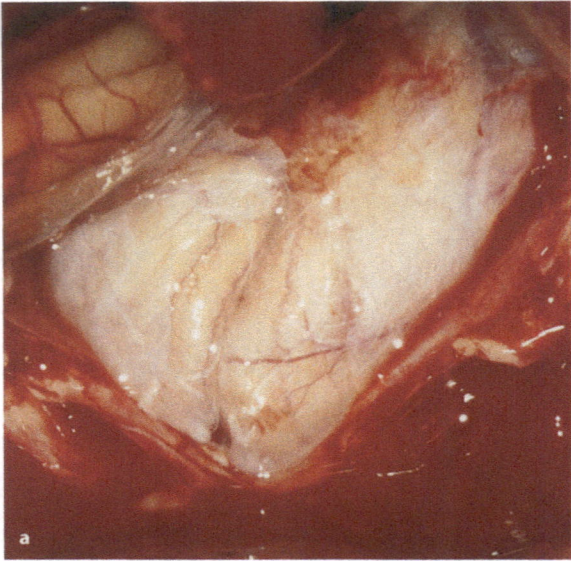

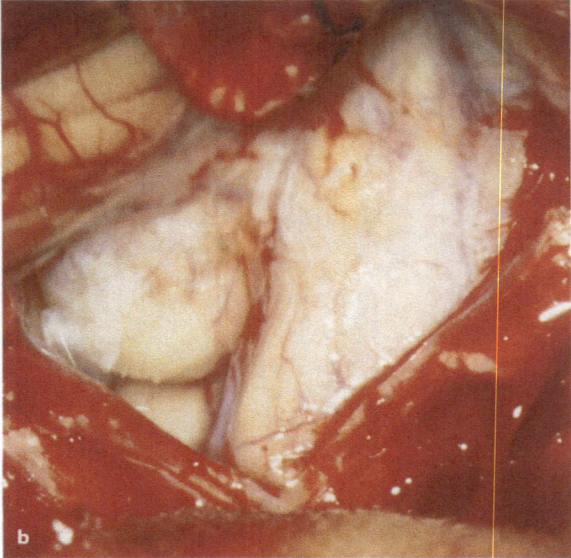

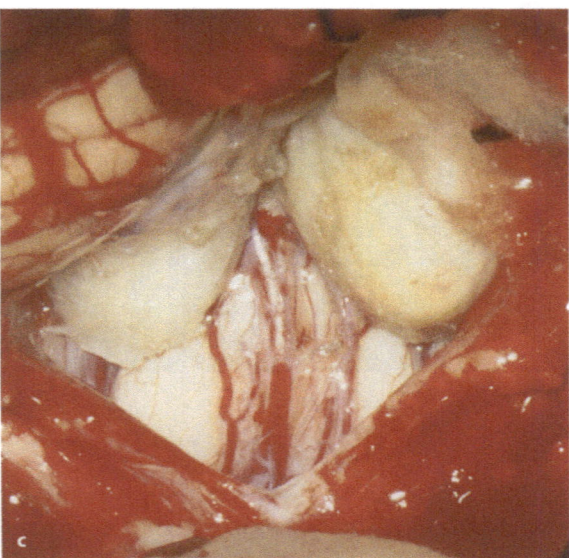

Fig. 3.24 a–c. These intraoperative photographs during surgery in semi-sitting position demonstrate how much space may be gained for the cisterna magna with coagulation of cerebellar tonsils. The situation is shown before coagulation (**a**), after coagulation of the left side (**b**), and after both sides have been done to reveal the now unobstructed foramen of Magendie (**c**)

Intraoperatively, arachnoid scarring associated with CMI was classified accordingly:

► Grade 0 = arachnoid translucent; normal appearing CSF flow after dura opening
► Grade 1 = arachnoid thickened; adhesions between tonsils and/or brainstem
► Grade 2 = arachnoid thickened; complete block of CSF flow at foramen magnum; foramen of Magendie closed

Clinically, a history of meningitis, previous surgery at the foramen magnum, or birth injury are indications that arachnoiditis at the foramen magnum might be present. Radiologically, hydrocephalus or arachnoid cysts are indicators of arachnoid pathology. For the individual patient, however, it is not possible to predict precisely what will be encountered intraoperatively in terms of arachnoid pathology.

3.1.4.3
Decompression for Chiari II Malformation

Surgery for CMII is indicated in patients with neurological symptoms of brainstem compression despite sufficient treatment of the hydrocephalus [52, 128, 156, 208]. It is estimated that approximately 20–33% of patients develop symptoms of brainstem compression that require decompression [208]. It is important to evaluate all neuroradiological studies and clinical data before this operation is indicated. Tethered cord release rather than decompression of the brainstem may be required in some of these patients [156, 273]. For patients with CMII, the same guidelines for positioning and monitoring apply. However, decompression has to be performed in the cervical canal and not at the level of the foramen magnum. In CMII the foramen magnum is enlarged. Compression of the brainstem occurs in the cervical spine [62, 189, 201, 208, 257]. Therefore, the extent of tonsillar herniation has to be precisely determined in order to correctly plan the extent of exposure. Imaging studies should be examined carefully to look for spina bifida in this region. Figures 3.25 and 3.26 provide examples for decompressions in an infant and adolescent patient, respectively. The exposure has to provide a clear view of the foramen magnum and all cervical laminae which

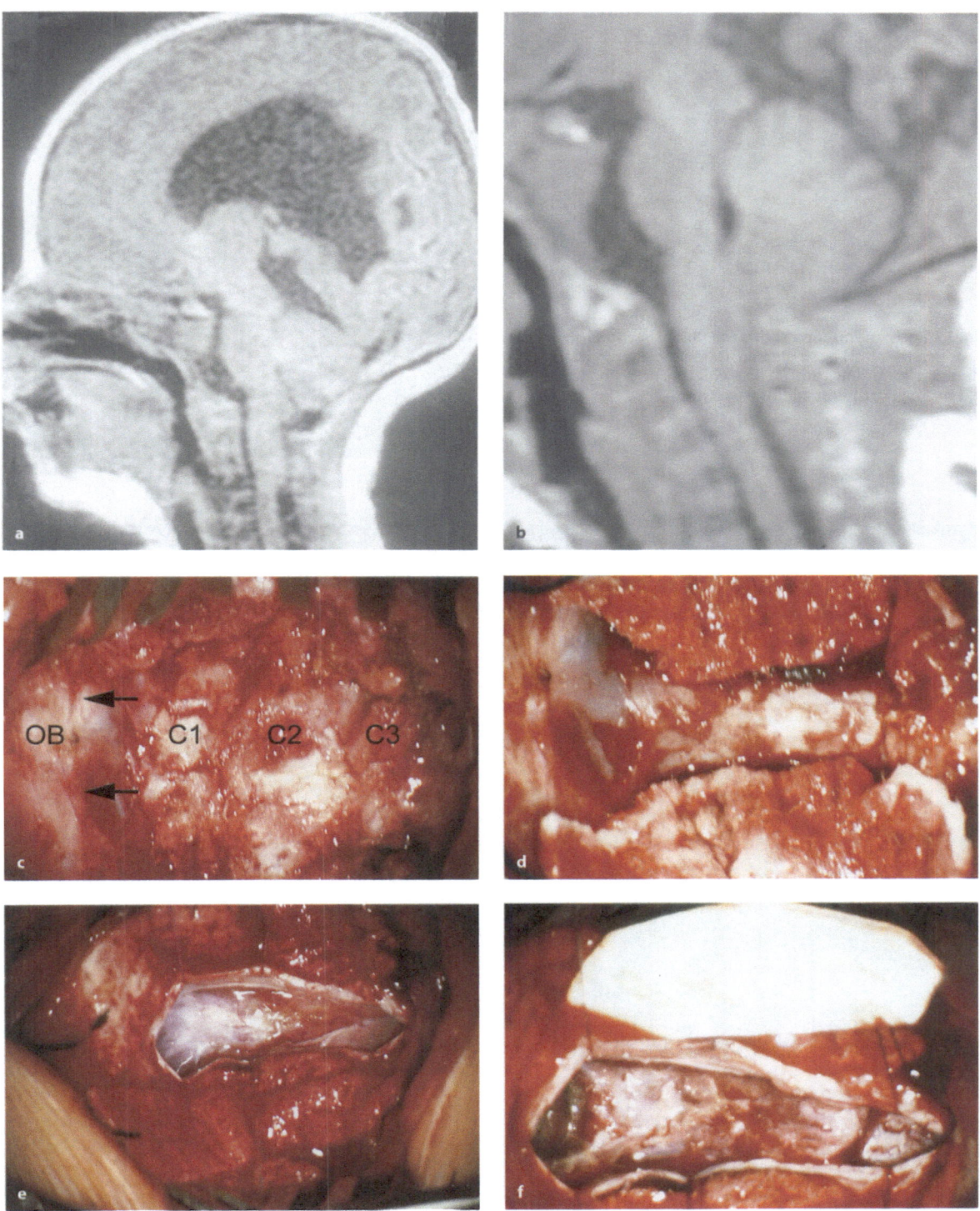

Fig. 3.25 a–h. a The sagittal T1-weighted MRI scan of this 4-month-old boy with apnea spells demonstrates Chiari II malformation with insertion of the tentorium at the posterior rim of the foramen magnum and hydrocephalus. **b** A closer look at the foramen magnum area reveals a tonsillar descent to C3. **c** This intraoperative picture was taken after soft tissue dissection of the craniocervical junction. Occipital bone (OB), C1, C2, and C3 are marked, as is the rim of the foramen magnum (*arrows*). **d** Upon removal of the medial parts of laminae C1 to C3, the dura bulges out. **e** After opening of the dura, thickened arachnoid is seen to cover the cerebellar tonsils. **f** With arachnoid dissection posteriorly, a free CSF pathway could be established between spinal and intracranial subarachnoid spaces. The foramen of Magendie could be opened and can be seen under the cranial edge of the dura opening. A Gore-Tex patch has been fashioned according to the dura opening (continued on next page)

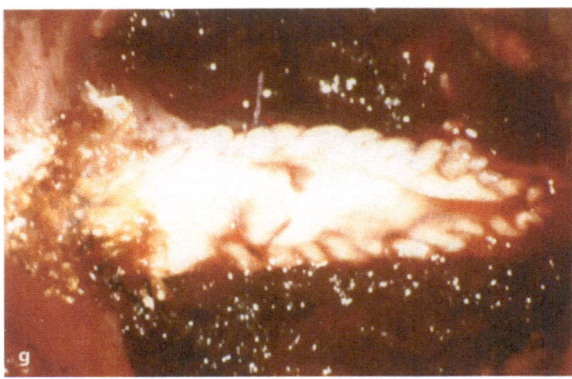

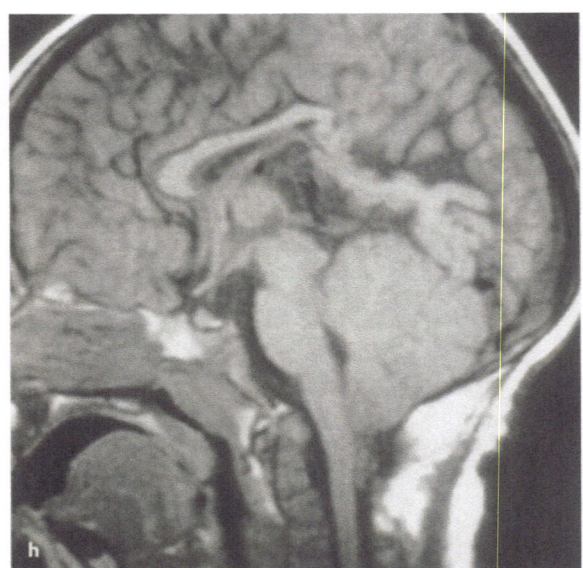

Fig. 3.25 g, h. g This view shows the duraplasty in place. **h** The postoperative MRI scan demonstrates the decompression of the brain stem down to C3. The child made a good recovery and no longer requires additional oxygen

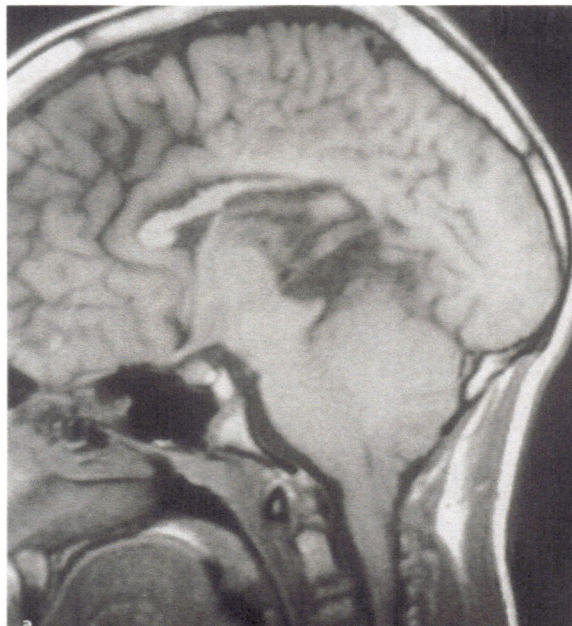

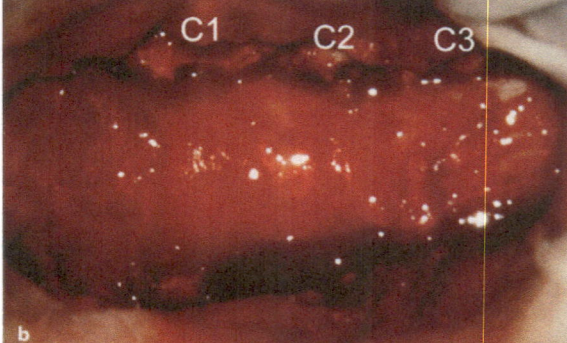

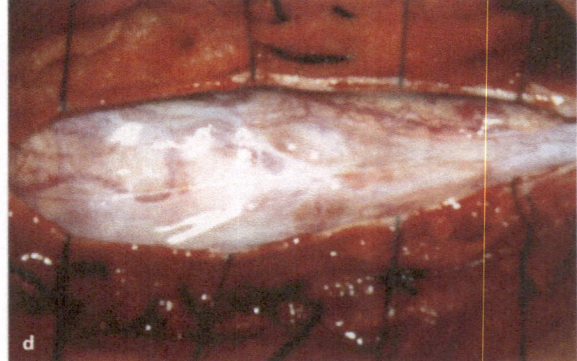

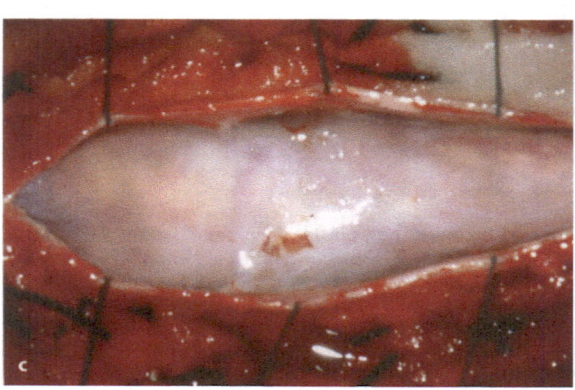

Fig. 3.26 a–i. a The T1-weighted MRI scan of this 11-year-old boy with scoliosis and progressive motor weakness of his right hand discloses Chiari II malformation with marked dysplasia of the midbrain and tonsillar descent to C3. **b** This intraoperative view after removal of laminae C1, C2, and C3 reveals a hyperemic dura mater, indicating the enormous pressure of central nervous structures at this level. The positions of the lateral remnants of the laminae are marked. **c** The situation after dura opening is revealed. The arachnoid is thickened. **d** After dissection of the outer layer of arachnoid, the cerebellar tonsils become visible underneath the inner arachnoid layer (continued on next page)

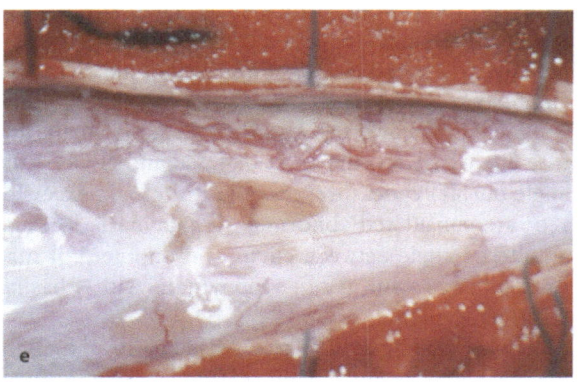

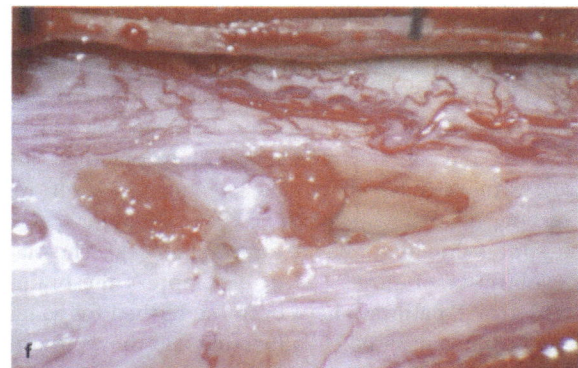

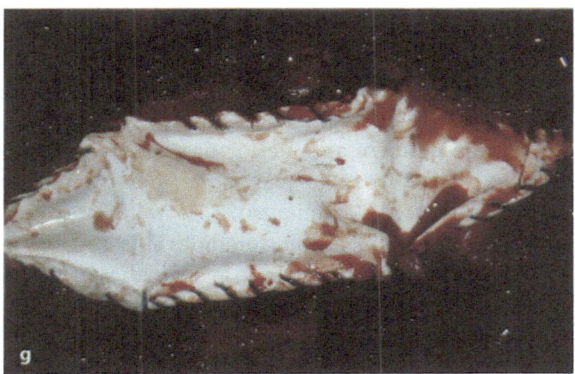

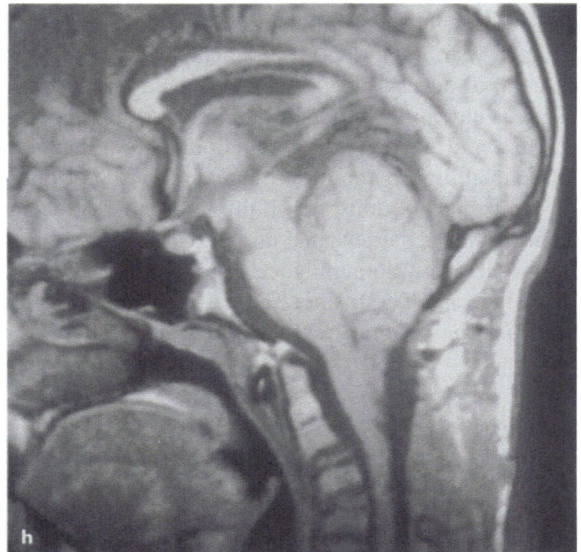

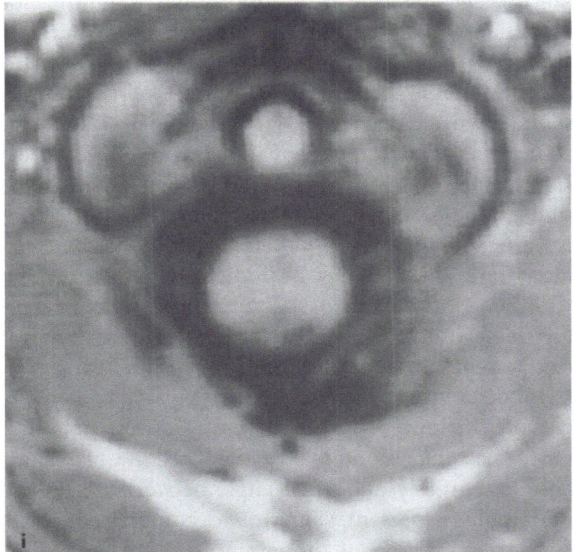

Fig. 3.26 e–i. e After incision of this arachnoidal sheath, the fourth ventricle is open. f With higher magnification and further dissection, a large opening of the fourth ventricle is achieved. Choroid plexus and the right PICA are visible. g The Gore-Tex duraplasty is in place. The postoperative sagittal (h) and axial (i) MRI scans after 3 months show the decompression of the brain stem with enlargement of the posterior subarachnoid space. The clinical condition is unchanged

cover cerebellar tissue. When performing the laminectomy, one should not use instruments for bone removal which need to be inserted underneath the lamina. Once the laminae are removed, one may observe the dural sac bulging out (Fig. 3.26b).

The next step is to open the dura in the midline in the cervical canal. It is not advised to enlarge the foramen magnum and to open the dura of the posterior fossa. The transverse sinus and torcula may be directly at the posterior rim of the foramen; profuse bleeding may be encountered. Dural opening in this region is not required and is hazardous. As for patients with CMI, an epidural band at the foramen magnum may compress the brainstem at this level and should be transected [208].

Once the dura is opened, the arachnoid should be opened over the spinal cord and tonsils to gain free CSF passage between intracranial and spinal subarachnoid space. In general, it is not advised to mobilize the tonsils off the brainstem. Usually, they are tightly adherent, so that such a maneuver may damage the brainstem or posterior inferior cerebellar arteries [201]. At the level of the foramen magnum, it may be possible to gain access to the fourth ventricle by spreading the tonsils apart in the midline with two mi-crodissectors. If communication between the fourth ventricle and subarachnoid space can be obtained this way, without much dissection and manipulation, we consider it worthwhile to do so (Figs. 3.25f and 3.26 e, f) – but it should not be attempted at all cost. The ma-jor objective of surgery is to decompress the brain-stem. If CSF pathways have been established for as far as possible, a dura patch is inserted and the wound is closed as described for CMI.

We have operated on 11 of 13 patients with CMII. The mean age was significantly lower than with CMI (11.5±10 years). Of these, 3 patients were less than 2 years of age – the youngest was approximately 4 weeks old, and 2 patients were in the group between 2 years and 12 years; the remainder were between 14 years and 27 years of age. One child was not oper-ated on due to additional multiple organ malforma-tions. All these patients had undergone closure of their lumbosacral myelomeningocele and ventriculoperito-neal shunting. The 11 operated patients demonstrated clinical progression, despite a functioning shunt and unrelated to re-tethering at the site of the myelome-ningocele repair.

It has to be emphasized, however, that treatment of CMII is by no means complete with adequate and suc-cessful decompression. Especially in children, spinal instability is very common after cervical laminectomy for decompression of the brainstem. Aronson et al. de-termined instability in 19 of 20 children examined. A close follow-up is mandatory for these children [16]. Patients need careful monitoring for spinal deformi-ties throughout adolescence.

3.1.4.4
Basilar Invagination and Chiari Malformation

Basilar invagination can be accompanied by CMI with or without a syrinx. It is characterized by protrusion of the odontoid peg into the foramen magnum and was originally described by Chamberlain. The key to diagnosis is the projection of the odontoid tip project-ing for more than 2.5 mm over Chamberlain's line, which is drawn between the tip of the hard palate and the posterior margin, i.e., opisthion, of the foramen magnum. Basilar invagination may be associated with a shortened basiocciput, shortened clivus, and platy-basia. This constellation leads to a shallow posterior fossa and elevation of the plane of the foramen mag-num, due to the higher position of its anterior rim [162]. Alternatively, basilar invagination may be caused by hypoplasia of the exoccipital bone. This is associated with a normal clivus, which is somewhat displaced posteriorly, and a downward curved squa-mous occipital bone, which is elevated toward the foramen magnum [162]. In most instances, individual patients will demonstrate combinations of these two extremes.

Platybasia, however, describes an abnormally ob-tuse angle between the anterior fossa and clivus. This angle normally measures 120–140°. Angles in excess of 140° are considered abnormal. As platybasia leads to an altered angle between clivus and odontoid, it may predispose to – but is not synonymous with – basilar invagination.

To be distinguished from basilar invagination, which is a congenital malformation, basilar impres-sion refers to acquired luxation of the odontoid into the foramen magnum. This is due to bone diseases such as Paget's disease or rheumatoid arthritis.

In patients with basilar invagination and CMI, planning of the surgical strategy can be quite difficult: should one perform an anterior or posterior decom-pression of the foramen magnum? Does the patient need craniocervical stabilization? Do we have to per-form a combined operation from both sides?

Only a thorough clinical and neuroradiological ex-amination can answer these questions [37, 56, 63, 66, 81, 94, 125, 133, 138, 163, 173, 233, 252, 253]. Clinically, neck pain and symptoms of brainstem or cervical cord compression predominate in most instances. A syrinx – if present – usually is of minor clinical significance in patients with basilar invagination. The surgical strategy – posterior decompression only or anterior decompression plus craniocervical stabilization – should be discussed with each patient in detail.

If the anterior component appears not to be of great significance on MRI and the craniocervical junction is stable, a posterior decompression as described above is sufficient (Fig. 3.21) [94]. If instability can be de-monstrated, which may be indicated by severe pain with neck movements or a significant soft tissue pan-nus adjacent to an incompetent joint, and the anterior component can be reduced or is not significant, pos-terior decompression and craniocervical fusion are ne-cessary. If, however, anterior compression predomi-nates, i.e., the odontoid peg deforms the brainstem and/or a grossly abnormal angle between clivus and odontoid is present, anterior decompression with transoral resection of the odontoid peg are required (Fig. 3.27) [94, 127, 160, 161, 162, 163, 196]. Approxi-mately two-thirds of the patients become unstable after transoral resection of the dens [67, 68, 253]. How-ever, some patients may demonstrate improvement of CMI and syringomyelia after anterior decompression alone [196]. This leaves two possibilities: anterior de-compression only or in combination with occipitocer-vical fusion and foramen magnum decompression. In patients without either CMI or anterior soft tissue pan-nus, anterior decompression alone may be sufficient. However, patients have to be examined carefully for

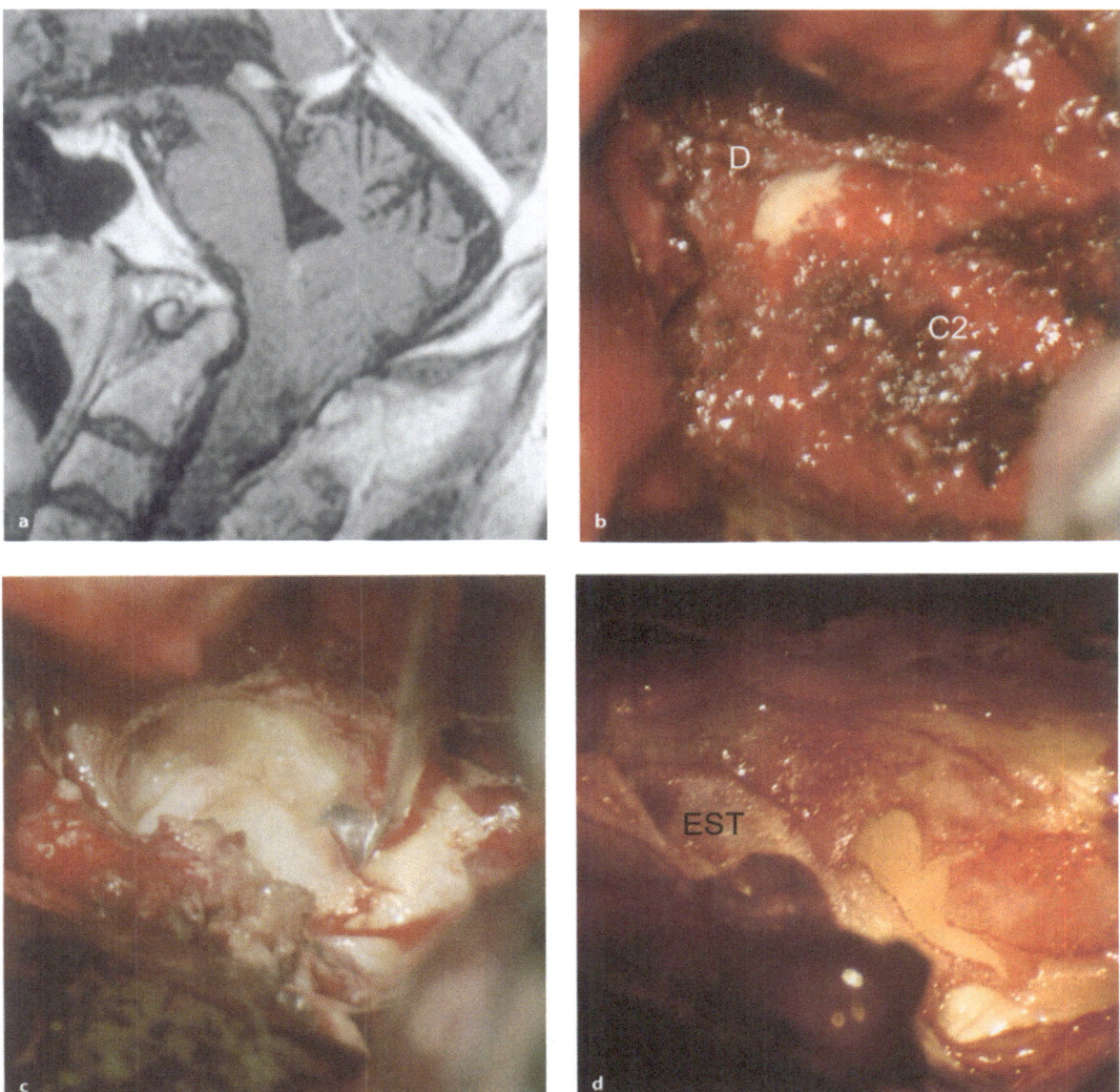

Fig. 3.27 a–i. This 37-year-old patient presented with a 1-year history of progressive gait ataxia and occipital pain. With ante-flexion of his head he could provoke gait problems, making it almost impossible for him to climb down stairs. Recently, he reported difficulties with swallowing and a hoarse voice. Neurological examination disclosed severe incompetence of vagus and glossopharyngus nerves, with no gag reflex bilaterally, but intact function of hypoglossal and accessory nerves. He complained about double vision with left lateral gaze. There were no signs of motor weakness but bilateral Babinski signs. On MRI (**a**), CT, and lateral tomograms, both basilar invagination and Chiari I malformation were evident (see also Fig. 3.7). There was no sign of instability on flexion extension scans nor indirect signs, such as soft tissue pannus. In a first step, the patient underwent anterior decompression with transoral resection of the odontoid. **b** The intraoperative view is shown after soft tissue dissection. The position of the vertebral body (*C2*) and dens (*D*) are marked. **c** The dens is gradually removed with sharp dissection. **d** Finally, the dura and epidural soft tissue (*EST*) become visible. Postoperatively, the patient was placed in a HALO vest after lateral tomographies in retro- (**e**) and anteflexion (**f**) showed instability of the C1/C2 segment. The decompressed anterior aspect of the foramen magnum with preservation of C1 is also demonstrated. The patient underwent posterior decompression and fusion in a second operation. **g** After soft tissue dissection, the medial part of C1 has been removed and the foramen magnum (*FM*) enlarged. The bony decompression was limited by the size of the Rands-ford Loop. **h** This view shows the Randsford Loop secured in place with soft wire. A small duraplasty was inserted to facilitate formation of a cisterna magna. **i** Postoperative X-ray shows the device in good position. Additionally, iliac crest bone was put between occiput and C2. The patient made a good recovery with improved gait, working gag reflexes, normal swallowing, and the disappearance of Babinski signs (**e–i** see next page)

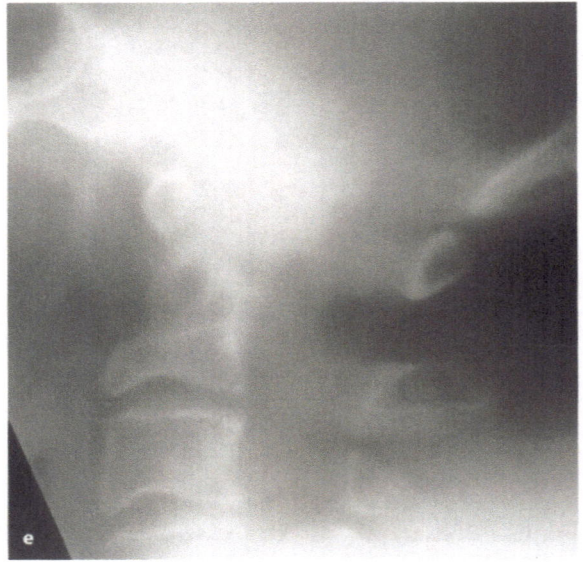

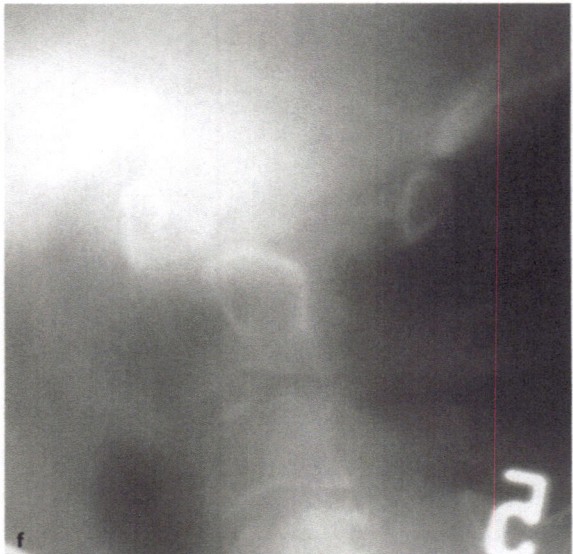

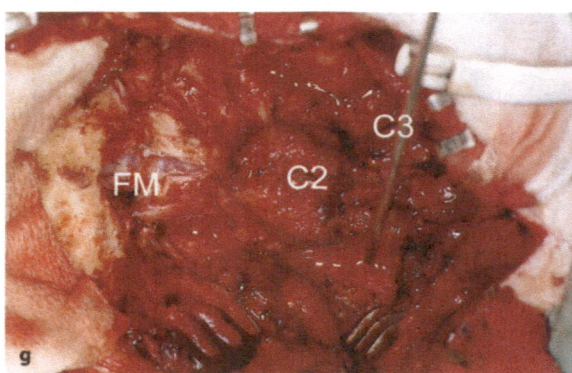

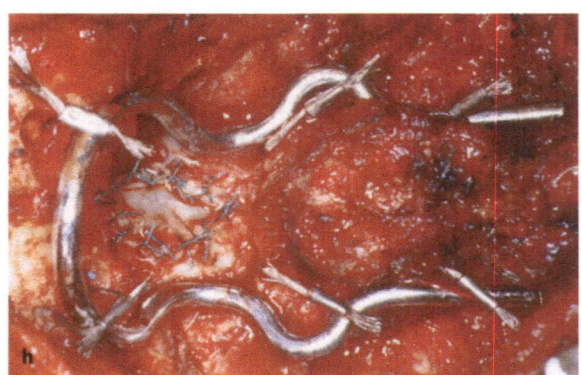

Fig. 3.27 e–i

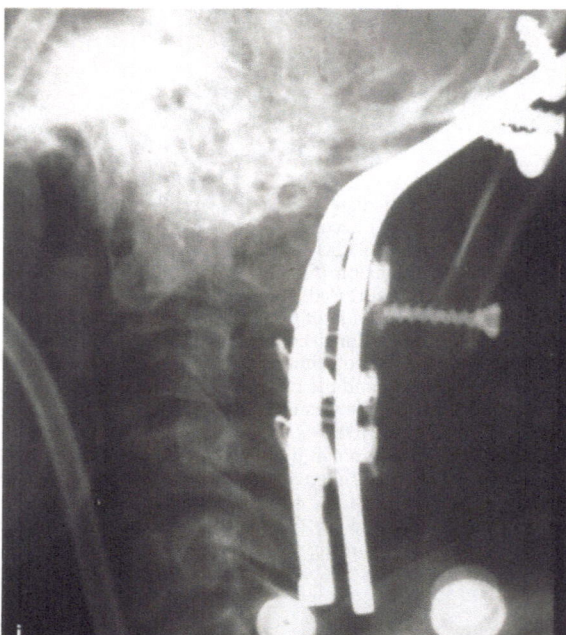

evidence of instability after transoral surgery. Pannus, however, is a result of chronic instability and indicates that fusion will be required. Likewise, concomitant Klippel-Feil syndrome or occipitalization of C1 should alert the surgeon that postoperative instability will be likely after anterior decompression alone. If CMI is combined with basilar invagination, anterior decompression should be followed by posterior decompression and fusion (Fig. 3.27). These patients should be put in a HALO vest after anterior surgery or undergo craniocervical stabilization in the same operation.

A patient with basilar invagination and CMI who is scheduled for transoral resection of the odontoid peg should be intubated with fiberoptic endoscopy to avoid undue movements of the neck during intubation. Any neck movement may cause significant brainstem compression. The positioning is done under SSEP monitoring for the same reason. During positioning, slight extension is applied and the head is fixed in a Mayfield clamp. The patient may be positioned on the side, so that both transoral and posterior approaches can be done without having to reposition the patient. Alternatively, the patient undergoes anterior decompression first and is then repositioned for the posterior decompression.

For the transoral decompression, topical steroids are applied to the tongue to minimize swelling, the retractor is inserted, and a sagittal incision is performed with C_1 as the center. In most instances, it is necessary to split the soft palate. Pharyngeal muscles and mucosa are reflected laterally and longus colli and longus capitis muscles are dissected free from their bony and fibrous attachments, so that the lower clivus, anterior part of C_1, the body of C_2, and the base of the odontoid become visible (Fig. 3.27b). To avoid injury of the hypoglossal nerve, Eustachian tube, or vertebral artery, lateral exposure is limited to approximately 1.5 cm to either side. The anterior atlas is removed with a high-speed drill as far as required for adequate access to the odontoid. Similarly, the lower clivus may be resected if necessary. Then the odontoid and soft tissue pannus can be removed (Fig. 3.27 c). To accomplish this safely, one may either start at the tip of the odontoid and proceed caudally in a piecemeal fashion or transect the base of the odontoid, pull the odontoid caudally with a toothed rongeur, and remove it in toto after transecting ligamentous attachments at the odontoid tip. To accomplish an adequate decompression, soft tissue pannus may also be removed. However, if pannus is densely adherent to the underlying dura, this should not be attempted vigorously. With appropriate fusion, pannus may regress spontaneously [141]. The transverse ligament and tectorial membrane can be removed to visualize the dura. Once dura pulsations are visible then the decompression is sufficient (Fig. 3.27d). Throughout the decompression, lateral radiographs can aid anatomical orientation. Contrast agent placed into the decompression site may be particularly helpful. Alternatively, navigation systems using bone CT can be used [200]. After decompression, muscles and mucosa may be sutured independently or in a single layer. If the dura was injured, it is covered with fascia and a lumbar drain is inserted and maintained for at least a week. The second step of the operation consists of the stabilization procedure posteriorly, combined with decompression of the foramen magnum (Fig. 3.27g–i).

The patient should not receive any food orally for approximately 3 days so the mucosa will heal. Intraoperatively, a nasogastric tube is inserted under direct vision. Intubation is maintained until swelling of the oral soft tissue has regressed sufficiently. Excellent papers on this subject were published by Menezes [161, 163, 196, 252, 253] and Crockard and coworkers [123, 233].

Two patients in our series required combined anterior and posterior decompression with craniocervical stabilization for CMI and basilar invagination. An-

other six patients demonstrated a less dramatic anterior compression associated with minor degrees of basilar invagination. These patients were exclusively decompressed from the posterior without additional fusion. None of them became unstable [94].

3.1.4.5
Craniocervical Instability and Chiari Malformation

Craniocervical instability may be observed with basilar invagination, Klippel-Feil syndrome, or occipitalization of C_1 [68]. Whenever any of these features are discovered on standard neuroradiological images, we would recommend additional studies be done as outlined earlier. Flexion-extension images may not disclose instability, as the patient may not allow any detectable range of movement due to muscular compensation and severe pain.

If instability is detected, occipitocervical fusion can be performed in the same procedure as was done for decompression of the foramen magnum. The exposure only needs to be extended further down the cervical spine. We advise to perform a lateral X-ray study of the head and cervical spine before surgery in exactly the position that the patient wants the fixation to be. With positioning of the patient in the Mayfield clamp, intraoperative X-ray control can achieve that desired angle precisely. Otherwise, the optimum angle of fixation may not be obtained and the patient may acquire kyphotic angulation below the level of fusion. Obviously, positioning should be done with monitoring of SSEPs.

In the past, the Ransford loop was used for stabilization [207]. In the meantime, new fixation systems have appeared which can be adapted much easier to the individual anatomy (Fig. 3.28) [76, 103]. After decompression and duraplasty are completed, the bone surfaces are decorticated and the fixation material is formed to fit the anatomy and secured to the occipital bone with screws. Depending on the system used, it may be fixed to the spine with transarticular screws or to vertebral arches with soft wires. CT analysis may be useful to determine the thickness of the occipital bone to help choose the right area for screw placement and ascertain abnormal positions of the vertebral artery. In general, occipital bone is thickest in the midline and along the nuchal line. Finally, bone material may be added to obtain a bony fusion [50, 145, 231].

3.1.4.6
Degenerative Changes of the Spine and Chiari Malformation

Five patients in our series presented with radicular symptoms due to degenerative disc disease (Figs. 3.29, 3.30) and underwent disc removal and ventral fusion in the affected spinal levels. Postoperative analysis revealed that only the radicular symptoms improved, as

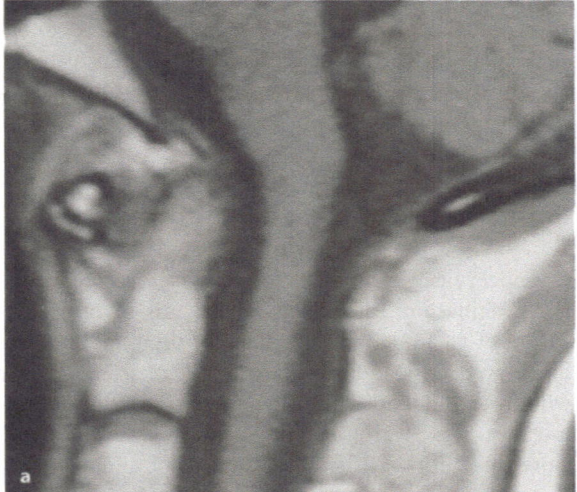

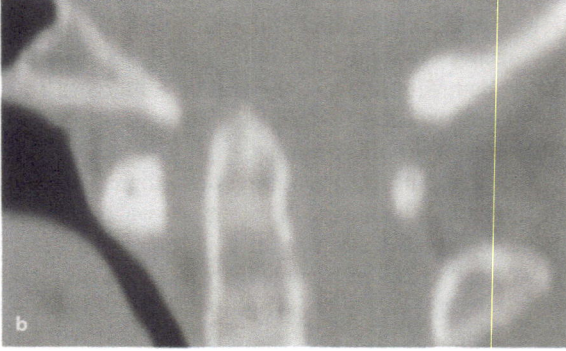

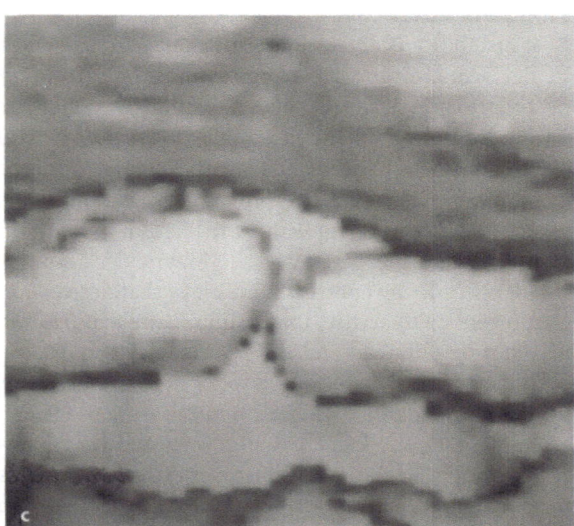

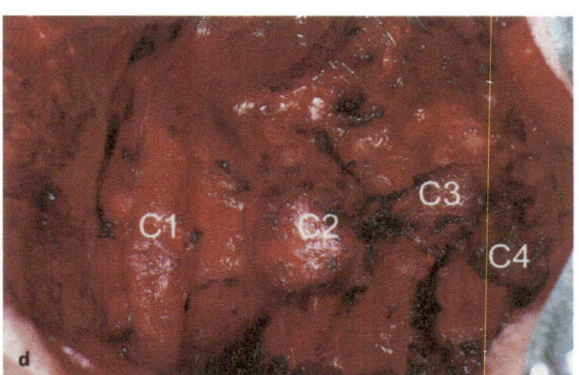

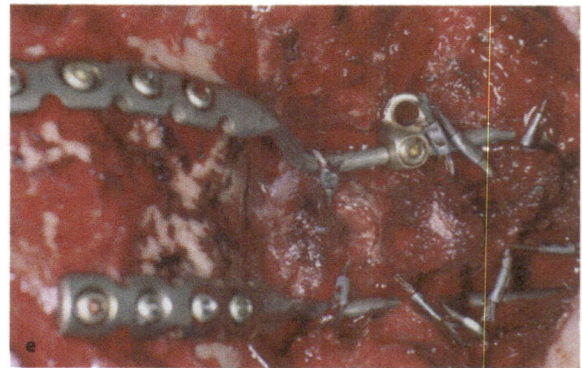

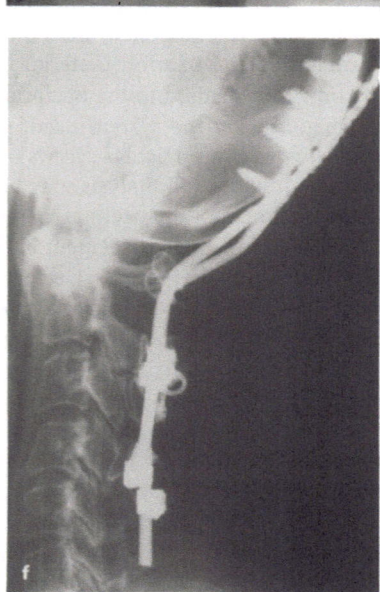

Fig. 3.28 a–f. a The preoperative T1-weighted MRI scan of this 64-year-old woman with occipital pain and no neurological deficits shows basilar invagination and forward luxation of C1, indicating instability. Sagittal (**b**) and 3D CT (**c**) disclose the bony anatomy and reveal an incomplete closure of C1. With no relevant compression from anterior, the decision was made to perform occipitocervical fusion only. **d** This intraoperative view shows the bony structures after soft tissue dissection. C1 and the spinous processes of C2 to C4 are marked. **e** The Cervifix fixation system (Mathys Synthes, Bochum, Germany) is shown in place. Screws secure the plates to the occiput while soft wires provide a firm connection to the upper cervical laminae. **f** Postoperative X-ray shows correct positioning of the instrumentation. The patient no longer complains about occipital headache

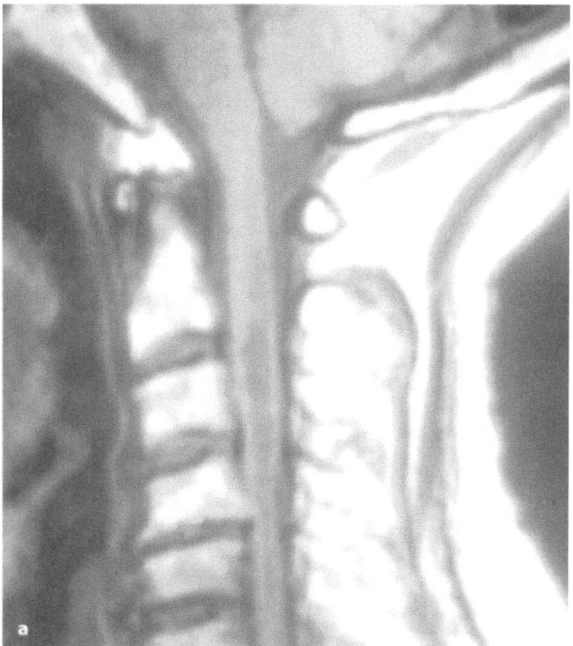

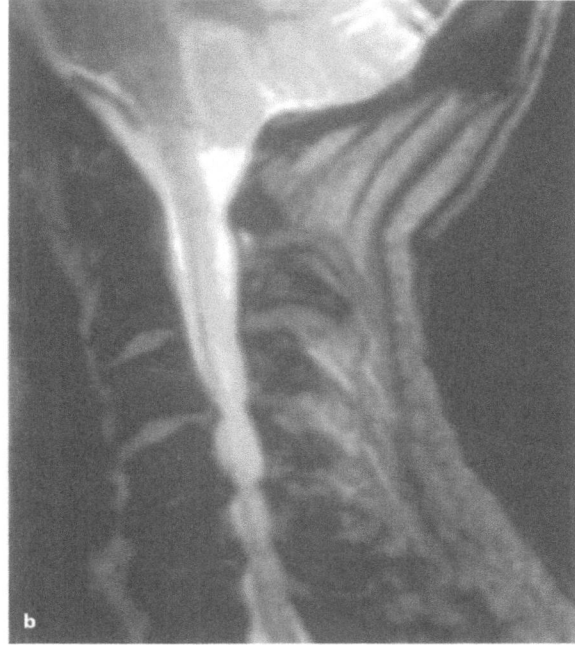

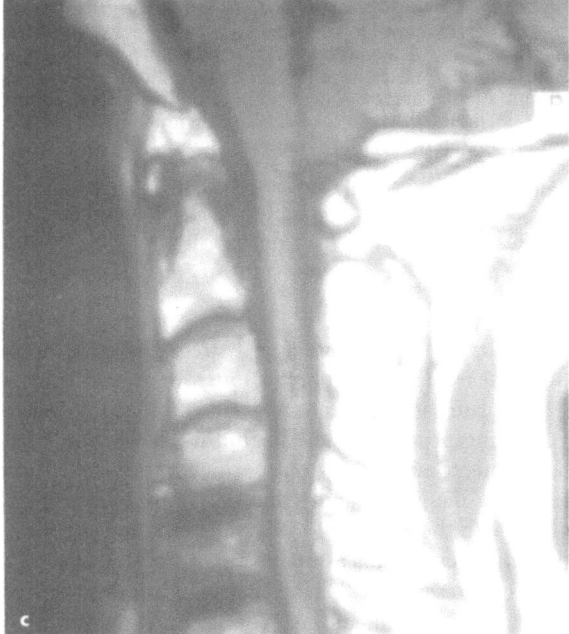

Fig. 3.29 a–c. This 68-year-old patient complained about a C6-radiculopathy on the right side for the past 8 years. Recently, he observed a weakness in his right leg and deterioration of fine finger movements of his right hand. On examination, weakness of his right arm was evident, with C6-innervated muscle groups affected predominantly. His gait was slightly ataxic with a right-sided positive Babinski sign. Neuroradiological examinations disclosed Chiari I malformation with syringomyelia and marked degenerative disease of his cervical spine in T1- (**a**) and T2-weighted MRI scans (**b**). The patient underwent a C4/5 and C5/6 discectomy and ventral fusion with iliac crest bone and plating. Postoperatively, the syrinx decreased in diameter (**c**) and the patient was discharged with improved gait and motor function of his right upper extremity

one would expect. Postoperative MRI, however, demonstrated a decrease of the syrinx size in three of four patients after cervical fusion (Fig. 3.29). We attribute this finding to improved CSF flow in the cervical subarachnoid space due to ventral decompression of the cord.

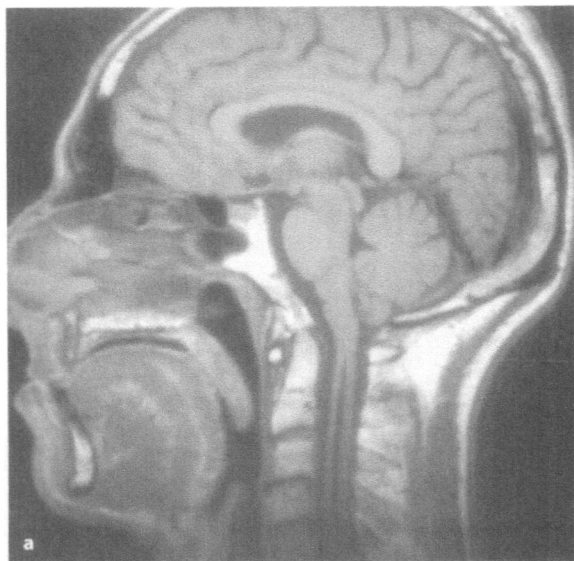

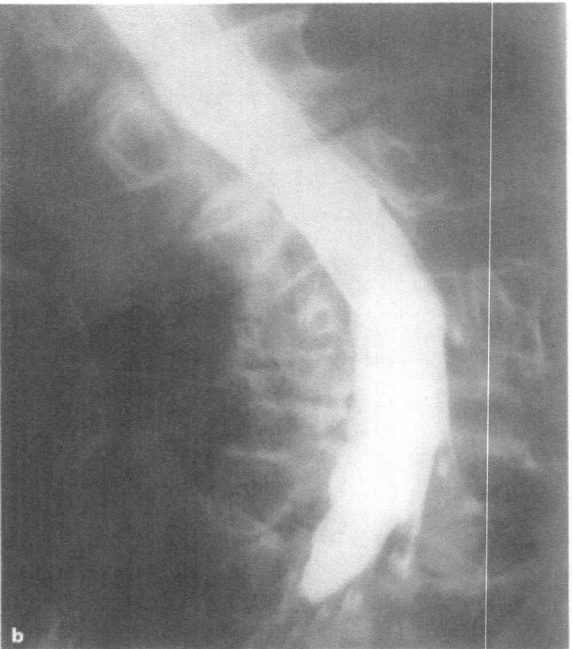

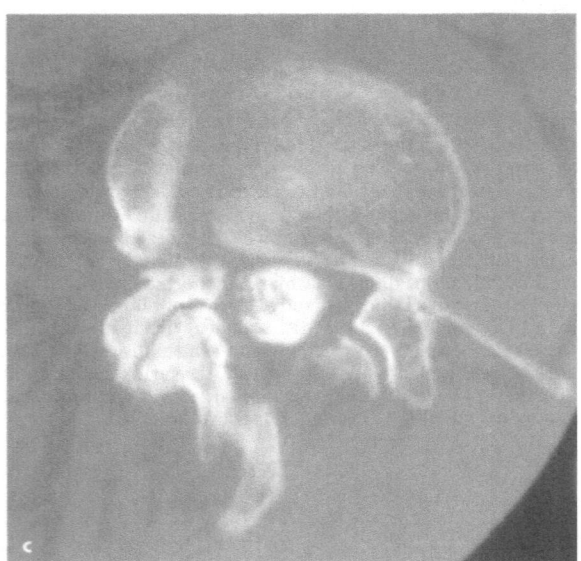

Fig. 3.30 a–c. This 52-year-old patient with Chiari I malformation and syringomyelia presented signs of spinal claudication and back pain for the past 5 years. His right leg was predominantly affected. There were no signs of spasticity or incompetence of cranial nerves. A detailed neuroradiological investigation – including MRI of the craniocervical junction (**a**), ascending myelography (**b**), and CT (**c**) – disclosed Chiari I malformation and syringomyelia and a stenosis at L3/4 and a significant scoliosis of his entire spine. A decompression at this level with hemilaminectomy L3 improved his gait substantially so that no further surgical intervention was necessary

3.1.5
Postoperative Outcome

Between 1978 and 2000, a total of 230 patients with CMI were treated. During these years, 202 patients underwent 223 surgeries and 28 patients were not operated on because they lacked any symptoms or refused surgery. We performed 196 foramen magnum decompressions, while 19 patients were treated by syringoperitoneal (n=12), syringopleural (n=2), or syringosubarachnoid shunting (n=5). Five patients underwent cervical fusions or lumbar disc surgery for associated degenerative disc diseases and two received a ventriculoperitoneal shunt for accompanying hydrocephalus. One patient was treated by sympathectomy for severe pain.

The different surgical methods employed represent a learning process. At the beginning, large suboccipital craniectomies were done for decompression of the foramen magnum, sometimes including obex plugging. With the advent of MRI, more detailed preoperative information was available and it became clear that a decompression of the foramen magnum did not require a large craniectomy. The second major line of treatment was shunting of the syrinx to the subarachnoid, pleural, or peritoneal space. Therefore, we can distinguish three major groups of patients with CMI who underwent surgery:

► Group A: Small craniectomy ≤ 3 cm in diameter, no obex plugging, duraplasty, i.e., foramen magnum decompression (n=141)
► Group B: Large craniectomy > 3 cm, with or without obex plugging, duraplasty, i.e., posterior fossa decompression (n=55)
► Group C: Syrinx shunting (n=19)

Table 3.5. Complications after surgery for Chiari I and II malformations

Complication	Decompression CMI	Shunt CMI	Decompression CMII
Infection	2 (1)	3 (3)	–
Aseptic meningitis	14	–	–
CSF fistula	15 (9)	1 (1)	1 (1)
Hydrocephalus	5 (5)	–	–
Cerebellar infarction	1 (1)	–	–
Cerebral infarction	1	–	–
Hemorrhage	1 (1)	–	–
Central dysregulation	2	–	2
Apnea spells	2	–	–
Swallowing dysfunction	3	–	–
Shunt malfunction	–	1 (1)	–
Dysesthesias	–	3	–
Pneumothorax	1	–	–
Pneumonia	3	–	1
Urinary tract infection	4	–	–
Total	54 (28%)	8 (42%)	4 (36%)

Numbers in brackets denote operative revisions.
CMI, Chiari I malformation; CMII, Chiari II malformation

The only variants in group A were the type of material used for duraplasty, amount of arachnoid dissection, and extent of tonsillar shrinking performed.

3.1.5.1
Complications

Complications were encountered in 28% of patients after decompression and in 42% after syrinx shunting in CMI; complications arose in 36% of patients after decompression for CMII (Table 3.5). Similar figures were given in the literature [5, 159, 273]. In CMI and decompression of the foramen magnum, the complication rate was higher for patients in whom the arachnoid was not opened than for patients undergoing arachnoid dissection (50% and 25%, respectively; Chi-square test: $P=0.017$). Three patients developed pseudomeningocele; three others developed transient caudal cranial nerve dysfunctions in the group without arachnoid opening, even though no arachnoid dissection had taken place and the duraplasty had been inserted with a running suture. For patients undergoing arachnoid dissection, the grade of arachnoid pathology had no significant influence on complication rates (26% for grade 0, 23% for grade I, and 26% for grade II, respectively; Chi-square test: not significant).

However, 17 patients developed serious complications worthy of further comment. Four patients showed transient postoperative brainstem dysfunction in the form of apnea or mesencephalic and hypothalamic dysfunctions, including electrolyte imbalances [64, 160]. Transient postoperative swallowing problems developed in three of our patients and had been reported previously [81, 159, 191]. To prevent these complications, we recommend that the arachnoid dissection not be extended too far laterally, especially when dealing with adhesions underneath the tonsils toward the brainstem, lest small perforating arteries may be compromised [159]. If in doubt, fiberoptic endoscopy after extubation is a valuable adjunct to investigate caudal cranial nerve dysfunction postoperatively. One patient developed a small postoperative cerebellar infarction with subsequent obstructive hydrocephalus. After insertion of an external ventricular drain, the hydrocephalus resolved and the patient recovered without additional neurological deficits or need for a permanent shunt. Presumably, vasospasm of the PICA was responsible for this complication. We observed PICA vasospasm during arachnoid dissection in one other patient. This responded to local application of nimodipine to the artery, without neurological sequelae. One patient developed a posterior cere-

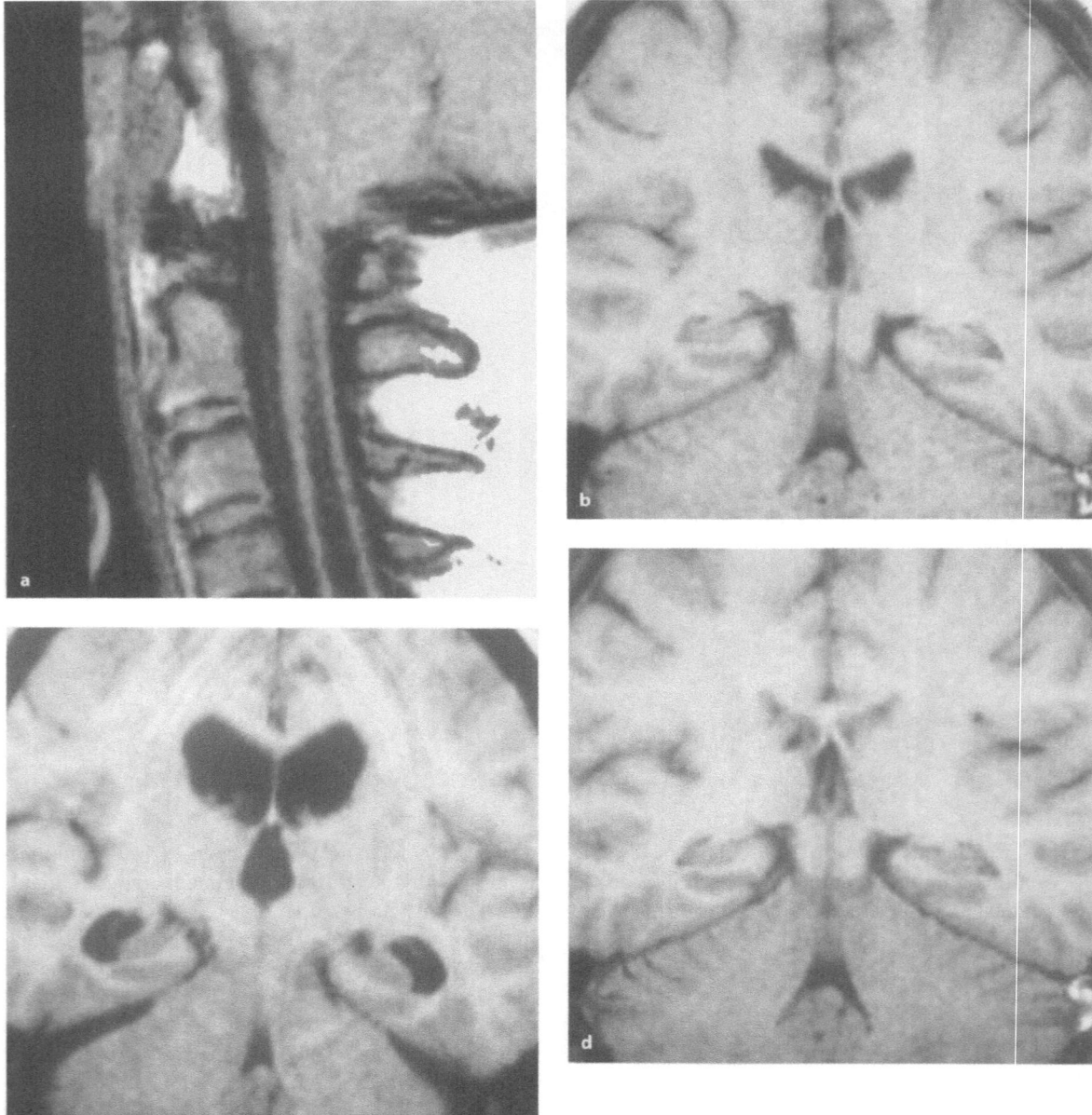

Fig. 3.31 a–e. a Preoperative T1-weighted MRI image of a 29-year-old man with Chiari I malformation and syringomyelia. There was no hydrocephalus (b). Postoperatively, the patient became gradually obtunded 2 weeks after surgery. MRI examination revealed hydrocephalus (c). After ventriculoperitoneal shunting, the ventricular size returned to normal (d) and the patient recovered with no further problems (e)

bral artery infarction due to embolization from a rheumatic mitral valve. Five patients developed postoperative hydrocephalus and a CSF fistula [159]. Use of neither MRI nor CT could identify an obstruction to CSF flow or any other explanation. Clinical symptoms, CSF fistula, and neuroradiological findings normalized

immediately after insertion of a medium-pressure ventriculo peritoneal shunt (Fig. 3.31). Eisenstat et al. [74] reported one instance of postoperative hydrocephalus among 47 operations, and Hankinson [101] described 3 patients with decompensated hydrocephalus among 84 who underwent foramen magnum decompression. Although the precise cause of hydrocephalus remains a matter of speculation, the most likely mechanism seems to be the postoperative alteration of CSF dynamics. One patient developed a pneumothorax due to high positive endexspiratory pressure (PEEP) ventilation in the semi-sitting position. This can be easily avoided by changing to the prone position.

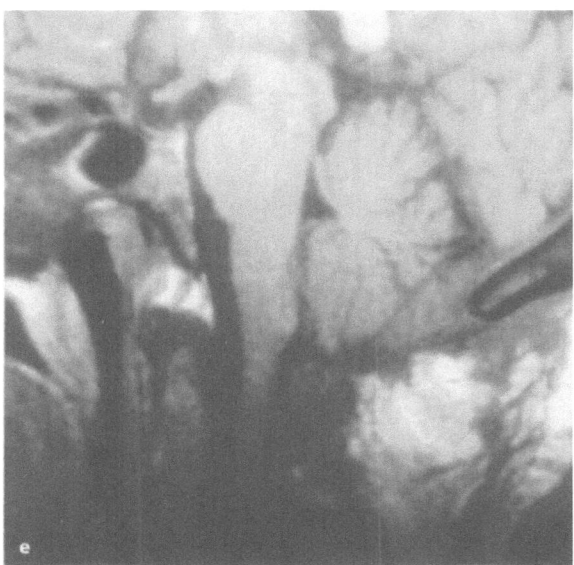

Fig. 3.31 e

In the literature, mortality rates vary from 0.7% [5] to 1.4% [191] and 12.1% [140].Two patients of our series died in the early postoperative period, indicating a surgical mortality of 1%. One patient was transferred to the normal ward on the day of surgery and died from cardiorespiratory arrest during a severe apnea attack. Therefore, we strongly recommend monitoring patients operated on at the foramen magnum in intensive care for at least 24 hours postoperatively. Finally, one patient died from a massive postoperative hemorrhage, despite early evacuation of the clot.

Compared with decompression at the foramen magnum, syrinx shunting procedures cannot be considered procedures of lower risk. The overall complication rate is similar, if one does not count postoperative sensory disturbances related to the myelotomy. Three patients reported new dysesthesias and pain related to shunt implantation. Postoperative MRI disclosed a tethered cord caused by arachnoid adhesions associated with the catheter position [194, 245]. After decompression of the foramen magnum in these patients, symptoms of cord and brainstem compression improved but the dysesthesias remained. Long-term complications such as displacement or blocking of the tube are responsible for a significant number of recurrences in patients with CMI and syrinx shunts.

3.1.5.2
Radiological Results for Chiari I Malformation

The postoperative radiological examination should demonstrate a sufficient decompression of the foramen magnum, a functioning cisterna magna, and a decrease in syrinx size. Standard MRI techniques are able to demonstrate adequacy of the decompression and changes in syrinx size. To evaluate the function of the cisterna magna, cardiac-gated cine MRI is the ideal technique [27, 36, 41, 42, 88, 134].

Adequate decompression was obtained in every patient who underwent a foramen magnum decompression. Long-term studies, however, revealed a tendency for recurrent brainstem and cervical cord compression due to herniation of the cerebellum in patients who had undergone a large oversized craniectomy (group B).

For patients with CMI and syringomyelia, the rates for postoperative decrease of syrinx size were significantly different, depending on the surgical technique employed. In group A, 85% demonstrated sustained postoperative decrease of syrinx size. Most of them showed this result within a few days of surgery, some only after several months. For 13% of patients, no change in syrinx diameter was detected during follow-up, while 2% experienced an increase of syrinx size some time after surgery [85, 106]. For patients with grade 0 or grade 1 arachnoid changes, 89% and 86% of patients, respectively, demonstrated a sustained postoperative decrease in syrinx size, compared with only 67% for grade 2 arachnoid scarring (r=–0.1989, P=0.027). In contrast, group B patients demonstrated decrease of the syrinx in just 64% of cases, no change in 14%, and an increase in 21%. After syrinx shunting, the syrinx immediately decreased postoperatively. However, during follow-up, just 14% of patients showed a sustained radiological effect of the shunt. While the great majority of 79% of patients developed a recurrent increase of syrinx size postoperatively (Chi-square-test: P<0.0001), 7% demonstrated no change.

3.1.5.3
Clinical Results for Chiari I Malformation

Postoperative outcome depends on three factors: preoperative symptoms, type of operation, and arachnoid scarring at the foramen magnum. In terms of preoperative symptoms, we have to separately analyze the results for symptoms related to brainstem and cervical cord compression and those symptoms related to syringomyelia. We have separately analyzed results for three types of operation (foramen magnum decompression – group A, posterior fossa decompression – group B, and syrinx shunting – group C) and, finally, correlated preoperative symptoms and outcome to the grade of arachnoid scarring as determined during surgery. Arachnoid changes at the foramen magnum were found to have a major influence on clinical presentation and postoperative result. The type of operation predominantly influenced long-term outcome.

Table 3.6. Percentage of CMI patients with preoperative neurological symptoms related to arachnoid scarring at the foramen magnum

Symptom	Grade 0, n=17	Grade 1, n=110	Grade 2, n =22	r-value	P-value
Sensory function	73%	75%	85%	−0.139	0.0461
Dysesthesias	60%	56%	60%	–	n.s.
Occipital pain	93%	78%	65%	+0.283	0.0003
Motor weakness	40%	47%	80%	−0.342	<0.0001
Gait ataxia	47%	61%	85%	−0.295	0.0001
Bladder function	27%	24%	40%	−0.155	0.03
Bowel function	13%	15%	20%	–	n.s.
Caudal cranial nerves	13%	18%	25%	–	n.s.

n.s., not significant

Looking at results in the literature is a very tedious task [131]. A lot of authors do not specify precisely which operative steps were taken, do not clarify their criteria for success or failure of treatment, and do not provide follow-up information for a long enough time period. Sometimes a postoperative improvement that was only short-lived is still considered a success, even though the patient again developed progressive symptoms postoperatively. However, there is general agreement now that foramen magnum decompression is the method of choice in CMI [5, 37, 38, 57, 65, 83, 85, 131, 137, 138, 139, 147, 214, 215, 245]. In terms of surgical details of this procedure, there still exists considerable controversy. Several studies emphasize the necessity of obex plugging [23, 45, 72, 74, 87, 140, 153, 192, 194, 195, 246] or an additional shunt of the syrinx [33, 153, 168, 169, 210]. From our experience, we advise against both of these maneuvers.

3.1.5.3.1
Preoperative Symptoms and Postoperative Clinical Results Related to Arachnoid Scarring

Arachnoid changes led to clinical manifestations [1, 5] due to CSF flow obstruction and tethering of the cervical cord. Site and extent of scarring determined site and extent of CSF flow obstruction, i.e., whether the patient developed a syrinx or hydrocephalus. Hydrocephalus was present in none of the patients without arachnoiditis at the foramen magnum, in 9% of patients with grade 1, and in 35% of patients with grade 2 arachnoid scarring (r=0.27, P=0.0004). Likewise, the percentage of patients with syringomyelia correlated significantly with the amount of arachnoid scarring (grade 0=70%, grade 1=74%, grade 2=94%; r=0.027, P=0.155). Preoperative diagnosis of hydrocephalus or dilated ventricles should alert the surgeon that he may

encounter significant arachnoid pathology at surgery [114, 181, 267], and that this aspect has to be recognized for planning adequate surgical treatment. Other indicators of arachnoid pathology may be an arachnoid cyst in the posterior fossa or craniocervical instability [5]. The latter may provoke arachnoid changes due to mechanical irritation.

Arachnoid pathology, however, not only causes these radiological features but also has a significant influence on clinical presentation [1, 2, 5]. Patients without arachnoid changes tend to present predominantly with occipital headaches, which can be attributed to compression at the foramen magnum. They are less likely to develop more severe neurological deficits or syringomyelia and constitute the group of patients with the best long-term prognosis after surgery.

However, motor weakness of the upper limbs, gait ataxia, sensory deficits, and bladder function demonstrate a significant correlation with the grade of arachnoid pathology at the foramen magnum. Dysesthesias, bowel function, and cranial nerve deficits did not show such a correlation (Table 3.6).

The preoperative Karnofsky score decreased significantly with the amount of arachnoid scarring found at surgery (grade 0=74±14, grade 1=73±15, grade 2=67±15; r=−0.242, P=0.002). These observations strongly suggest that arachnoid changes at the foramen magnum may cause symptoms independently from other pathomechanisms, such as brainstem or cervical cord compression. If this is the case, we have to conclude that arachnoid pathology – if present – needs to be addressed at surgery. If this aspect is neglected, the long-term result of treatment may be less satisfactory.

Table 3.7 gives an overview for the percentages of patients with residual symptoms after 1 year, in relation to grade of arachnoid scarring at the foramen

Table 3.7. Percentage of Chiari I malformation patients with postoperative neurological symptoms related to arachnoid scarring at the foramen magnum

Symptom	Grade 0	Grade 1	Grade 2	r-value	P-value
Sensory function	71%	71%	70%	–	n.s.
Dysesthesias	43%	52%	40%	–	n.s.
Occipital pain	86%	45%	60%	–	n.s.
Motor weakness	14%	38%	60%	−0.241	0.014
Gait ataxia	14%	38%	80%	−0.309	0.002
Bladder function	29%	18%	30%	–	n.s.
Bowel function	0%	11%	30%	−0.259	0.009
Caudal cranial nerves	14%	16%	30%	–	n.s.

n.s., not significant

magnum. As was the case with preoperative symptoms, a significant correlation between the degree of motor weakness and gait ataxia to grade of arachnoid scarring could be identified. Additionally, sphincter disturbances were more likely to persist in patients with severe arachnoiditis. No significant correlation was found for the remainder of neurological symptoms and signs. However, occipital headaches due to compression at the foramen magnum regularly improve postoperatively, regardless of arachnoid pathology (Table 3.8).

The grade of arachnoid scarring correlated with the Karnofsky score at 1 year after surgery (r=−0.191, P=0.041). Patients without arachnoiditis (Grade 0) improved their high preoperative Karnofsky score during this time (71±20 and 80±19, respectively; $P < 0.0001$). Patients with grade 1 improved from 74±13 to 80±14 ($P<0.0001$), and patients with grade 2 from 71±13 to 74±15 (not significant) (Table 3.8). For patients in whom the arachnoid was not opened, the Karnofsky score also improved significantly during the first postoperative year (63±26 to 70±24, P=0.013).

3.1.5.3.2
Postoperative Clinical Results Related to Preoperative Symptoms

Overall, the best postoperative effect of foramen magnum decompression was demonstrated for occipital headaches, which almost always improved [5, 26, 61, 72, 90, 91, 173, 180, 182, 214, 246, 259]. Likewise, other symptoms of brainstem compression, such as swallowing or gait problems, regularly got better [5, 38, 180, 214, 259, 267]. Less positive effects were obtained for symptoms primarily related to the syrinx, such as sensory changes, dysesthesias, or motor weakness [5, 38, 259].

Burning type dysesthesias pose a special therapeutic problem. Even in patients with otherwise very satisfactory outcome – improved gait, decrease of syrinx size, etc. – this symptom may persist. Williams observed postoperative aggravations even despite a complete postoperative collapse of the syrinx (personal communication). Only half of the patients report some postoperative improvement of dysesthesias in our series [24, 170]. Milhorat et al. [170] considered burning type dysesthesias to be a sign of deafferentiation. They showed a high concentration of substance P in the spinal cord of syringomyelia patients below the lower pole of the cyst [171]. Nevertheless, pathophysiology of this symptom remains unclear. Beric et al. [32] hypothesized that this symptom is of central origin, due to a mismatch of preserved posterior column signals and missing spinothalamic afferents.

Drug treatment of this problem is very difficult. Some patients report improvement with carbamazepine, clonidine, or phenytoin. Sometimes this improvement also causes some decrease of spasticity, which patients may experience as a loss of motor power and, for that reason, discontinue the medication. A similar effect was reported by a patient after implantation of a spinal cord stimulator. The only other effective alternative at the moment seems to be opiate therapy.

3.1.5.3.3
Postoperative Clinical Results Related to Type of Operation

Overall in group A, 61% of patients reported sustained improvement, while 34% were stabilized in their clinical course, and 4% deteriorated. In group B, 55% observed improvement, 29% were stabilized, and 16% deteriorated. With syrinx shunting, 21% were better or

Table 3.8. Preoperative and postoperative symptoms related to grade of arachnoid scarring for patients with Chiari I malformation after foramen magnum decompression

Group	Preop.	Postop.	3 months	6 months	1 year	P
Sensory deficits						
Grade 0	3.9±1.1	4.1±0.9	4.1±0.9	4.1±0.9	4.1±0.9	n.s.
Grade 1	3.5±1.1	3.7±1.0	3.8±1.0	3.9±1.0	3.9±1.0	<0.01
Grade 2	3.4±1.1	3.5±1.2	3.5±1.2	3.5±1.2	3.5±1.2	n.s.
Dysesthesias						
Grade 0	4.1±0.7	4.6±0.5	4.6±0.5	4.7±0.5	4.6±0.5	0.04
Grade 1	4.0±1.0	4.3±0.9	4.3±0.9	4.3±0.9	4.3±0.9	<0.01
Grade 2	4.0±0.9	4.1±0.8	4.3±0.9	4.3±0.9	4.3±0.9	n.s.
Pain						
Grade 0	3.4±1.0	4.1±0.7	4.3±0.5	4.6±0.5	4.3±0.8	<0.01
Grade 1	3.6±1.0	4.2±0.7	4.4±0.7	4.4±0.8	4.4±0.8	<0.01
Grade 2	3.9±0.8	4.3±0.5	4.5±0.5	4.5±0.5	4.5±0.5	0.03
Motor power						
Grade 0	4.6±0.8	4.7±0.8	4.9±0.4	4.9±0.4	4.9±0.4	n.s.
Grade 1	4.3±0.9	4.4±0.8	4.5±0.8	4.5±0.8	4.5±0.8	<0.01
Grade 2	3.3±1.2	3.4±1.3	3.5±1.2	3.5±1.2	3.5±1.2	n.s.
Gait ataxia						
Grade 0	4.1±1.0	4.3±1.1	4.4±1.1	4.4±1.1	4.6±0.8	0.04
Grade 1	3.9±1.0	4.0±1.0	4.2±1.0	4.3±0.9	4.3±1.0	<0.01
Grade 2	3.8±1.0	3.8±1.0	3.8±1.0	3.8±1.0	3.8±1.0	n.s.
Bladder function						
Grade 0	4.7±0.5	4.1±1.2	4.7±0.5	4.7±0.5	4.7±0.5	n.s.
Grade 1	4.6±0.8	4.7±0.5	4.8±0.5	4.8±0.5	4.8±0.4	<0.01
Grade 2	4.4±0.7	4.5±0.8	4.5±0.8	4.5±0.8	4.5±0.8	n.s.
Bowel function						
Grade 0	4.7±0.5	4.7±0.5	4.7±0.5	4.7±0.5	4.7±0.5	n.s.
Grade 1	4.8±0.7	4.9±0.4	4.9±0.3	4.9±0.3	4.9±0.3	0.04
Grade 2	4.8±0.5	4.5±0.8	4.5±0.8	4.5±0.8	4.5±0.8	n.s.
Swallowing function						
Grade 0	4.4±1.0	4.6±0.8	4.6±0.8	4.6±0.8	4.6±0.8	n.s.
Grade 1	4.7±0.7	4.8±0.5	4.8±0.4	4.8±0.5	4.8±0.5	<0.01
Grade 2	4.9±0.4	4.9±0.4	4.9±0.4	4.9±0.4	4.9±0.4	n.s.
Karnofsky score						
Grade 0	71±20	74±21	77±17	80±19	80±19	<0.01
Grade 1	74±13	76±13	79±13	79±14	80±14	<0.01
Grade 2	71±15	74±15	74±15	74±15	74±15	n.s.

Preop., preoperative; Postop., postoperative; P P-value for comparison of preoperative and postoperative status after 1 year; n.s., not significant

Table 3.9. Preoperative and postoperative clinical symptoms related to type of operation for patients with Chiari I malformation

Group	Preop.	Postop.	3 months	6 months	1 year	P
Sensory deficits						
Group A	3.5±1.1	3.7±1.1	3.8±1.0	3.8±1.0	3.8±1.0	<0.01
Group B	3.6±1.1	3.7±1.0	4.0±1.0	4.0±1.1	4.0±1.0	<0.01
Group C	2.6±0.5	2.6±0.5	2.7±0.5	2.7±0.5	2.6±0.5	n.s.
Dysesthesias						
Group A	4.0±1.0	4.3±0.8	4.3±0.8	4.3±0.9	4.3±0.9	<0.01
Group B	4.1±0.9	4.3±0.8	4.4±0.7	4.4±0.7	4.4±0.8	<0.01
Group C	3.6±1.1	3.8±0.9	4.0±0.7	4.1±0.8	3.9±0.9	n.s.
Pain						
Group A	3.6±1.0	4.2±0.7	4.4±0.7	4.4±0.7	4.4±0.8	<0.01
Group B	3.8±1.1	4.1±0.8	4.4±0.7	4.4±0.8	4.4±0.8	<0.01
Group C	3.9±1.1	4.0±0.7	4.4±0.8	4.4±0.8	4.2±0.8	n.s.
Motor power						
Group A	4.2±1.0	4.3±0.9	4.4±0.9	4.4±0.9	4.4±0.9	<0.01
Group B	4.3±0.8	4.4±0.9	4.5±0.8	4.5±0.8	4.4±0.8	0.03
Group C	3.5±1.1	3.6±1.1	3.9±1.1	4.0±1.2	3.7±1.3	n.s.
Gait ataxia						
Group A	3.9±1.0	4.0±1.0	4.2±1.0	4.3±1.0	4.3±1.0	<0.01
Group B	3.9±1.0	4.1±1.0	4.2±1.0	4.2±1.0	4.2±1.0	n.s.
Group C	4.0±1.0	3.9±1.2	4.3±1.0	4.4±0.9	4.2±1.0	n.s.
Bladder function						
Group A	4.6±0.7	4.7±0.6	4.8±0.5	4.8±0.5	4.8±0.5	<0.01
Group B	4.4±1.2	4.4±1.0	4.5±1.0	4.5±1.0	4.5±1.0	n.s.
Group C	4.1±1.4	4.2±1.4	4.4±0.8	4.3±0.9	4.2±0.9	n.s.
Bowel function						
Group A	4.8±0.6	4.8±0.5	4.8±0.4	4.8±0.4	4.8±0.4	n.s.
Group B	4.8±0.6	4.8±0.6	4.8±0.5	4.8±0.5	4.8±0.5	n.s.
Group C	4.4±0.9	4.5±0.8	4.7±0.6	4.7±0.6	4.6±0.8	n.s.
Swallowing function						
Group A	4.7±0.7	4.8±0.5	4.8±0.5	4.8±0.5	4.8±0.5	<0.01
Group B	4.3±1.0	4.5±0.8	4.6±0.7	4.7±0.7	4.7±0.7	<0.01
Group C	4.6±0.8	4.7±0.6	4.7±0.6	4.7±0.6	4.7±0.6	<0.01
Karnofsky score						
Group A	74±13	76±13	78±13	79±14	80±14	<0.01
Group B	73±11	73±15	77±14	78±15	77±15	<0.01
Group C	69±13	70±14	74±13	75±10	72±12	n.s.

Preop., preoperative; Postop., postoperative; *P* *P*-value for comparison of preoperative and postoperative status after 1 year; n.s., not significant

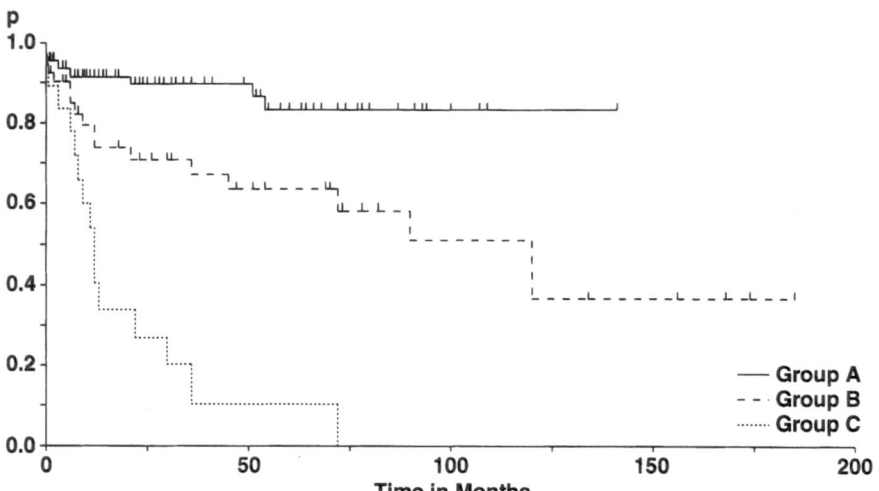

Fig. 3.32. Kaplan-Meier analysis of clinical recurrence rates for patients with Chiari I malformation, depending on the type of surgery performed (log-rank test: $P<0.0001$)

unchanged, respectively, and 58% observed clinical progression, regardless of whether a shunt had been placed as the first line of treatment or as a secondary procedure (Chi-square-test: $P<0.0001$). In their multicenter study, Aghakhani et al. [5] determined a postoperative rate for clinical stabilization of 87% after foramen magnum decompression, whereas a figure of 71% was given after syrinx shunting.

Looking at the postoperative course of particular symptoms (Table 3.9) reveals steady postoperative improvement for almost every symptom in group A with a small craniectomy, i.e., foramen magnum decompression and a spacious duraplasty. In group B, a similar postoperative result is obtained within the first postoperative year. Group B consists of patients in whom the craniectomy was significantly larger and various maneuvers such as obex plugging or leaving the dura open had been performed, which could be shown by multiple regression analysis to put patients at an increased risk for recurrence. With shunting of the syrinx (group C), however, symptoms start to deteriorate toward the end of the first postoperative year. In other words, shunting of a syrinx provides a preliminary benefit, but does not stabilize the clinical situation.

Looking at postoperative clinical recurrence rates, significant differences were detected between the three treatment groups of our series (log-rank test: $P<0.0001$; Fig. 3.32).

The best long-term results were obtained in group A. In group B, patients with a large craniectomy are at risk for downward herniation of the cerebellum into the spinal canal [5, 29, 65, 109, 110, 267]. This may cause spinal cord compression and adherence of the cerebellum to the dura (i.e., obliteration of the cisterna magna and CSF flow obstruction) and, thus, lead to clinical deterioration [109, 110].

The worst results were seen for patients after syrinx shunting. Apart from the fact, that syrinx shunting cannot influence symptoms and pathomechanisms of brainstem and cervical cord compression, the most common causes for shunt failure were dislocation, obstruction due to glial tissue, syrinx septations, and a postoperative tethered cord due to arachnoid scarring related to the shunt insertion [30, 245]. Due to increasingly reported problems with syrinx drainage [30, 147, 226, 251, 254], pure syrinx shunting is no longer recommended as the first line of treatment for CMI, even though a recent report claimed very good postoperative results provided that the distal end of the catheter was placed in the anterior part of the cervical subarachnoid space [120]. Avoiding contact between the catheter and dural suture may indeed limit problems of postoperative tethering. However, all other points of criticism against this technique still remain.

Among patients in group A, we saw a trend to higher clinical recurrence rates according to the grade of arachnoid scarring [2, 5, 216]. With an overall surgical morbidity of 4.6%, we observed clinical recurrences in 5% of patients after arachnoid opening, but without arachnoid changes at the foramen magnum. With grade 1, the recurrence rate after 5 years was 16%. The corresponding figure for grade 2 was 47% (log-rank test: not significant) (Fig. 3.33).

In 21 patients of group A, the arachnoid was not opened at surgery. Comparing these patients with those of grade 0 or 1 arachnoiditis, who underwent arachnoid dissection, revealed a significantly higher recurrence rate for the former group (17% with arachnoid opening and 41% without arachnoid opening; log-rank test: $P=0.0369$) (Fig. 3.34). Also revealed was the trend for a lower rate of postoperative decrease in syrinx size (67% and 86%, respectively; not significant).

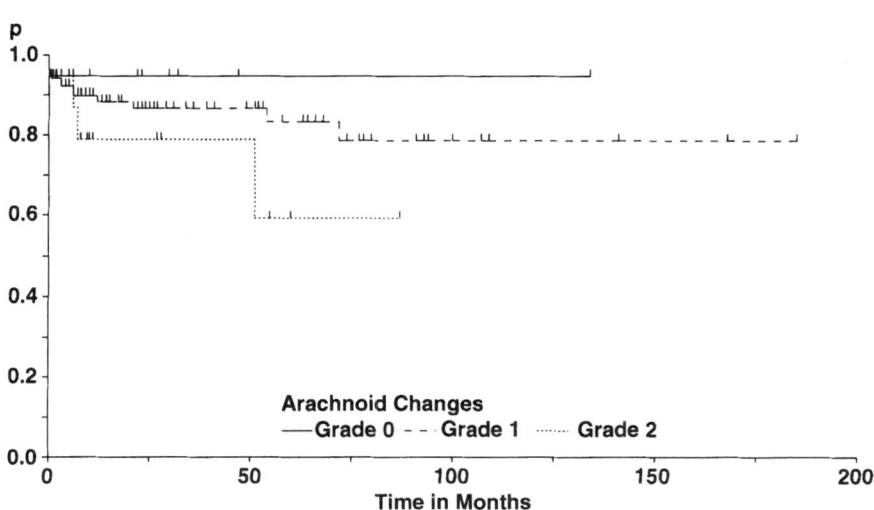

Fig. 3.33. Kaplan-Meier analysis for patients with Chiari I malformation who underwent a small foramen magnum decompression (group A) but with different grades of arachnoid pathology (log-rank test: not significant)

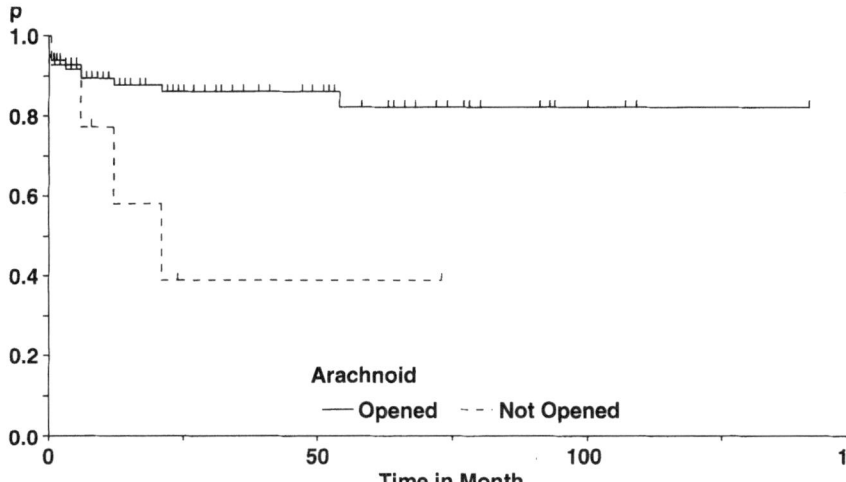

Fig. 3.34. Kaplan-Meier analysis for patients with Chiari I malformation who underwent a small foramen magnum decompression (group A) with or without arachnoid dissection (log-rank test: $P=0.0369$)

Valentine Logue [138, 139] originally recommended that the arachnoid be left intact during decompression for CMI. This came at a time when surgical mortalities for the Gardner operation were quite high. Recently, this method has been proposed again by a number of authors. In fact, early postoperative results are quite in favor of this strategy. However, most of the studies recommending this method analyze a small number of patients with a rather short period of follow-up [69, 89, 116, 118, 206, 215, 216]. This method does have some appeal – without arachnoid opening, the risk of complications should be lower. In particular, CSF fistulas should be avoidable and there is no spillage of blood into the subarachnoid space. Arachnoid dissection, however, offers the potential risk of damaging small perforating arteries or even the PICA [131, 159, 267, 268]. Therefore, if similar or even better clinical results can be obtained using a more limited procedure, there would be no justification to extend the operation into the subarachnoid space. Other authors, however, have pointed out the value of arachnoid dissection [5, 196, 250, 273] and reduction of tonsillar volume [99].

Our own experience clearly shows that long-term results are worse if the arachnoid is not opened and the arachnoid pathology is not treated. It was the general policy to open the arachnoid and to inspect the fourth ventricle, unless the arachnoid was considered absolutely normal. Therefore, those 21 patients in whom the arachnoid was left intact, resemble a group which should have had no arachnoid changes, or only very discrete ones, and be associated with a particularly favorable prognosis. The results show that the immediate postoperative outcome for patients without arachnoid opening was quite satisfactory. However, analysis of clinical recurrence rates indicates a significantly worse long-term result for this group compared with patients in whom the arachnoid was opened [99].

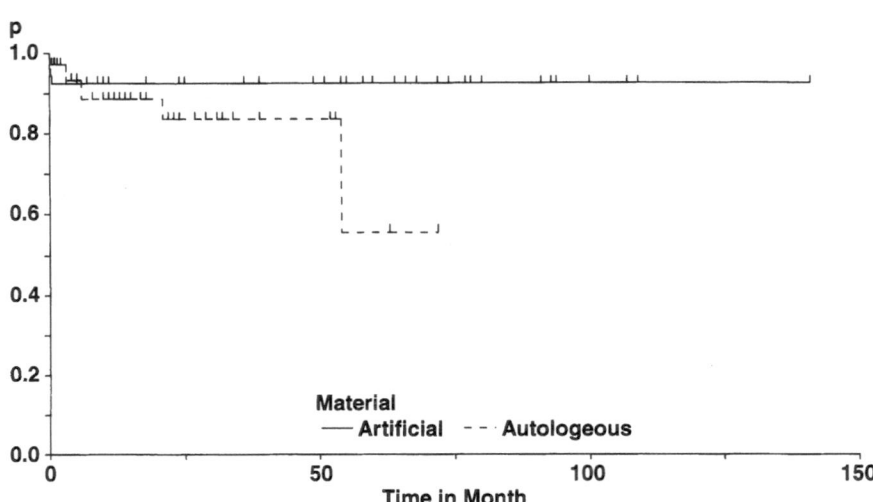

Fig. 3.35. Kaplan-Meier analysis for patients with Chiari I malformation who underwent a small foramen magnum decompression (group A) with a duraplasty of artificial or autologous material (log-rank test: $P=0.05$)

In other words, a certain percentage of patients with CMI is not sufficiently treated with bony decompression and dural grafting alone. Without arachnoid opening, some degree of arachnoid pathology may be overlooked intraoperatively. Inspection of the arachnoid after dura opening may not be sufficient to evaluate the adequacy of CSF flow [250].

Oldfield et al. [185] suggested the use of intraoperative ultrasound to study CSF flow at the foramen magnum. However, it is debatable whether CSF flow is adequate once pulsations are detectable. Such pulsations may just resemble movements of the cerebellar tonsils related to volume changes due to arterial filling and may not represent adequate CSF flow.

Finally, higher clinical recurrence rates were observed for group A patients in whom autologous material – fascia lata or galea – was used for the duraplasty, compared with patients in whom artificial material was employed (37% and 9% after 5 years, respectively; log-rank test: $P=0.05$) (Fig. 3.35). This tendency for higher clinical recurrence rates, regarding patients in whom autologous material was employed as a dura substitute, is related to formation of arachnoid adhesions between duraplasty and underlying cerebellar tonsils and brainstem, as witnessed during secondary operations in these patients. Therefore, the long-term prognosis of patients with CMI is influenced significantly by arachnoid pathology – whether already present at surgery or developed postoperatively.

Several authors emphasized that postoperative improvements may be observed after foramen magnum decompression, provided the operation was done early enough. Patients with long-standing symptoms and atrophic cords do not experience postoperative improvements [10, 37, 39, 101, 259]. This may also be related to the course of the disease; at the beginning, signs of cord and brainstem compression predominate, while symptoms due to the syrinx appear later.

As signs of the syrinx generally not improve postoperatively, while those due to compression do, this observation may be explained. From our experience, recurrence rates are not influenced by the preoperative status of the patient.

3.1.5.4
Postoperative Results for Chiari II Malformation

Of 11 patients with CMII and functioning ventricular shunts undergoing decompression, 6 demonstrated permanent postoperative improvements, 3 remained unchanged, while 2 patients deteriorated further. One of these was operated on a second time and improved; the other declined a further intervention. In the literature, it is reported that postoperative results depend on patient age [31]. This may be related to the less dramatic clinical course in adult patients versus young children. Possibly, the indication for decompression has been considered too late for infants in the past [110, 198, 201, 257]. Neuropathological changes in the brainstem of infants with CMII (which demonstrate areas of demyelination, small hemorrhages, and necrotic areas) may be secondary events provoked by respiratory problems and repeated hypoxic episodes during apnea attacks [75, 198, 208, 257]. In our series, young infants showed dramatic postoperative improvement of respiratory problems in particular. Likewise, swallowing difficulties and dysarthria had a good postoperative prognosis. Provided that shunt infections can be avoided, these children may achieve normal intellectual standards [208, 244]. Therefore, we are strictly opposed against therapeutic nihilism in these children. We would recommend decompressing children with CMII early, if neurological symptoms persist or progress further despite a functioning ventricular shunt, unless severe multiple malformations provide a bad prognosis regardless of the problem at the foramen magnum [242, 255]; children who breathe normally and then deteriorate to respiratory insufficiency are good candidates for decompression [115]. In 80% of children, Teo et al. [242] found a complete resolution of preoperative symptoms within 1 year of decompression. Vandertop et al. [255] observed an excellent result in 15 of 17 infants decompressed for CMII, while 2 infants subsequently died. Zerah [273] operated on 22 children with progressive neurological signs, from a total of 204 with CMII. Of these, 10 underwent revision of the ventriculoperitoneal shunt, 12 were operated on at the level of the myelomeningocele for re-tethering, 2 received a syrinx shunt, while 8 underwent decompression of the brain stem. After surgery, 90% of operated children stabilized or improved. Pollack et al. [201] found 10 of 13 children improved after decompression in a prospective study. Once bilateral vocal cord palsies were present, surgery no longer had a beneficial effect. In other words, it is essential to perform decompression early enough.

In adults with CMII, occipital pain, gait problem, and sensory disturbances also demonstrated some postoperative improvement comparable with adults who had CMI. In this age group, preoperative history and postoperative outcome after decompression are quite similar to CMI.

3.1.6
Management of Clinical Recurrences of Chiari Malformations

Foramen magnum decompression is widely recognized as the procedure of choice for treatment of CMI patients with or without syringomyelia [2, 5, 38, 65, 93, 99, 160]. However, what should be done if a foramen magnum decompression has not stabilized the clinical course postoperatively?

The pathology in patients with CMI is located at the foramen magnum. If a foramen magnum decompression did not produce a favorable outcome, this area needs to be explored again. Additionally, the craniocervical junction and cervical spine need to be carefully evaluated for evidence of instability [122] or degenerative problems (Fig. 3.36). Concomitant degenerative changes may produce cervical myelopathy, which may present with similar signs and symptoms.

In patients with CMII and a neurological recurrence, the ventricular shunt needs to be checked, and the clinical examination has to distinguish whether the clinical deterioration is related to the craniocervical junction or to the repair site of the lumbar myelomeningocele. For instance, a gait problem may be caused by lumbar re-tethering, rather than a craniocervical problem [46, 273].

What may be the reasons for failure of a foramen magnum decompression in CMI? In children, new

bone formation has been shown to cause recurrent brainstem compression [12, 112, 273]. Another possible cause is herniation of the cerebellum due to an oversized craniectomy, so-called cerebellar ptosis [109]. The most common cause of clinical deterioration in adults, however, is arachnoid scarring at this level (Figs. 3.37, 3.38, 3.39) [216]. This may be difficult to demonstrate radiologically. Therefore, all information on the first operation and neuroradiological studies need to be examined carefully. The operation notes should be studied. Was a duraplasty inserted? What material was used? Was the obex plugged? Did the surgeon comment on arachnoid changes? How was the arachnoid dealt with?

Autologous material for duraplasty has the advantage of lower complication rates in terms of CSF fistulas [250], but carries a significant risk of adherence to brainstem or cerebellar tonsils [268]. This may interfere with CSF circulation in such a manner that neurological symptoms and syringomyelia reappear (Fig. 3.37) [196]. Likewise, obex plugging may cause severe arachnoid scarring at the foramen of Magendie and brainstem (Fig. 3.38) [131, 216, 250]. If no duraplasty was inserted, postoperative arachnoid scarring may cause adherence of the dura to the underlying nervous tissue and, thus, recurrent CSF flow obstruction [179, 196]. Likewise, pseudomeningocele may lead to the same situation if the duraplasty is pushed anteriorly, leading to arachnoid adhesions (Fig. 3.39) [188].

In our series, 20 patients underwent 21 secondary operations. Compared with patients undergoing a first decompression at the foramen magnum, patient age for secondary surgeries was similar at 43±16 years, whereas the clinical history (32±52 months and 76±106 months, respectively; $P<0.01$) and follow-up (17±25 months and 34±45 months, respectively; $P<0.05$) time periods were significantly shorter. The average interval between first and second operation at the foramen magnum was 40±34 months (range 1–121 months). Table 3.10 gives an overview on clinical and radiological data.

In terms of clinical symptoms, patients undergoing a first or secondary operation at the foramen magnum were similarly affected for sensory problems, dysesthesias, pain, affections of caudal cranial nerves, or sphincter functions. However, patients for secondary foramen magnum decompressions demonstrated significantly worse motor power of upper extremities ($P<0.0001$) and gait ataxia ($P=0.03$). Consequently, the average preoperative Karnofsky score was significantly lower in this group (59±18 and 73±14, respectively; $P=0.004$).

Only two patients undergoing a secondary foramen magnum decompression presented with evidence of brainstem compression, which was due to either herniation of the cerebellum into the enlarged foramen

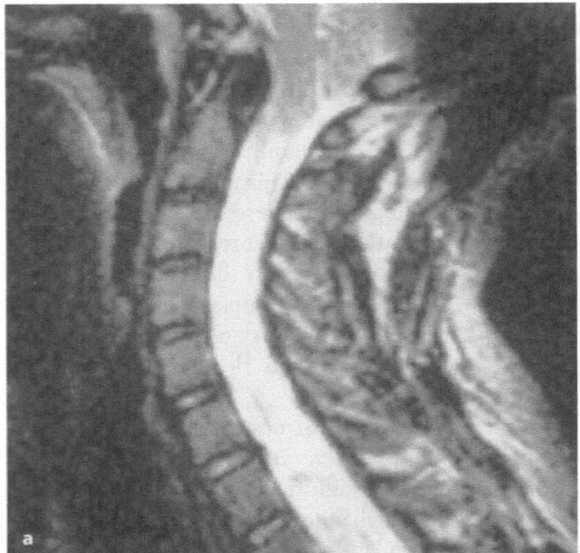

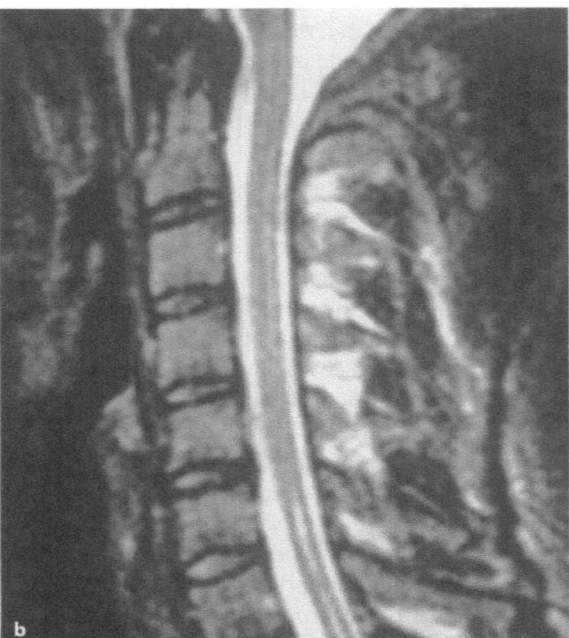

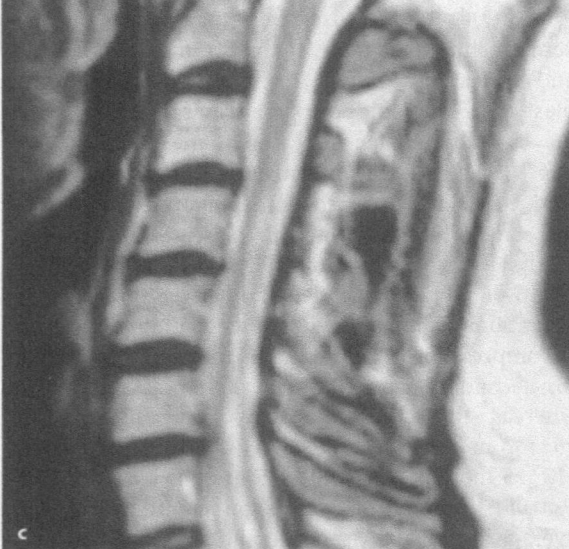

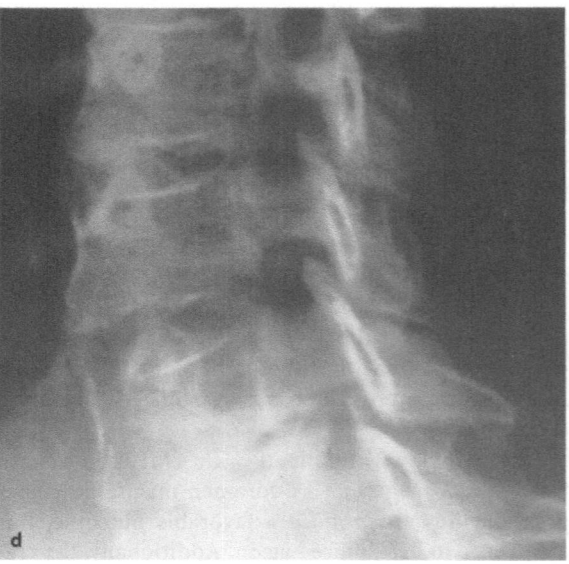

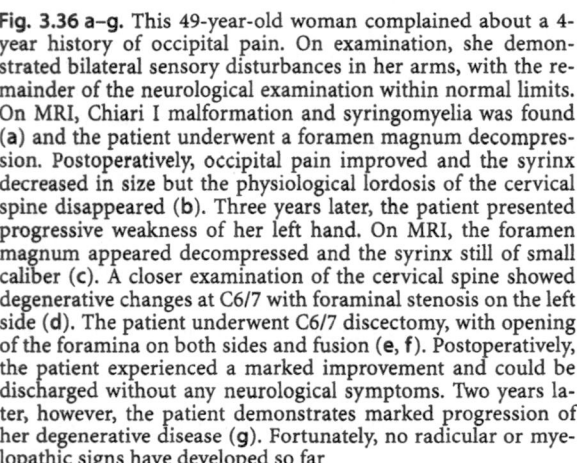

Fig. 3.36 a–g. This 49-year-old woman complained about a 4-year history of occipital pain. On examination, she demonstrated bilateral sensory disturbances in her arms, with the remainder of the neurological examination within normal limits. On MRI, Chiari I malformation and syringomyelia was found (**a**) and the patient underwent a foramen magnum decompression. Postoperatively, occipital pain improved and the syrinx decreased in size but the physiological lordosis of the cervical spine disappeared (**b**). Three years later, the patient presented progressive weakness of her left hand. On MRI, the foramen magnum appeared decompressed and the syrinx still of small caliber (**c**). A closer examination of the cervical spine showed degenerative changes at C6/7 with foraminal stenosis on the left side (**d**). The patient underwent C6/7 discectomy, with opening of the foramina on both sides and fusion (**e, f**). Postoperatively, the patient experienced a marked improvement and could be discharged without any neurological symptoms. Two years later, however, the patient demonstrates marked progression of her degenerative disease (**g**). Fortunately, no radicular or myelopathic signs have developed so far

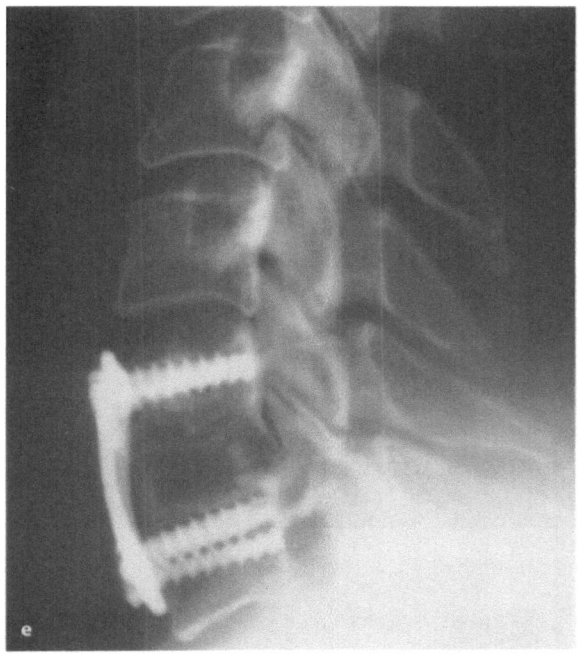

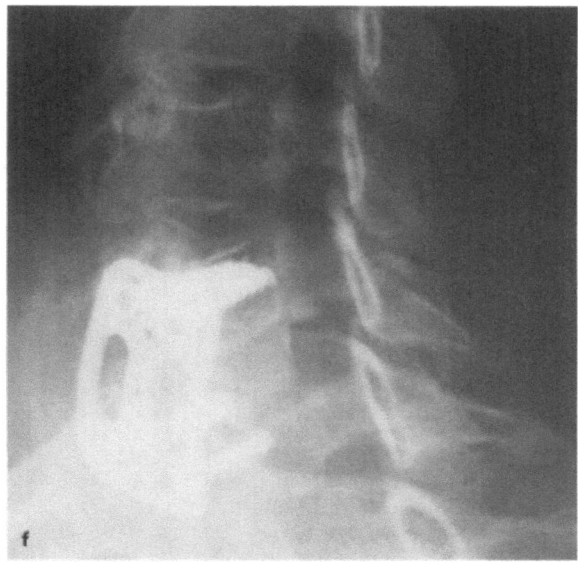

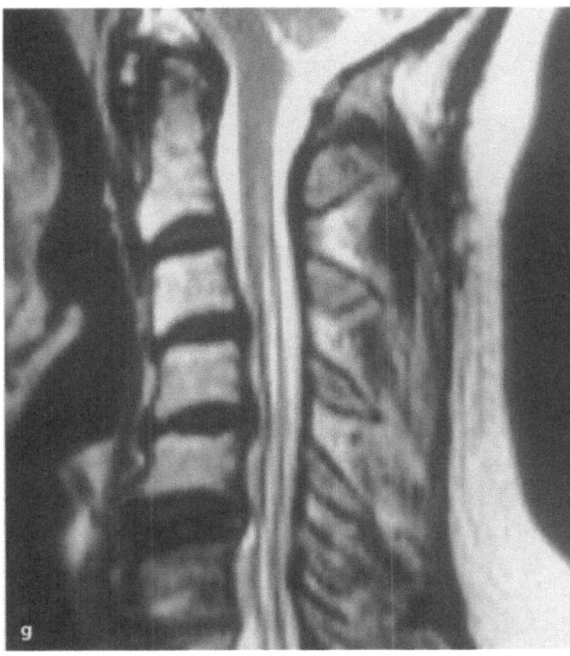

Fig. 3.36 e–g

magnum after an oversized craniectomy (no. 15) or insufficient decompression (no. 6) (Table 3.11). In all other instances, standard MRI studies demonstrated an adequately sized foramen magnum with no apparent compression at this level. In five instances, patients underwent a syringosubarachnoid or syringoperitoneal shunt elsewhere after the initial foramen magnum decompression because the postoperative result at the foramen magnum was either interpreted to be adequate or revision surgery was judged to be too hazardous. None of these syrinx-shunting operations were clinically successful.

Once operative notes have been evaluated, neuroradiological imaging becomes a crucial part in the decision process of how to treat a patient with CMI or CMII and progressive symptoms after foramen magnum decompression. The imaging methods of choice are standard and, especially, cardiac-gated MRI [5, 41, 42, 65, 216]. The former may indicate brainstem compression due to an oversized craniectomy with downward herniation of the cerebellum [109] or to insufficient decompression [131, 267]. This, however, is the exception. Neuroradiological studies must try to find evidence for CSF flow obstruction due to arachnoid scarring at the foramen magnum in this patient group. Standard MRI studies may indicate arachnoid scarring by adherence of the dura or dura graft to brainstem or cerebellar tonsils (Figs. 3.37, 3.39) [188]. Mechanical irritation of the arachnoid at those points may then lead to arachnoid adhesions and CSF flow obstruction. If present, hydrocephalus may be interpreted as an indicator of a more generalized arachnoid

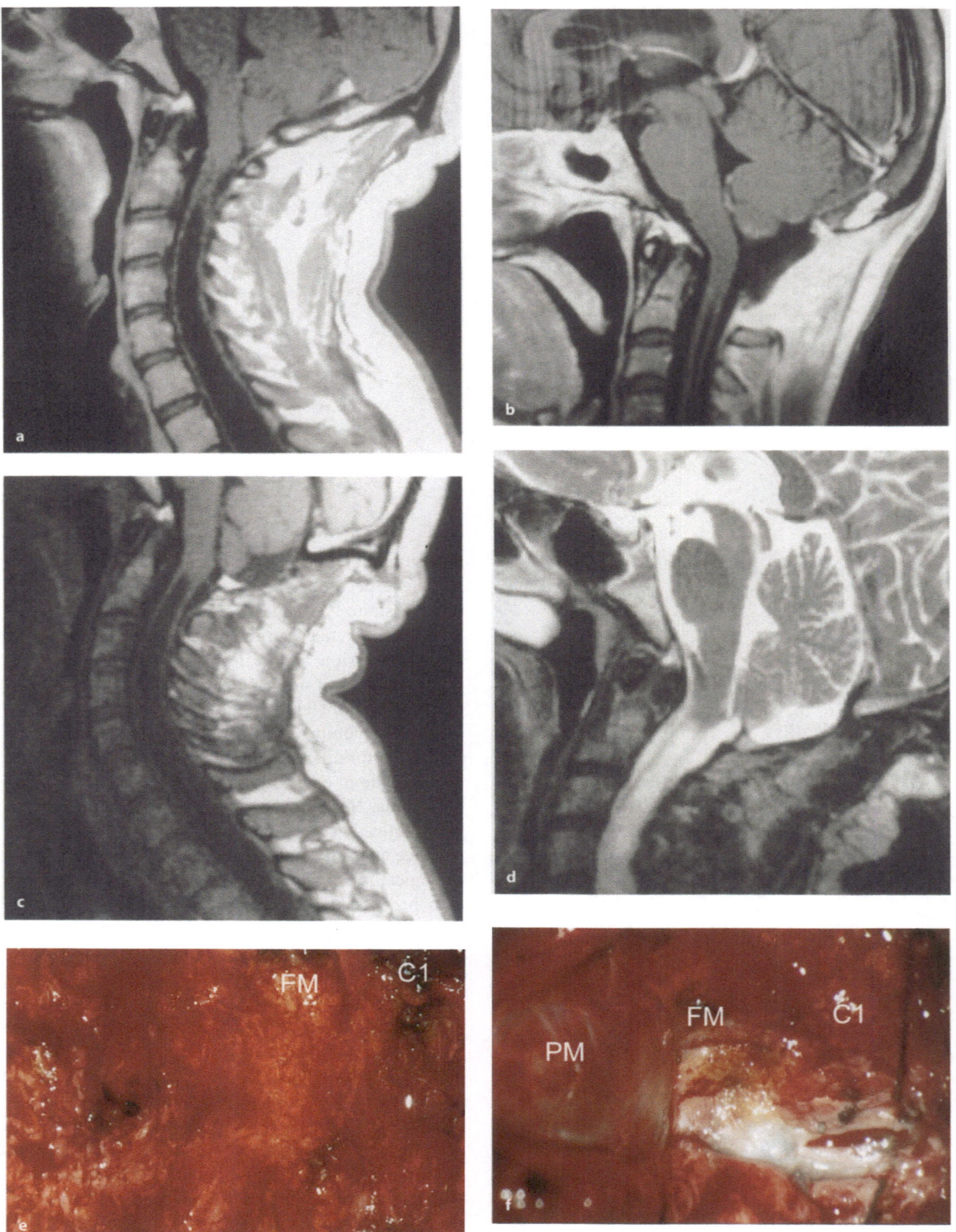

Fig. 3.37 a–f

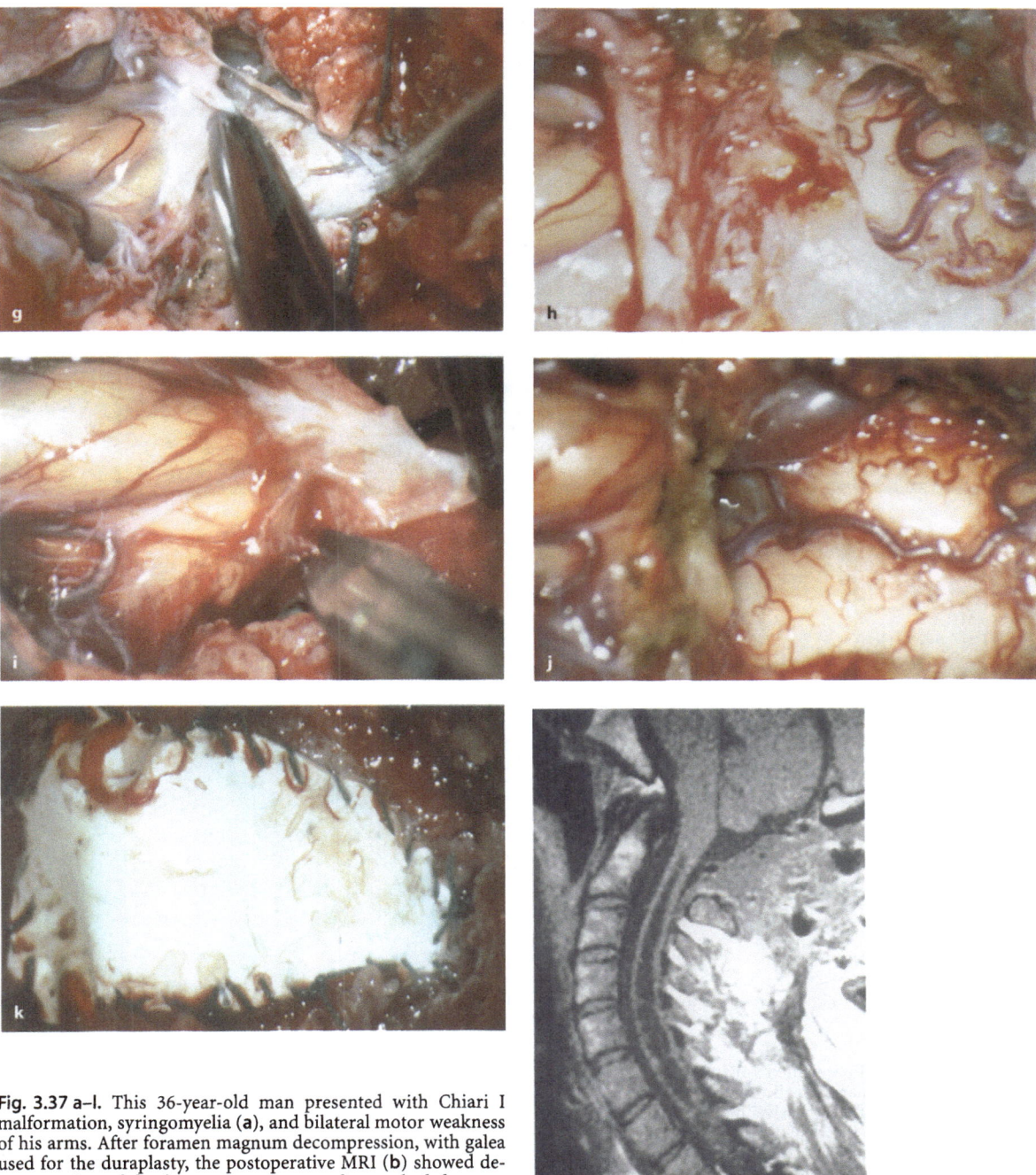

Fig. 3.37 a–l. This 36-year-old man presented with Chiari I malformation, syringomyelia (**a**), and bilateral motor weakness of his arms. After foramen magnum decompression, with galea used for the duraplasty, the postoperative MRI (**b**) showed decompression of the foramen magnum and a marked decrease of the syrinx. One year later, the patient again experienced progressive motor weakness of his arms and hands. The T1- (**c**) and T2-weighted (**d**) MRI scans show reappearance of the syrinx and adhesion of the duraplasty to the tonsillar tips, obstructing CSF flow at this level. **e** The intraoperative view after soft tissue dissection shows the duraplasty at the craniocervical junction exposed. For better orientation, the levels of the foramen magnum (FM) and C1 are marked. **f** This view demonstrates the situation at the beginning of the dura incision. With opening of the duraplasty in the midline above the level of the FM, a pseudomembrane (PM) bulges out, indicating a block of CSF flow between the intracranial and spinal subarachnoid space. At the level of C1, arachnoid scarring is less severe and veins of the posterior cord surface are already visible. **g** After resection of the PM above the level of obstruction, the area of

adhesion between tonsils and duraplasty is clearly visible. **h** After dissection of the spinal arachnoid, the small area of CSF flow obstruction is shown. It requires sharp dissection (**i**) until the fourth ventricle is open, the right PICA is visible, and all CSF pathways are open again (**j**). **k** The Gore-Tex duraplasty has been inserted. **l** The postoperative T1-weighted MRI scan 2 weeks after surgery demonstrates ascension of the cerebellar tonsils, which are no longer adherent to the duraplasty. The cisterna magna is functional and the syrinx has started to decrease in size. The patient's motor weakness has slightly improved

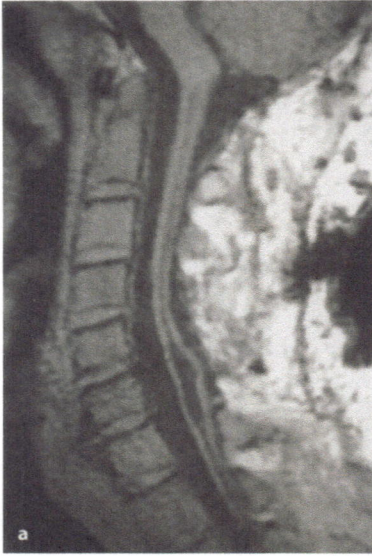
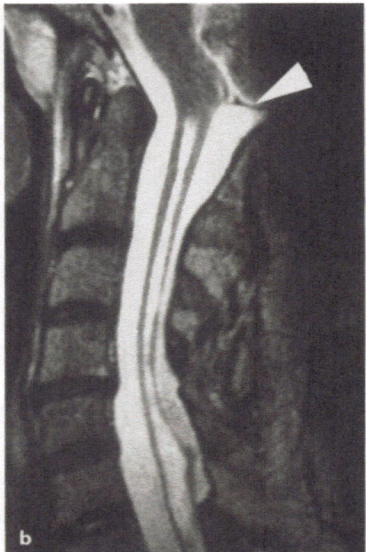
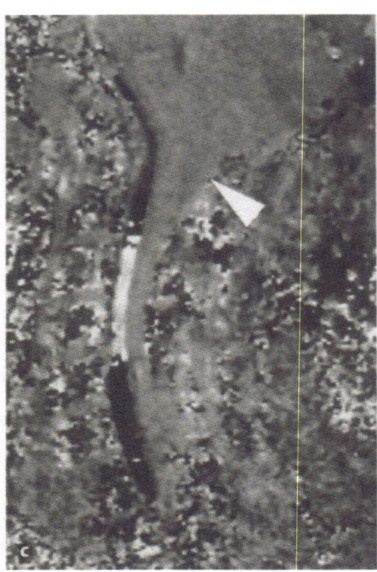

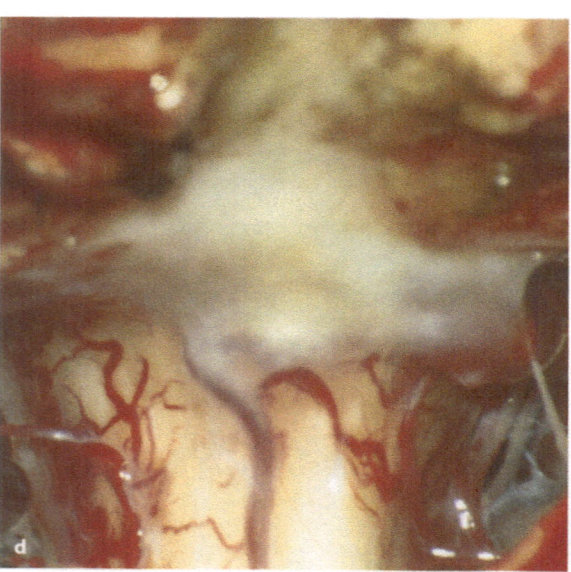
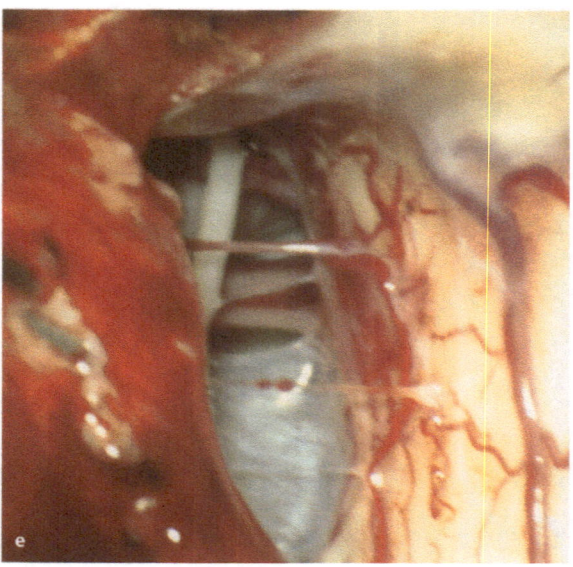

Fig. 3.38 a–i. a This T1-weighted MRI scan of a 44-year-old male patient with Chiari I malformation and syringomyelia was taken because of progressive motor weakness of both upper extremities. At the depicted stage, the patient had already undergone two surgical attempts at the foramen magnum and syringosubarachnoid shunting at C6 for treatment of his syrinx, and also ventriculoperitoneal shunting for his hydrocephalus. This scan demonstrates no apparent reason for this clinical recurrence. The tethering of the cord due to the syringosubarachnoid shunt could not explain the clinical negative progression, as shoulder muscles were also affected. **b** The T2-weighted image also reveals a wide cisterna magna and sufficient space at the foramen magnum. However, a small membrane appears to block the foramen of Magendie (*arrow*). **c** The phase-contrast cine MRI shows an absent flow signal in the cisterna magna (*arrow*), suggesting some block of CSF flow at this level. As significant arachnoid changes were expected, surgery was planned in the semi-sitting position. **d** After dura opening, a complete block of the foramen of Magendie became apparent. The left PICA is completely embedded in scar tissue, while the right PICA is partly visible. **e** Toward both cerebellopontine cisterns no further arachnoid scars were to be found. Therefore, we attribute obstruction of the foramen of Magendie to muscle plugging of the obex performed at the first operation. With careful sharp dissection (**f**), the fourth ventricle is finally opened wide (**g**). To avoid problems of CSF leakage we chose fascia lata for the duraplasty (**h**). Postoperatively, neurological symptoms remained stable with slight improvement of motor power. The T2-weighted scan after 1 year shows a wide cisterna magna, with no apparent membrane occluding the foramen of Magendie any more (**i**)

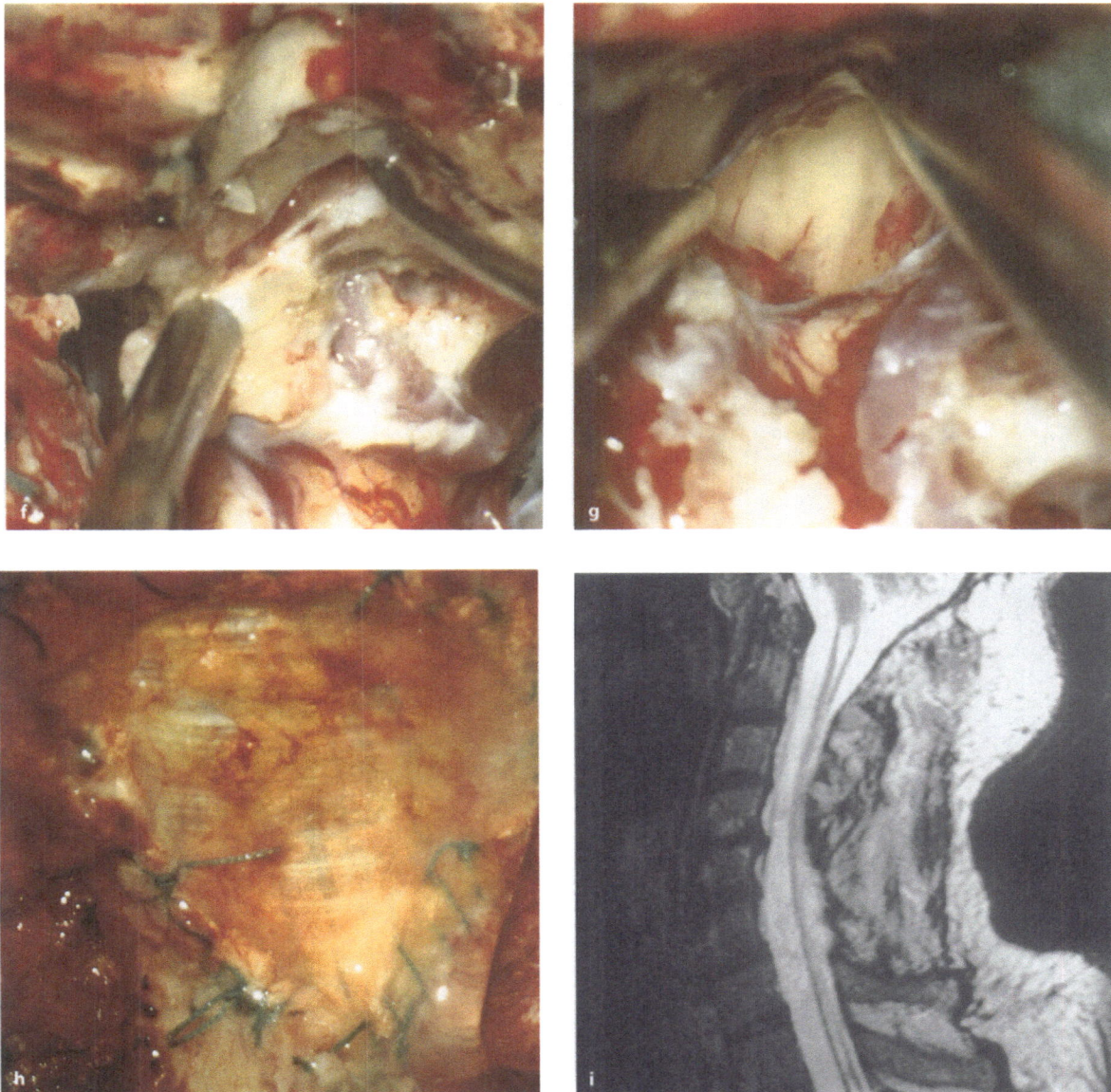

Fig. 3.38 f–i

pathology, due to a subarachnoid hemorrhage or meningitis, for instance.

The modality of choice to demonstrate CSF flow obstruction at the foramen magnum, however, is phase-contrast cine MRI [41, 42]. Even in patients with an adequately decompressed foramen magnum and an apparently normal cisterna magna, CSF flow obstructions may be present which would be missed otherwise (Fig. 3.38). From our experience, analysis of CSF flow at the foramen magnum with phase-contrast cine MRI is the best way to control the postoperative result after foramen magnum decompression and to identify the cause for failure after a foramen magnum procedure.

In our series of 20 patients, 5 patients demonstrated concomitant hydrocephalus, suggesting a more general arachnoid pathology. In 13 patients, the dura graft appeared to be in direct contact to the underlying brainstem or cerebellar tissue. In 5 of these, a pseudomeningocele appeared to have pushed the dura graft anteriorly (Table 3.10).

Once the cause of failure has been determined, these questions need to be answered. How significant are the clinical symptoms for the patient? Is a second operation warranted? If so, how severe is the arachnoid pathology? Can we expect to produce a better result than the first time, in terms of improving CSF circulation?

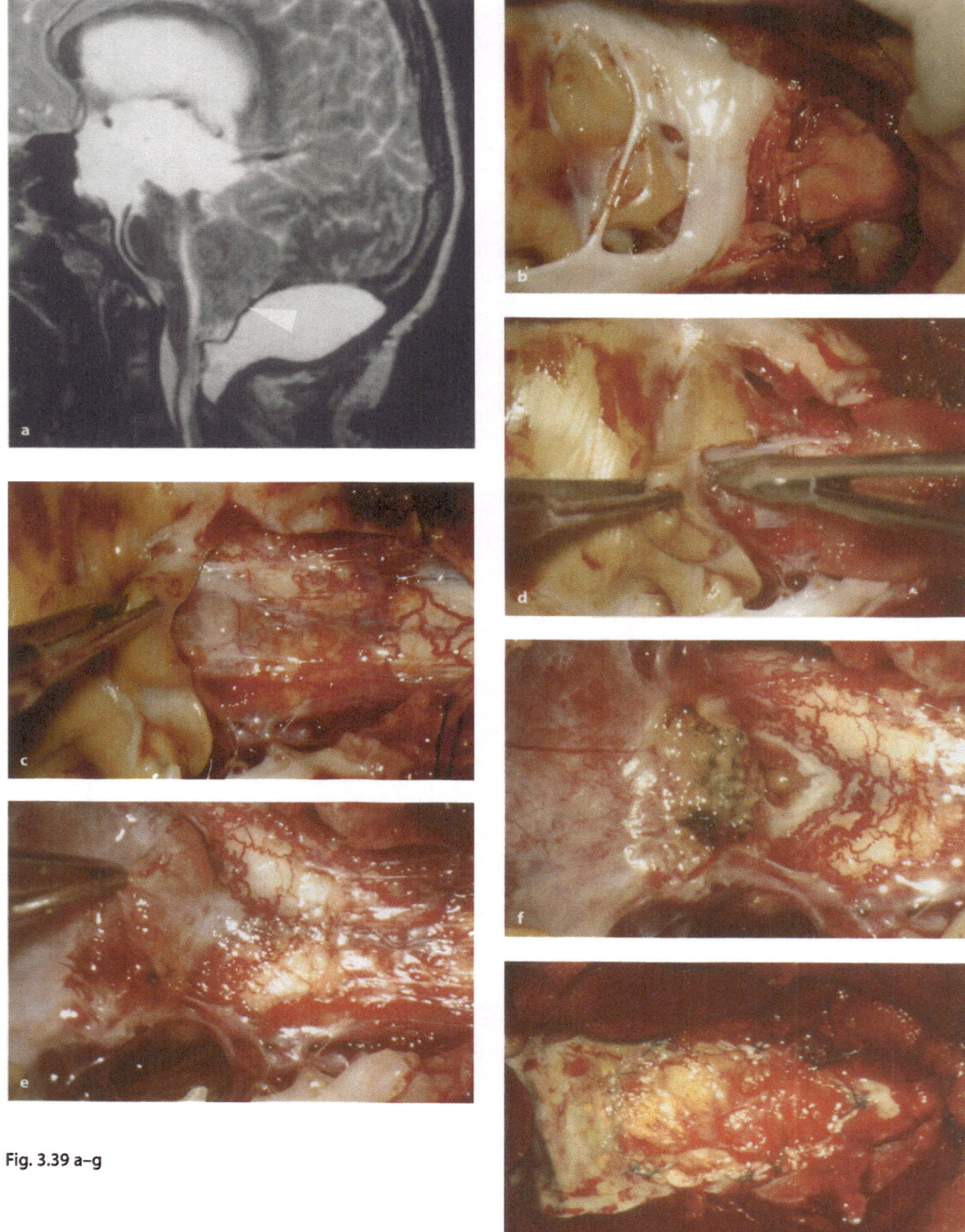

Fig. 3.39 a–g

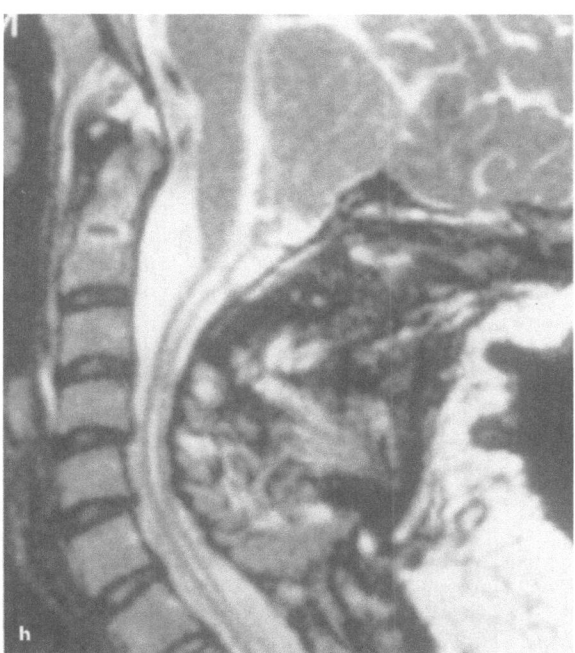

Fig. 3.39 a–h. **a** This T2-weighted MRI image of a 27-year-old woman with Chiari II malformation, syringomyelia, and a feeling of pressure in the occipitocervical region discloses a pseudomeningocele which pushed the dura graft anteriorly, causing adhesions between cerebellar tonsils and graft (*arrow*) so that a block of CSF flow resulted, despite a wide bony decompression. **b** This intraoperative view demonstrates the situation after epidural soft tissue dissection and opening of the pseudomeningocele. The yellowish colored duraplasty appeared to be inserted with single sutures only. Part of the white pseudomembrane still covers the duraplasty. **c** The duraplasty was adherent to cerebellar cortex and spinal cord and had to be dissected sharply (**d**) until the occluded foramen of Magendie was exposed (**e**). The remainder of the duraplasty was not dissected away from the cerebellar cortex, as this would have resulted in a large wound area and risked formation of further adhesions. The obstructed foramen of Magendie was opened (**f**) and a new duraplasty was inserted with a tight running suture (**g**). Again, fascia lata was used for this purpose. Postoperatively, the patient's condition improved. **h** The postoperative MRI scan shows a well-healed surgical wound with no sign of epidural CSF collection. However, the cisterna magna is somewhat smaller than desired

In patients with an associated hydrocephalus, the function of the ventriculoperitoneal shunt should be checked before a second operation at the foramen magnum is considered. Once hydrocephalus has been ruled out and CSF flow obstruction at the foramen magnum has been demonstrated, the strategy of treatment becomes obvious: revision at the foramen magnum with the objective to improve CSF circulation. However, revision surgery with significant arachnoid pathology at this level is certainly more hazardous than the routine of a first decompression. Shunting of the syrinx may be considered to be a less risky option.

However, our experience suggests that syrinx-shunting procedures do not produce any benefit in these patients – similar to our findings for patients with CMI in whom syrinx shunting was performed as the initial surgical procedure [131].

The major problem of preoperative evaluation is the judgement of the severity of arachnoiditis. The more extensive and dense the arachnoid pathology, the lesser the probability that another operation will produce a lasting benefit and the higher the risk of surgery [160]. Unless there is a history of meningitis or a clear description of severe arachnoid changes in the operation notes, it is almost impossible to foresee exactly what will be discovered after opening of the dura. Thus, it is difficult to judge the prognosis for a patient before revision surgery. This needs to be discussed with the patient. Reexploration of the foramen magnum is, to some degree, a diagnostic procedure to find out why the first operation did not provide the desired result. Depending on the intraoperative findings, a surgical strategy has to be adopted which improves CSF flow but minimizes the risk of postoperative arachnoid scarring, which may again lead to CSF flow obstruction and prevent long-term benefit.

Figures 3.37–3.39 provide examples of secondary foramen magnum decompressions. The dura is dissected free after reopening of the midline incision and detachment of the neck muscles from the remaining occipital bone, epidural scar, and the arch of C2. This requires some further bony removal in some instances to identify the dural layer. The epidural scar is dissected off the dura and the dura patch. The dura is then incised under the microscope. It is advisable to avoid the old suture line for incision as that area tends to be the most adherent to underlying meningeal and nervous tissue. In most instances, we incise the dura in a Y-shape with the suboccipital dura incisions placed a little more laterally or medially than the previous one (Figs. 3.38, 3.39). Alternatively, the dura-patch may be incised in the midline (Fig. 3.37). The spinal dura is incised first in the area immediately below the cerebellar tonsils. Dura retention sutures are applied next. If an autologous dura graft was inserted the graft may be densely adherent to the underlying cerebellar cortex, even with vascular supply from the pia mater. If this is the case, we do not attempt to dissect the graft off the underlying tissue but circumcise the adherent part, leaving it on the cerebellar cortex.

First, the arachnoid is opened sharply and resected in the midline to ensure free passage of CSF toward the spinal canal. Once this is achieved, the tonsils are identified and spread apart in the midline with two microdissectors. This usually requires some further arachnoid dissection in the midline toward the foramen of Magendie. The PICA on both sides is identified and the foramen of Magendie inspected. If obstructed,

Table 3.10. Overview of patients with secondary foramen magnum decompressions

	Overall history (months)	Interval (months)	Syrinx drainage	Grade of scarring	Cause	Outcome
No. 1	68	12	–	2	Fascia dura graft adherent to tonsils and brainstem	Impr.
No. 2	240	4	–	2	Pseudomeningocele, graft adherent to tonsils and brainstem	Impr.
No. 3	18	12	–	2	Generalized arachnoiditis, hydrocephalus	Worse
No. 4	11	8	–	2	Generalized arachnoiditis, hydrocephalus	Impr.
No. 5	36	20	Two syringoperitoneal shunts	2	Generalized arachnoiditis, hydrocephalus	Impr.
No. 6	72	62	–	2	No duraplasty at first surgery, brainstem compression	Impr.
No. 7	144	96	Syringosubarachnoid shunt	2	Obex plugging, generalized arachnoiditis, hydrocephalus	Rec.
No. 7	204	60	Syringosubarachnoid shunt	2	Obex plugging, generalized arachnoiditis, hydrocephalus	Impr.
No. 8	65	60	Syringoperitoneal + syringosubarachnoid shunts	1	Obex plugging	Impr.
No. 9	60	48	–	2	Pseudomeningocele, graft adherent to tonsils and brainstem	Impr.
No. 10	32	15	–	1	Arachnoid not opened at first surgery, pseudomeningocele, graft adherent to tonsils and brainstem	Impr.
No. 11	96	1	–	1	Arachnoiditis, arachnoid not opened at first surgery	Impr.
No. 12	36	11	–	2	Pseudomeningocele, graft adherent to tonsils and brainstem	Impr.
No. 13	99	75	–	2	Fascia dura graft adherent to tonsils	Stable
No. 14	129	33	–	2	Generalized arachnoiditis, hydrocephalus	Stable
No. 15	6	5	–	1	Large craniectomy at first surgery, tonsils adherent to graft, brainstem compression	Impr.
No. 16	144	39	–	2	Pseudomeningocele, graft adherent to tonsils and brainstem	Impr.
No. 17	141	121	–	2	Arachnoiditis, graft adherent to tonsils and brainstem	Impr.
No. 18	96	72	Syringosubarachnoid shunt	2	Arachnoiditis, graft adherent to tonsils and brainstem	Stable
No. 19	29	24	–	2	Arachnoiditis, no duraplasty at first surgery, dura adherent to brainstem	Impr.
No. 20	84	32	Syringoperitoneal shunt	2	Arachnoiditis, graft adherent to tonsils and brainstem	Impr.

Interval, interval between foramen magnum decompressions; Impr., improved; Rec., clinical recurrence

Table 3.11. Preoperative and postoperative clinical symptoms after primary and secondary foramen magnum decompression for Chiari I malformation

Group	Preop.	Postop.	3 months	6 months	P
Sensory deficits					
Primary	3.6±1.0	3.8±1.0	3.9±1.0	3.9±1.0	
Secondary	2.9±1.1	2.9±1.1	2.9±1.1	2.9±1.1	<0.001
Dysesthesias					
Primary	4.0±1.0	4.3±0.8	4.4±0.8	4.4±0.8	
Secondary	4.0±0.9	4.0±0.9	4.1±0.8	4.0±1.0	n.s.
Pain					
Primary	3.6±1.0	4.1±0.7	4.4±0.7	4.4±0.7	
Secondary	4.4±0.5	4.3±0.5	4.6±0.5	4.6±0.5	n.s.
Motor power					
Primary	4.3±0.9	4.4±0.8	4.5±0.8	4.5±0.8	
Secondary	2.9±1.4	2.9±1.4	3.0±1.3	3.0±1.3	<0.001
Gait ataxia					
Primary	3.9±1.0	4.0±1.1	4.2±1.1	4.3±1.0	
Secondary	2.7±1.2	2.7±1.2	2.8±1.2	2.8±1.2	<0.001
Bladder function					
Primary	4.6±0.9	4.6±0.9	4.7±0.8	4.7±0.8	
Secondary	3.6±1.9	3.9±1.4	3.9±1.4	3.9±1.4	<0.05
Bowel function					
Primary	4.7±0.8	4.8±0.7	4.8±0.7	4.8±0.7	
Secondary	4.0±1.4	3.8±1.4	3.9±1.4	3.9±1.4	<0.001
Swallowing function					
Primary	4.5±0.8	4.7±0.6	4.7±0.6	4.7±0.6	
Secondary	4.6±0.7	4.6±0.7	4.6±0.7	4.6±0.7	n.s.
Karnofsky score					
Primary	73±14	75±14	78±14	79±15	
Secondary	59±18	60±19	62±18	62±18	<0.001

Preop., preoperative; Postop., postoperative; P P-value for comparison of preoperative and postoperative status after 1 year; n.s., not significant

the foramen is opened. In order to gain a good overview of the foramen of Magendie and to ensure good outflow from the fourth ventricle, the size of the tonsils may be reduced by bipolar coagulation or subpial suction [28, 29, 100]. Concluding the intradural part of the surgery, the pathway toward the cerebellopontine cisterns is inspected. However, dense adhesions lateral to the brainstem are not dissected, as this would carry considerable risk of injury to perforating vessels or caudal cranial nerves which may be very difficult to identify and preserve. Blunt dissection of

arachnoid adhesions should be avoided for the same reason [132, 160]. After providing a free CSF pathway from the fourth ventricle and the cerebellopontine cisterns toward the spinal canal, a cisterna magna is created with a spacious dura graft. To minimize the risk of postoperative adhesion of the graft (Fig. 3.39), we avoid autologous material and use either Gore-Tex (Gore and Associates GmbH, Putzbrunn, Germany) (Fig. 3.37) or a Neuropatch (Braun Melsungen, Germany). Finally, great care is taken to get a good soft tissue closure, which is mandatory to avoid postoperative CSF leaks. With extensive soft tissue scarring from the first operation, this may be difficult to achieve in some patients. If this is the case, a lumbar drain is inserted for a few days.

Obstruction of CSF pathways could be found in every patient undergoing revision surgery at the foramen magnum. In each case, this obstruction was directly caused or accompanied by arachnoid scarring, either between dura graft and cerebellum and brainstem or arachnoiditis at the foramen of Magendie. Arachnoiditis at the foramen of Magendie was encountered after obex plugging with muscle, whereas adherence of the dura graft to underlying tissue with resulting obstruction of CSF flow at the cisterna magna was due to pseudomeningocele formation pushing the dura graft anteriorly, an oversized craniectomy with cerebellar herniation, autologous graft material, or insufficient arachnoid dissection at the first operation (Table 3.9).

When comparing complication rates for first and secondary foramen magnum procedures, we found almost identical values, i.e., 29% and 30% for the secondary and primary group, respectively. In the group of secondary operations, the rate for CSF fistulas was higher due to significant soft tissue scarring from the previous operation.

Of 80% of patients with syringomyelia, 73% demonstrated a decrease in syrinx size postoperatively, while the remainder of patients showed no postoperative change in the appearance of syringomyelia. Fourteen patients demonstrated some sustained postoperative clinical improvement while three patients stabilized their course after the second surgery at the foramen magnum. Two patients deteriorated postoperatively, of whom one was revised again at the foramen magnum and demonstrated some improvement of hand function after this third foramen magnum operation. The other patient declined any further operation.

Table 3.11 gives an overview of postoperative outcomes for each clinical symptom and the related Karnofsky score. Even though both primary and secondary operations at the foramen magnum led to postoperative improvements for the majority of patients, this effect was significantly reduced in the secondary group, because these patients had significantly worse neurological deficits preoperatively and postoperative improvements were less pronounced than in the group for primary surgeries. For symptoms such as pain, dysesthesias, and swallowing problems, preoperative symptoms and postoperative outcomes were similar.

Even though clinical improvements were reported by most patients after revision surgery, they tended to be marginal and of little functional significance. Similar experiences have been made for patients with severe foramen magnum arachnoiditis of other causes [2]. The realistic outlook for patients undergoing a second foramen magnum procedure is clinical stabilization of the previously progressive course. Three major reasons may account for this outcome. First, the overall history is longer than in patients undergoing a first operation. The disease process is further advanced, as indicated by more severe motor deficits and a reduced Karnofsky score [39, 147]. Second, the more severe arachnoid pathology in this patient group may prohibit a better postoperative result [2]. In spinal arachnoid scarring and syringomyelia, the postoperative outcome correlated directly to the extent and severity of arachnoid scarring [132]. A similar effect can also be expected for the foramen magnum. Third, postoperative clinical improvements for patients with CMI and CMII are predominantly observed for symptoms of brainstem compression [38, 131, 250, 267], which no longer poses a problem in the majority of patients requiring a second intervention.

3.1.7
Conclusions for Patients with Chiari Malformations

Patients with neurological symptoms attributable to CMI or CMII should undergo decompression once hydrocephalus has been ruled out or treated. Arachnoid adhesions are common in patients with CMI or CMII and contribute to the severity of preoperative neurological symptoms. Without opening and dissection of the arachnoid during foramen magnum decompression, it may not be possible to assess the adequacy of CSF flow in this region to ensure a good long-term result. We recommend opening of the arachnoid during foramen magnum procedures in every patient, to inspect and if necessary to open the foramen of Magendie, and to ensure a free CSF pathway by placing an artificial dura graft. Provided no arachnoid dissection lateral of the brainstem is performed and tonsillar coagulation is limited to gain access to the foramen of Magendie, this policy is not associated with higher complication or surgical morbidity rates but with lower clinical recurrence rates, if compared with patients in whom the arachnoid was left intact.

In patients with CMI or CMII and neurological deterioration after foramen magnum decompression should be evaluated for evidence of CSF flow obstruction at the foramen magnum. If clinical symptoms progress, reexploration at the foramen magnum should be recommended. In patients with cerebellar ptosis, a recent report has mentioned favorable results with reconstructive cranioplasty [109]. In patients with adequate decompression, revision surgery should primarily aim to establish free CSF pathways between the fourth ventricle, cerebellopontine cisterns, and spinal canal with careful sharp arachnoid dissection and creation of a cisterna magna by a spacious dura graft. Stabilization of the clinical course is the realistic postoperative perspective for these patients. Syrinx-shunting procedures are not indicated.

References

1. Abe T, Tashibu K, Onoue H, Watanabe R, Nakamura N (1992) [The pattern of neurological deterioration and the mechanism of neurological deficit in syringomyelia.] Rinsho Shinkeigaku 32:979–983
2. Abe T, Okudo Y, Nagashima H, Isojima A, Tani S (1995) [Surgical treatment of syringomyelia.] Rinsho Shinkeigaku 35:1406–1408
3. Aboulezz AO, Sartor K, Geyer CA, Gado MH (1985) Position of cerebellar tonsils in the normal population and in patients with Chiari malformation: a quantitative approach with MR imaging. J Comput Assist Tomogr 9:1033–1036
4. Aboulker J (1979) La syringomyélie et les liquides intra-rachidiens. Neurochirurgie 25 [Suppl 1]:1–144
5. Aghakhani N, Parker F, Tadie M (1999) [Syringomyelia and Chiari abnormality in the adult. Analysis of the results of a cooperative series of 285 cases.] Neurochirurgie 45 [Suppl 1]:23–36
6. Alegre S, Garcia-Rubira JC, Patrignani G (1994) Cardiac arrest in 31-year-old man because of the Arnold-Chiari malformation. Int J Cardiol 46:286–288
7. Alvarez D, Requena I, Arias M, Valdes L, Pereiro I, De la Torre R (1995) Acute respiratory failure as the first sign of Arnold-Chiari malformation associated with syringomyelia. Eur Respir J 8:661–663
8. Alvisi C, Cerisoli M (1984) Long-term results of the surgical treatment of syringohydromyelia. Acta Neurochir (Wien) 71:133–140
9. Aminoff MJ, Wilcox CS (1972) Autonomic dysfunction in syringomyelia. Postgrad Med J 48:113–115
10. Anderson NE, Willoughby EW, Wrightson P (1985) The natural history and the influence of surgical treatment in syringomyelia. Acta Neurol Scand 71:472–479
11. Anderson NE, Willoughby EW, Wrightson P (1986) The natural history of syringomyelia. Clin Exp Neurol 22:71–80
12. Aoki N, Oikawa A, Sakai T (1995) Spontaneous regeneration of the foramen magnum after decompressive suboccipital craniectomy in Chiari malformation: case report. Neurosurgery 37:340–342
13. Arai S, Ohtsuka Y, Moriya H, Kitahara H, Minami S (1993) Scoliosis associated with syringomyelia. Spine 18:1591–1592
14. Arcaya J, Cacho J, DelCampo F, Grande J, Maillo A (1993) Arnold-Chiari malformation associated with sleep apnea and central dysregulation of arterial pressure. Acta Neurol Scand 88:224–226
15. Armonda RA, Citrin CM, Foley KT, Ellenbogen RG (1994) Quantitative cine-mode magnetic resonance imaging of Chiari I malformations: an analysis of cerebrospinal fluid dynamics. Neurosurgery 35:214–224
16. Aronson DD, Kahn RH, Canady A, Bollinger RO, Towbin R (1991) Instability of the cervical spine after decompression in patients who have Arnold-Chiari malformation. J Bone Joint Surg Am 73:898–906
17. Aubin ML, Baleriaux D, Cosnard G, Crouzet G, Doyon D, Halimi P, Manelfe C (1987) MRI in syringomyelia of congenital, infectious, traumatic or idiopathic origin. A study of 142 cases. J Neuroradiol 14:313–336
18. Avellino AM, Kim DK, Weinberger E, Roberts TS (1996) Resolution of spinal syringes and Chiari malformation in a child. Case illustration. J Neurosurg 84:708
19. Avellino AM, Britz GW, McDowell JR, Shaw DW, Ellenbogen RG, Roberts TS (1999) Spontaneous resolution of a cervicothoracic syrinx in a child. Case report and review of the literature. Pediatr Neurosurg 30:43–46
20. Azimullah PC, Smit LMF, Rietveld-Knol E, Valk J (1991) Malformations of the spinal cord in 53 patients with spina bifida studied by magnetic resonance imaging. Child's Nerv Syst 7:63–66
21. Babcook CJ, Goldstein RB, Barth RA, Damato NM, Callen PW, Filly RA (1994) Prevalence of ventriculomegaly in association with myelomeningocele: correlation with gestational age and severity of posterior fossa deformity. Radiology 190:703–707
22. Badie B, Mendoza D, Batzdorf U (1995) Posterior fossa volume and response to suboccipital decompression in patients with Chiari I malformation. Neurosurgery 37:214–218
23. Ballantine HT Jr, Ojemann RG, Drew JH (1971) Syringohydromyelia. Prog Neurol Surg 4:227–245
24. Banerji NK, Millar JHD (1974) Chiari malformation presenting in adult life: its relationship to syringomyelia. Brain 97:157–168
25. Bannister CM, Russell SA, Rimmer S (1998) Pre-natal brain development of fetuses with a myelomeningocele. Eur J Pediatr Surg 8 [Suppl 1]:15–17
26. Barbaro NM, Wilson CB, Gutin PH, Edwards MSB (1984) Surgical treatment of syringomyelia. J Neurosurg 61:531–538
27. Barkovich AJ, Sherman JL, Citrin CM, Wippold FJ II (1987) MR of postoperative syringomyelia. AJNR Am J Neuroradiol 8:319–327
28. Batzdorf U (1991) Syringomyelia related to abnormalities at the level of the craniocervical junction. In: Batzdorf U (ed) Syringomyelia. Current concepts in diagnosis and treatment. Williams and Wilkins, Baltimore, pp 163–182
29. Batzdorf U (1993) Chiari malformation and syringomyelia. In: Apuzzo M (ed) Brain surgery, Williams and Wilkins, Baltimore, pp 1985–2001
30. Batzdorf U, Klekamp J, Johnson JP (1998) A critical appraisal of syrinx cavity shunting procedures. J Neurosurg 89:382–388
31. Bell WO, Charney EB, Bruce DA, Sutton LN, Schut L (1987) Symptomatic Arnold-Chiari malformation: review of experience with 22 cases. J Neurosurg 66:812–816
32. Beric A, Dimitrijevic MR, Lindblom U (1988) Central dysesthesia syndrome in spinal cord injury patients. Pain 34:109–116
33. Bertalanffy H, Eggert HR (1990) Microsurgical treatment of syringomyelia: intraoperative findings and results. Adv Neurosurg 16:137–140
34. Bertrand SL, Drvaric DM, Roberts JM (1989) Scoliosis in syringomyelia. Orthopedics 12:335–337
35. Beuls EAM, Vandersteen MAM, Vanormelingen LM, Adriaensens PJ, Freling G, Herpers MJHM, Gelan JM (1996) Deformation of the cervicomedullary junction and spinal cord in surgically treated adult Chiari I hindbrain hernia associated with syringomyelia: a magnetic resonance microscopic and neuropathological study. Case report. J Neurosurg 85:701–708
36. Bhadelia RA, Bogdan AR, Wolpert SM, Lev S, Appigna-

ni BA, Heilman CB (1995) Cerebrospinal fluid flow waveforms: analysis in patients with Chiari I malformation by means of gated phase-contrast MR imaging velocity measurements. Radiology 196:195–202

37. Bidzinski J (1988) Late results of the surgical treatment of syringomyelia. Acta Neurochir (Wien) [Suppl 43]:29–31

38. Bindal AK, Dunsker SB, Tew JM (1995) Chiari I malformation: classification and management. Neurosurgery 37:1069–1074

39. Boiardi A, Munari L, Silvani A, Porta E, Scuratti A, Lodrini S (1991) Natural history and postsurgical outcome of syringomyelia. Ital J Neurol Sci 12:575–579

40. Bokinsky GE, Hudson LD, Weil JV (1973) Impaired peripheral chemosensitivity and acute respiratory failure in Arnold-Chiari malformation and syringomyelia. N Engl J Med 288:947–948

41. Brugieres P, Iffenecker C, Hurth M, Parker F, Fuerxer F, Idy-Peretti I, Bittoun J (1999) [Dynamic MRI in the evaluation of syringomyelic cysts.] Neurochirurgie 45 [Suppl 1]:115–129

42. Brugieres P, Idy-Peretti I, Iffenecker C, Parker F, Jolivet O, Hurth M, Gaston A, Boutton J (2000) CSF flow measurement in syringomyelia. AJNR Am J Neuroradiol 21:1785–1792

43. Bullock R, Todd NV, Easton J, Hadley D (1988) Isolated central respiratory failure due to syringomyelia and Arnold-Chiari malformation. BMJ 297:1448–1449

44. Cai C, Oakes WJ (1997) Hindbrain herniation syndromes: the Chiari malformations (I and II). Semin Pediatr Neurol 4:179–191

45. Cahan LD, Bentson JR (1982) Considerations in the diagnosis and treatment of syringomyelia and the Chiari malformation. J Neurosurg 57:24–31

46. Caldarelli M, Di Rocco C, Colosimo C Jr, Fariello G, Di Gennaro M (1995) Surgical treatment of late neurological deterioration in children with myelodysplasia. Acta Neurochir (Wien) 137:199–206

47. Cama A, Tortori-Donati P, Piatelli GL, Fondelli MP, Andreussi L (1995) Chiari complex in children – neuroradiological diagnosis, neurosurgical treatment and proposal of a new classification (312 cases). Eur J Pediatr Surg 5 [Suppl 1]:35–38

48. Caraceni TA, Celano J, Borghi P (1978) Evaluation of the results obtained from the surgical treatment of patients affected by syringomyelia associated with Chiari type I malformation. Acta Neurochir (Wien) 44:257

49. Carmel PW (1983) Management of the Chiari malformation in childhood. Clin Neurosurg 30:385–406

50. Casey AT, Hayward RD, Harkness WF, Crockard HA (1995) The use of autologous skull bone grafts for posterior fusion of the upper cervical spine in children. Spine 20:2217–2220

51. Castillo M, Wilson JD (1995) Spontaneous resolution of a Chiari malformation: MR demonstration. AJNR Am J Neuroradiol 16:1158–1160

52. Charney EB, Rorke LB, Sutton LN, Schut L (1987) Management of Chiari II complications in infants with myelomeningocele. J Pediatr 111:364–371

53. Charry O, Koop S, Winter R, Lonstein J, Denis F, Bailey W (1994) Syringomyelia and scoliosis: a review of twenty-five pediatric patients. J Pediatr Orthop 14:309–317

54. Chiari H (1891) Veränderungen des Kleinhirns infolge von Hydrocephalie des Grosshirns. Dtsch Med Wochenschr 17:1172–1175

55. Chiari H (1896) Über Veränderungen des Kleinhirns, des Pons und der Medulla oblongata infolge von congenitaler Hydrocephalie des Grosshirns. Denkschr Akad Wiss Wien 63:71–116

56. Chopra JS, Sawhney IMS, Kak VK, Khosla VK (1988) Craniovertebral anomalies: a study of 82 cases. Br J Neurosurg 2:455–464

57. Chumas PD, Armstrong DC, Drake JM, Kulkarni AV, Hoffman HJ, Humphreys RP, Rutka JT, Hendrick EB (1993) Tonsillar herniation: the rule rather than the exception after lumboperitoneal shunting in the pediatric population. J Neurosurg 78:568–573

58. Cinalli G, Renier D, Sebag G, Sainte-Rose C, Arnaud E, Pierre-Kahn A (1995) Chronic tonsillar herniation in Crouzon's and Apert's syndrome: the role of premature synostosis of the lambdoid suture. J Neurosurg 83:575–582

59. Cleland J (1883) Contribution to the study of spina bifida, encephalocele, and anencephalus. J Anat Physiol 17:257–291

60. Cochrane DD, Adderley R, White CP, Norman M, Steinbok P (1990) Apnea in patients with myelomeningocele. Pediatr Neurosurg 16:232–239

61. Cristante L, Westphal M, Herrmann HD (1994) Cranio-cervical decompression for Chiari I malformation. A retrospective evaluation of functional outcome with particular attention to motor deficits. Acta Neurochir (Wien) 130:94–100

62. Curnes JT, Oakes WJ, Boyko OB (1989) MR imaging of hindbrain deformity in Chiari II patients with and without symptoms of brian stem compression. AJNR Am J Neuroradiol 10:293–302

63. Da Silva JAG (1993) Basilar impression and Arnold-Chiari malformation. Surgical findings in 209 cases. Neurochirurgia 35:189–195

64. Da Silva JAG, De Farias Brito JC, Da Nobrega PV (1992) Autonomic nervous system disorders in 230 cases of basilar impression and Arnold-Chiari deformity. Neurochirurgia 35:183–188

65. David P, Tadie M (1999) [Treatment of syringomyelia.] Neurochirurgie 45 [Suppl 1]:130–137

66. De Barros MC, Farias W, Atiade L, Lins S (1968) Basilar impression and Arnold-Chiari malformation. A study of 66 cases. J Neurol Neurosurg Psychiatry 31:596–605

67. Dickman CA, Locantro J, Fessler RG (1992) The influence of transoral odontoid resection on stability of the craniovertebral junction. J Neurosurg 77:525–530

68. Di Lorenzo N (1992) Craniocervical junction malformation treated by transoral approach. A survey of 25 cases with emphasis on postoperative instability and outcome. Acta Neurochir (Wien) 118:112–116

69. Di Lorenzo N, Palma L, Palatinsky E, Fortuna A (1995) "Conservative" cranio-cervical decompression in the treatment of syringomyelia-Chiari I complex. A prospective study of 20 adult cases. Spine 20:2479–2483

70. Du Boulay G, Shah SH, Currie JC, Logue V (1974) The mechanism of hydromyelia in Chiari type I malformations. Br J Radiol 47:579–587

71. Du Boulay GH, O'Connell JEA, Cume J, Bostik T, Ver-

ity P (1972) Further investigations on pulsatile movements of the cerebrospinal fluid pathways. Acta Radiol 13:496–523

72. Dyste GN, Menezes AH, Van Gilder JC (1989) Symptomatic Chiari malformations. An analysis of presentation, management, and long-term outcome. J Neurosurg 71:159–168

73. Edelman RR, Wedeen VJ, Davis KR, Widder D, Hahn P, Shoukimas G, Brady TJ (1986) Multiphase MR imaging: a new method for direct imaging of pulsatile CSF flow. Radiology 161:779–783

74. Eisenstat DDR, Bernstein M, Fleming JFR, Vanderlinden RG, Schutz HI (1986) Chiari malformation in adults: a review of 40 cases. Can J Neurol Sci 13:221–228

75. El Gammal T, Mark EK, Brooks BS (1988) MR imaging of Chiari II malformation. AJR Am J Roentgenol 150:163–170

76. Ellis PM, Findlay JM (1994) Craniocervical fusion with contoured Luque rod and autogeneic bone graft. Can J Surg 37:50–54

77. Elster AD, Chen MYM (1992) Chiari I malformations: clinical and radiologic reappraisal. Radiology 183:347–353

78. Ely EW, McCall WV, Haponik EF (1994) Multifactorial obstructive sleep apnea in a patient with Chiari malformation. J Neurol Sci 126:232–236

79. Enzmann DR, Pelc NJ (1991) Normal flow patterns with phase-contrast cine MRI imaging. Radiology 178:467–474

80. Enzmann DR, O'Donehue J, Rubin JB, Shuer L, Cogen P, Silverberg G (1987) CSF pulsations within nonneoplastic spinal cord cysts. AJR Am J Roentgenol 149:149–157

81. Erbengi A, Öge HK (1994) Congenital malformations of the craniovertebral junction: classification and surgical treatment. Acta Neurochir (Wien) 127:180–185

82. Farley FA, Song KM, Birch JG, Browne R (1995) Syringomyelia and scoliosis in children. J Pediatr Orthop 15:187–192

83. Faulhauer K, Loew K (1978) The surgical treatment of syringomyelia. Long-term results. Acta Neurochir (Wien) 44:215–222

84. Feinberg DA, Mark AS (1987) Human brain motion and cerebrospinal fluid circulation demonstrated with MR velocity imaging. Radiology 163:793–799

85. Filizzolo F, Versari P, D'Aliberti G, Arena O, Scotti G, Mariani C (1988) Foramen magnum decompression versus terminal ventriculostomy for treatment of syringomyelia. Acta Neurochir (Wien) 93:96–99

86. Forcadas I, Hurtado P, Madoz P, Zarranz JJ (1988) [Somatosensory evoked potentials in syringomyelia and in Arnold-Chiari anomaly. Clinical and imaging correlations.] Neurologia 3:172–175

87. Freckmann N, Westphal M, Winkler D, Valdueza JM, Herrmann HD (1993) Neurosurgical management of the syringohydromyelia-complex. Acta Neurochir (Wien) 123:201–203

88. Fukushima T, Matsuda T, Tsuchinochi H, Yamamoto M, Tsuga H, Tomonaga M, Mitsudome A, Utsunomiya H, Asakawa K (1994) Symptomatic Chiari malformation and associated pathophysiology in pediatric and adult patients without myelodysplasia. Neurol Med Chir (Tokyo) 34:738–743

89. Gambardella G, Caruso G, Caffo M, Germano A, La Rosa G, Tomasello F (1998) Transverse microincisions of the outer layer of the dura mater combined with foramen magnum decompression as treatment for syringomyelia with Chiari I malformation. Acta Neurochir (Wien) 140:134–139

90. Garcia-Uria J, Leunda G, Carrillo R, Bravo G (1981) Syringomyelia: long-term results after posterior fossa decompression. J Neurosurg 54:380–383

91. Gardner WJ (1965) Hydrodynamic mechanism of syringomyelia: its relationship to myelocele. J Neurol Neurosurg Psychiatry 28:247–259

92. Girard N, Lasjaunias P, Taylor W (1994) Reversible tonsillar prolapse in vein of Galen aneurysmal malformations: report of eight cases and pathophysiological hypothesis. Child's Nerv Syst 10:141–147

93. Goel A, Desai K (2000) Surgery for syringomyelia: an analysis based on 163 surgical cases. Acta Neurochir (Wien) 142:293–301; discussion 301–302

94. Goel A, Bhatjiwale M, Desai K (1998) Basilar invagination: a study based on 190 surgically treated patients. J Neurosurg 88:962–968

95. Grant R, Hadley DM, Lang D, Condon B, Johnston R, Bone I, Teasdale GM (1987) MRI measurement of syrinx size before and after operation. J Neurol Neurosurg Psychiatry 50:1685–1687

96. Greitz D (1993) Cerebrospinal fluid circulation and associated intracranial dynamics. A radiologic investigation using MR imaging and radionuclide cisternography. Acta Radiol Suppl 386:1–23

97. Greitz D, Franck A, Nordell B (1993) On the pulsatile nature of intracranial and spinal CSF-circulation demonstrated by MR imaging. Acta Radiol 34:321–328

98. Gunberg DL (1956) Spina bifida and Arnold-Chiari malformation in the progeny of trypan blue injected rats. Anat Rec 126:343–367

99. Guyotat J, Bret P, Jouanneau E, Ricci AC, Lapras C (1998) Syringomyelia associated with type I Chiari malformation. A 21-year retrospective study on 75 cases treated by foramen magnum decompression with a special emphasis on the value of tonsils resection. Acta Neurochir (Wien) 140:745–754

100. Halamandaris GG, Batzdorf U (1989) Adult Chiari malformation. Contemp Neurosurg 11:1–6

101. Hankinson J (1978) The surgical treatment of syringomyelia. In: Krayenbuehl H (ed) Advances and technical standards in neurosurgery, vol 5. Springer, New York Berlin Heidelberg, pp 127–151

102. Haponik EF, Givens D, Angelo J (1983) Syringobulbiamyelia with obstructive sleep apnea. Neurology 33:1046–1049

103. Heidecke V, Rainov NG, Burkert W (1998) Occipitocervical fusion with the cervical Cotrel-Dubousset rod system. Acta Neurochir (Wien) 140:969–976

104. Hertel G, Kramer S, Placzek E (1973) Die Syringomyelie. Klinische Verlaufsbeobachtungen bei 323 Patienten. Nervenarzt 44:1–13

105. Hida K, Iwasaki Y, Imamura H, Abe H (1994) Birth injury as a causative factor of syringomyelia with Chiari type I deformity. J Neurol Neurosurg Psychiatry 57:373–374

106. Hida K, Iwasaki Y, Koyanagi I, Sawamura Y, Abe H (1995) Surgical indication and results of foramen magnum decompression versus syringosubarachnoid

shunting for syringomyelia associated with Chiari I malformation. Neurosurgery 37:673–679

107. Hofmann E, Warmuth-Metz M, Bendszus M, Solymosi L (2000) Phase-contrast MR imaging of the cervical CSF and spinal cord: volumetric motion analysis in patients with Chiari I malformation. AJNR Am J Neuroradiol 21:151–158

108. Holliday PO, Pillsbury D, Kelly DL Jr, Dillard R (1985) Brain stem auditory evoked potentials in Arnold-Chiari malformation: possible prognostic value and changes with surgical decompression. Neurosurgery 16:48–53

109. Holly LT, Batzdorf U (2001) Management of cerebellar ptosis following craniovertebral decompression for Chiari I malformation. J Neurosurg 94:21–96

110. Holschneider AM, Bliesener JA, Abel M (1990) [Brain stem dysfunction in Arnold-Chiari II syndrome.] Z Kinderchir 45:67–71

111. Hort-Legrand C, Emery E (1999) [Evoked motor and sensory potentials in syringomyelia.] Neurochirurgie 45 [Suppl 1]:95–104

112. Hudgins RJ, Boydston WR (1995) Bone regrowth and recurrence of symptoms following decompression in the infant with Chiari II malformation [see comments]. Pediatr Neurosurg 23:323–327

113. Huebert HT, MacKinnon WB (1969) Syringomyelia and scoliosis. J Bone Joint Surg Br 51:338–343

114. Hurth M, Parker F (1999) Histoire, controverses et pathogénie. Neurochirurgie 45 [Suppl 1]:138–157

115. Ishak BA, McLone D, Seleny FL (1980) Intraoperative autonomic dysfunction associated with Arnold-Chiari malformation. Child's Brain 7:146–149

116. Isu T, Sasaki H, Takamura H, Kobayashi N (1993) Foramen magnum decompression with removal of the outer layer of the dura as treatment for syringomyelia occurring with Chiari I malformation. Neurosurgery 33:844–849; discussion 849–850

117. Itabashi T (1990) Quantitative analysis of cervical CSF and syrinx fluid pulsations. Nippon Seikeigeka Gakkai Zasshi 64:523–533

118. Iwasaki Y, Hida K, Koyanagi I, Kuroda S, Abe H (1995) [Surgical treatment for syringomyelia associated with Chiari malformation.] Rinsho Shinkeigaku 35:1409–1411

119. Iwasaki Y, Hida K, Koyanagi I, Abe H (2000) Re-evaluation of syringosubarachnoid shunt for syringomyelia with Chiari malformation. Neurosurgery 46:407–412

120. Jabbari B, Geyer C, Gunderson C, Chu A, Brophy J, McBurney JW, Jonas B (1990) Somatosensory evoked potentials and magnetic resonance imaging in syringomyelia. Electroencephalogr Clin Neurophysiol 77:277–285

121. Jack CR Jr, Kokmen E, Onofrio BM (1991) Spontaneous decompression of syringomyelia: magnetic resonance imaging findings. J Neurosurg 74:283–286

122. Jacob RP, Rhoton AL Jr (1997) The Chiari I malformation. In: Anson JA, Benzel EC, Awad IA (eds) Syringomyelia and the Chiari malformations. American Association of Neurological Surgeons, Park Ridge, pp 57–67

123. James D, Crockard HA (1991) Surgical access to the base of skull and upper cervical spine by extended maxillotomy. Neurosurgery 29:411–416

124. James DS (1995) Significance of chronic tonsillar herniation in sudden death. Forensic Sci Int 75:217–223

125. Jones DN, Davies R, Sage MR, Hanieh A, Morris L (1992) Assimilation of the atlas with associated syringomyelia and Chiari I malformation (Klippel-Feil type 2). Australas Radiol 36:339–342

126. Keefover R, Sam M, Bodensteiner J (1995) Hypersomnolence and pure central sleep apnea associated with Chiari I malformation. J Child Neurol 10:65–67

127. Kingdom TT, Nockels RP, Kaplan MJ (1995) Transoral-transpharyngeal approach to the craniocervical junction. Otolaryngol Head Neck Surg 113:393–400

128. Kirsch WM, Duncan BR, Black FO, Stears JC (1968) Laryngeal palsy in association with myelomeningocele, hydrocephalus, and the Arnold-Chiari malformation. J Neurosurg 28:207–214

129. Klekamp J, Riedel A, Harper C, Kretschmann HJ (1989) Morphometric study on the growth of non-cortical brain regions in Australian Aborigines and Caucasians. Brain Res 485:79–88

130. Klekamp J, Samii M, Tatagiba M, Sepehrnia A (1995) Syringomyelia in association with tumours of the posterior fossa: pathophysiological considerations, based on observations on three related cases. Acta Neurochir (Wien) 137:38–43

131. Klekamp J, Batzdorf U, Samii M, Bothe HW (1996) The surgical treatment of Chiari I malformation. Acta Neurochir (Wien) 138:788–801

132. Klekamp J, Batzdorf U, Samii M, Bothe HW (1997) Treatment of syringomyelia associated with arachnoid scarring caused by arachnoiditis or trauma. J Neurosurg 86:233–240

133. Kohno K, Sakaki S, Nakamura H, Sakoh M, Takeda S, Sadamoto K (1991) Foramen magnum decompression for syringomyelia associated with basilar impression and Chiari I malformation. Report of three cases. Neurol Med Chir (Tokyo) 31:715–719

134. Kuroda S, Matsuzawa H, Iwasaki Y, Hida K, Imamura H, Abe H, Saito H (1994) [CSF dynamics in the patients with syringomyelia associated with Chiari's malformation – quantitative analysis on cine MRI.] No To Shinkei 46:59–64

135. Lee BCP, Zimmerman RD, Manning JJ, Deck MDF (1985) MR imaging of syringomyelia and hydromyelia. AJR Am J Roentgenol 144:1149–1156

136. Levy MR, Di Chiro G (1990) MR phase imaging and cerebrospinal fluid flow in the head and spine. Neuroradiology 32:399–406

137. Levy WJ, Mason L, Hahn JF (1983) Chiari malformation presenting in adults: a surgical experience in 127 cases. Neurosurgery 12:377–390

138. Logue V (1971) Syringomyelia: a radiodiagnostic and radiotherapeutic saga. Clin Radiol 22:2–16

139. Logue V, Edwards MR (1981) Syringomyelia and its surgical treatment – an analysis of 75 patients. J Neurol Neurosurg Psychiatry 44:273–284

140. Lorenzo DN, Fortuna A, Guidetti B (1982) Craniovertebral junction malformations. Cranioradiological findings, long term results and surgical indications in 63 cases. J Neurosurg 57:603–608

141. Lu K, Lee TC (1999) Spontaneous regression of periodontoid pannus mass in psoriatic atlantoaxial subluxation. Case report. Spine 24:578–581

142. Lui TN, Lee ST (1993) Surgical treatment of type I Chiari malformation with syringomyelia in adults. Chung Hua I Hsueh Tsa Chih 51:61–67

143. Madsen JR, Scott RM (1993) Chiari malformations, syringomyelia, and intramedullary spinal cord tumors. Curr Opin Neurol Neurosurg 6:559–563

144. Magnaes B (1989) Clinical studies of cranial and spinal compliance and the craniospinal flow of cerebrospinal fluid. Br J Neurosurg 3:659–668

145. Malcolm GP, Ransford AO, Crockard HA (1994) Treatment of non-rheumatoid occipitocervical instability. Internal fixation with the Hartshill-Ransford loop. J Bone Joint Surg Br 76:357–366

146. Mampalam TJ, Andrews BT, Gelb D, Ferriero D, Pitts LH (1988) Presentation of type I Chiari malformation after head trauma. Neurosurgery 23:760–762

147. Mariani C, Cislaghi MG, Barbieri S, Filizzolo F, Di Palma F, Farina E, D'Alberti G, Scarlato G (1991) The natural history and results of surgery in 50 cases of syringomyelia. J Neurol 238:433–438

148. Marin-Padilla M, Marin-Padilla TM (1981) Morphogenesis in experimentally induced Arnold-Chiari malformation. J Neurol Sci 50:29–55

149. Mark AS, Feinberg DA, Brant-Zawadzki MN (1987) Changes in size and magnetic resonance signal intensity of the cerebral CSF spaces during the cardiac cycle as studied by gated, high-resolution magnetic resonance imaging. Invest Radiol 22:290–297

150. Masur H, Nedjat S, Elger CE, Ludolph AC (1990) SEPs and evoked muscle responses after noninvasive magnetic stimulation in patients with syringomyelia. Adv Neurosurg 18:141–148

151. Masur H, Oberwittler C, Fahrendorf G, Heyen P, Reuther G, Nedjat S, Ludolph AC, Brune GG (1992) The relation between functional deficits, motor and sensory conduction times and MRI findings in syringomyelia. Electroencephalogr Clin Neurophysiol 85:321–330

152. Masur H, Oberwittler C, Reuther G, Heyen P (1995) Cerebellar herniation in syringomyelia: relation between tonsillar herniation and the dimensions of the syrinx and the remaining spinal cord. A quantitative MRI study. Eur Neurol 35:162–167

153. Matsumoto T, Symon L (1989) Surgical management of syringomyelia – current results. Surg Neurol 32:258–265

154. Matsuzawa H, Hida K, Houkin K, Yoshinobu I, Abe H, Akino M, Saito H (1992) [Quantitative analysis of cerebrospinal fluid dynamics in syringomyelia using cine MRI with pre-saturation.] No To Shinkei 44:24–29

155. Mayr U, Aichner F, Menardi G, Hager J (1986) Computer-tomographical appearances of the Chiari malformations of the posterior fossa. Z Kinderchir 41 [Suppl 1]:33–35

156. McLone DG (1997) The Chiari II malformation of the hindbrain and the associated hydromyelia. In: Anson JA, Benzel WC, Awad IA (eds) Syringomyelia and the Chiari malformations. American Association of Neurological Surgeons, Park Ridge, pp 69–82

157. McLone DG, Knepper PA (1989) The cause of Chiari II malformation: a unified theory. Pediatr Neurosci 15:1–12

158. Meadows J, Kraut M, Guarnieri M, Haroun RI, Carson BS (2000) Asymptomatic Chiari Type I malformations identified on magnetic resonance imaging. J Neurosurg 92:920–926

159. Menezes AH (1991/1992) Chiari I malformations and hydromyelia – complications. Pediatr Neurosurg 17:146–154

160. Menezes AH (1995) Primary craniovertebral anomalies and the hindbrain herniation syndrome (Chiari I): data base analysis. Pediatr Neurosurg 23:260–269

161. Menezes AH, VanGilder JC (1988) Transoral-transpharyngeal approach to the anterior craniocervical junction. Ten-year experience with 72 patients. J Neurosurg 69:895–903

162. Menezes AH, Van Gilder JC (1990) Anomalies of the craniocervical junction. In: Youmans JR (ed) Neurological surgery. Saunders, Philadelphia, pp 1359–1420

163. Menezes AH, Van Gilder JC, Graf CJ, McDonnell DE (1980) Craniocervical abnormalities. A comprehensive surgical approach. J Neurosurg 53:444–455

164. Meuli M, Meuli-Simmen C, Yingling CD, Hutchins GM, Timmel GB, Harrison MR, Adzick NS (1996) In utero repair of experimental myelomeningocele saves neurological function at birth. J Pediatr Surg 31:397–402

165. Meuli-Simmen C, Meuli M, Hutchins GM, Harrison MR, Buncke HJ, Sullivan KM, Adzick NS (1995) Fetal reconstructive surgery: experimental use of the latissimus dorsi flap to correct myelomeningocele in utero. Plast Reconstr Surg 96:1007–1011

166. Mikulis DJ, Diaz O, Egglin TK, Sanchez R (1992) Variance of the cerebellar tonsils with age: preliminary report. Radiology 183:725–728

167. Milerad J, Lagercrantz H, Johnson P (1992) Obstructive sleep apnea in Arnold-Chiari malformation treated with acetazolamide. Acta Paediatr 81:609–612

168. Milhorat TH, Johnson WD, Miller JI, Bergland RM, Hollenberg-Sher J (1992) Surgical treatment of syringomyelia based on magnetic resonance imaging criteria. Neurosurgery 31:231–245

169. Milhorat TH, Johnson WD, Miller JI (1992) Syrinx shunt to posterior fossa cisterns (syringocisternostomy) for bypassing obstructions of upper cervical theca. J Neurosurg 77:871–874

170. Milhorat TH, Kotzen RM, Mu HTM, Capocelli AL, Milhorat RH (1996) Dysesthetic pain in patients with syringomyelia. Neurosurgery 38:940–947

171. Milhorat TH, Mu HTM, LaMotte CC, Milhorat AT (1996) Distribution of substance P in the spinal cord of patients with syringomyelia. J Neurosurg 84:992–998

172. Milhorat TH, Chou MW, Trinidad EM, Kula RW, Mandell M, Wolpert C, Speer MC (1999) Chiari I malformation redefined: clinical and radiographic findings for 364 symptomatic patients. Neurosurgery 44:1005–1017

173. Mohr PD, Strang FA, Sambrook MA, Boddie HG (1977) The clinical and surgical features in 40 patients with primary cerebellar ectopia (adult Chiari malformation). Q J Med 46:85–96

174. Mori K, Uchida Y, Nishimura T, Eghwrudjakpor P (1988) Brainstem auditory evoked potentials in Chiari II malformation. Child's Nerv Syst 4:154–157

175. Morioka T, Shono T, Nishio S, Yoshida K, Hasu o K, Fukui M (1995) Acquired Chiari I malformation and syringomyelia associated with bilateral chronic subdural hematoma. Case report. J Neurosurg 83:556–558

176. Moriwaka F, Tashiro K, Tachibana S, Yada K (1995) [Epidemiology of syringomyelia in Japan – a nationwide survey.] Rinsho Shinkeigaku 35:1395–1397

177. Muhonen MG, Menezes AH, Sawin PD, Weinstein SL (1992) Scoliosis in pediatric Chiari malformations without myelodysplasia. J Neurosurg 77:69–77

178. Mullan S, Raimondi AJ (1962) Respiratory hazards of the surgical treatment of the Arnold-Chiari malformation. J Neurosurg 19:675–678

179. Munshi I, Frim D, Stine-Reyes R, Weir BK, Hekmatpanah J, Brown F (2000) Effects of posterior fossa decompression with and without duraplasty on Chiari malformation-associated hydromyelia. Neurosurgery 46:1384–1389

180. Nagib MG (1994) An approach to symptomatic children (ages 4–14 years) with Chiari type I malformation. Pediatr Neurosurg 21:31–35

181. Newman PK, Terenty TR, Foster JB (1981) Some observations on the pathogenesis of syringomyelia. J Neurol Neurosurg Psychiatry 44:964–969

182. Nohria V, Oakes WJ (9091) Chiari I malformation: a review of 43 patients. Pediatr Neurosurg 16:222–227

183. Nomura S, Akimura T, Eguchi Y, Shiroyama Y, Ito H, Saito T (1993) Apnea associated with Chiari malformation: medullary hemorrhage revealed by MRI. Child's Nerv Syst 9:348–349

184. Nyland H, Krogness KG (1978) Size of posterior fossa in Chiari type I malformation in adults. Acta Neurochir (Wien) 40:233–242

185. Oldfield EH, Muraszko K, Shawker TH, Patronas NJ (1994) Pathophysiology of syringomyelia associated with Chiari I malformation of the cerebellar tonsils. Implications for diagnosis and treatment. J Neurosurg 80:3–15

186. Olivero WC, Dinh DH (1992) Chiari I malformation with traumatic syringomyelia and spontaneous resolution: case report and literature review. Neurosurgery 30:758–760

187. Papasozomenos S, Roessmann U (1981) Respiratory distress and Arnold-Chiari malformation. Neurology 31:97–100

188. Pare LS, Batzdorf U (1998) Syringomyelia persistence after Chiari decompression as a result of pseudomeningocele formation: implications for syrinx pathogenesis: report of three cases. Neurosurgery 43:945–948

189. Park TS, Hoffman HJ, Hendrick EB, Humphreys RP (1983) Experience with surgical decompression of the Arnold-Chiari malformation in young infants with myelomeningocele. Neurosurgery 13:147–152

190. Pascuail J, Oterino A, Berciano J (1992) Headache in type I Chiari malformation. Neurology 42:1519–1521

191. Paul KS, Lye RH, Strang FA, Dutton J (1983) Arnold-Chiari malformation. Review of 71 cases. J Neurosurg 58:183–187

192. Peerless SJ, Durward QJ (1982) Management of syringomyelia: a pathophysiological approach. Clin Neurosurg 30:531–576

193. Pierallini A, Ferone E, Colonnese C (1997) [Magnetic resonance imaging of a case of spontaneous resolution of syringomyelia associated with type I Chiari malformation.] Radiol Med (Torino) 93:621–622

194. Pillay PK, Awad IA, Little JR, Hahn JF (1991) Surgical management of syringomyelia: a five year experience in the era of magnetic resonance imaging. Neurol Res 13:3–9

195. Pillay PK, Awad IA, Little JR, Hahn JF (1991) Symptomatic Chiari malformation in adults: a new classification based on magnetic resonance imaging with clinical and prognostic significance. Neurosurgery 28:639–645

196. Piper JG, Menezes AH (1997) The relationship between syringomyelia and the Chiari malformation. In: Anson JA, Benzel EC, Awad IA (eds) Syringomyelia and the Chiari malformations. American Association of Neurological Surgeons, Park Ridge, pp 91–104

197. Pojunas K, Williams AL, Daniels DL, Haughton VM (1984) Syringomyelia and hydromyelia: magnetic resonance evaluation. Radiology 153:679–683

198. Pollack IF, Pang D, Albright AL, Krieger D (1992) Outcome following hindbrain decompression of symptomatic Chiari malformations in children previously treated with myelomeningocele closure and shunts. J Neurosurg 77:881–888

199. Pollack IF, Pang D, Kocoshis S, Putnam P (1992) Neurogenic dysphagia resulting from Chiari malformations. Neurosurgery 30:709–719

200. Pollack IF, Welch W, Jacobs GB, Janecka IP (1995) Frameless stereotactic guidance. An intraoperative adjunct in the transoral approach for ventral cervicomedullary junction decompression. Spine 20:216–220

201. Pollack IF, Kinnunen D, Albright AL (1996) The effect of early craniospinal decompression on functional outcome in neonates and young infants with myelodysplasia and symptomatic Chiari II malformations: results from a prospective series. Neurosurgery 38:703–710

202. Pravda J, Ghelman B, Levine DB (1992) Syringomyelia associated with congenital scoliosis. A case report. Spine 171:372–374

203. Pujol J, Roig C, Capdevila A, Pon A, Marti-Vilalta JL, Kulisevsky J, Escartin A, Zannoli G (1995) Motion of the cerebellar tonsils in Chiari type I malformation studied by cine phase-contrast MRI. Neurology 45:1746–1753

204. Quencer RM, Ayyar DR, Angus E, Green BA (1988) Somatosensory evoked potential measurements in percutaneous fluid aspiration from intraspinal cystic lesions. AJNR Am J Neuroradiol 9:551–555

205. Quencer RM, Post MJD, Hinks RS (1990) Cine MRI in the evaluation of normal and abnormal CSF flow: intracranial and intraspinal studies. Neuroradiology 32:371–391

206. Raftopoulos C, Sanchez A, Matos C, Baleriaux D, Bank WO, Brotchi J (1993) Hydrosyringomyelia-Chiari I complex. Prospective evaluation of a modified foramen magnum decompression procedure: preliminary results. Surg Neurol 39:163–169

207. Ransford AO, Crockard HA, Pozo JL, Thomas NP, Nelson IW (1986) Craniocervical instability treated by contoured loop fixation. J Bone Joint Surg Br 68:173–177

208. Rauzzino M, Oakes WJ (1995) Chiari II malformation and syringomyelia. Neurosurg Clin N Am 6:293–309

209. Restuccia D, Manguiere F (1991) The contribution of median nerve SEPs in the functional assessment of the cervical spinal cord in syringomyelia. Brain 114:361–379

210. Rhoton AL Jr (1976) Microsurgery of Arnold-Chiari malformation in adults with and without hydromyelia. J Neurosurg 45:473–483

211. Riedel A, Klekamp J, Harper C, Kretschmann HJ (1989) Morphometric study on the growth of the cerebellum in Australian Aborigines and Caucasians. Brain Res 499:333–343

212. Rocker GM, MacAnlay MA, Sangalang V (1995) Sudden death and Chiari malformations. Intensive Care Med 21:621

213. Ruge JR, Masciopinto J, Storrs BB, McLone DG (1992) Anatomical progression of the Chiari II malformation. Child's Nerv Syst 8:86–91

214. Saez RJ, Onofrio BM, Yanagihara T (1976) Experience with Arnold-Chiari malformation, 1960–1970. J Neurosurg 45:416–422

215. Sahuquillo J, Rubio E, Poca MA, Rovira A, Rodriguez-Baeza A, Cervera C (1994) Posterior fossa reconstruction: a surgical technique for the treatment of Chiari I malformation and Chiari I/syringomyelia complex – preliminary results and magnetic resonance imaging quantitative assessment of hindbrain migration. Neurosurgery 35:874–885

216. Sakamoto H, Nishikawa M, Hakuba A, Yasui T, Kitano S, Nakanishi N, Inoue Y (1999) Expansive suboccipital cranioplasty for the treatment of syringomyelia associated with Chiari malformation. Acta Neurochir (Wien) 141:949–960; discussion 960–961

217. Santoro A, Delfini R, Innocenzi G, Di Biasi C, Trasimeni G, Gualdi G (1993) Spontaneous drainage of syringomyelia. Report of two cases. J Neurosurg 79:132–134

218. Sathi S, Stieg PE (1993) "Acquired" Chiari I malformation after multiple lumbar punctures: case report. Neurosurgery 32:306–309

219. Sattar TS, Bannister CM, Russell SA, Rimmer S (1998) Pre-natal diagnosis of occult spinal dysraphism by ultrasonography and post-natal evaluation by MR scanning. Eur J Pediatr Surg 8 [Suppl 1]:31–33

220. Schady W, Metcalfe RA, Butler P (1987) The incidence of craniocervical bony anomalies in the adult Chiari malformation. J Neurol Sci 82:193–203

221. Schliep G, Ritter U (1971) Klinik der Syringomyelie. Fortschr Neurol Psychiatr 39:53–82

222. Schroth G (1991) Physiologie und Pathologie der intrakraniellen Liquordynamik. Jahrbuch der Radiologie, pp 287–290

223. Schroth G, Palmbach M (1988) Syringomyelie: Korrelation kernspintomographischer und klinischer Befunde vor und nach Operation. ROFO 149:587–593

224. Schroth G, Klose U (1992) Cerebrospinal fluid flow. II. Physiology of respiration-related pulsations. Neuroradiology 35:10–15

225. Selmi F, Davies KG, Weeks RD (1995) Type I Chiari deformity presenting with profound sinus bradycardia: case report and literature review. Br J Neurosurg 9:543–545

226. Sgouros S, Williams B (1995) A critical appraisal of drainage in syringomyelia. J Neurosurg 82:1–10

227. Sherman JL, Barkovich AJ, Citrin CM (1987) The MR appearance of syringomyelia: new observations. AJR Am J Roentgenol 148:381–391

228. Sjaastad O, Frederikson TA, Pfaffenrath V (1990) Cervicogenic headache: diagnostic criteria. Headache 30:725–726

229. Smith J, Ridley A (1969) Cerebellar ectopia presenting in adult life. Br Med J 1:353–355

230. Snyder WE Jr, Luerssen TG, Boaz JC, Kalsbeck JE (1998) Chiari III malformation treated with CSF diversion and delayed surgical closure. Pediatr Neurosurg 29:117–120

231. Sonntag VK, Dickman CA (1993) Craniocervical stabilization. Clin Neurosurg 40:243–272

232. Stevens JM, Serva WAD, Kendall BE, Valentine AR, Ponsford JR (1993) Chiari malformation in adults: relation of morphological aspects to clinical features and operative outcome. J Neurol Neurosurg Psychiatry 56:1072–1077

233. Stevens JM, Chong WK, Barber C, Kendall BE, Crockard HA (1994) A new appraisal of abnormalities of the odontoid process associated with atlanto-axial subluxation and neurological disability. Brain 117:133–148

234. Stovner LJ (1993) Headache asociated with Chiari type I malformation. Headache 33:175–181

235. Stovner LJ, Rinck P (1992) Syringomyelia in Chiari malformation: relation to extent of cerebellar tissue herniation. Neurosurgery 31:913–917

236. Stovner LJ, Bergan U, Nilsen G, Sjaastad O (1993) Posterior cranial fossa dimensions in the Chiari I malformation: relation to pathogenesis and clinical presentation. Neuroradiology 35:113–118

237. Sudo K, Doi S, Maruo Y, Tashiro K, Terae S, Miyasaka K, Isu T (1990) Syringomyelia with spontaneous resolution. J Neurol Neurosurg Psychiatry 53:437–438

238. Sun JCL, Steinbok P, Cochrane DD (2000) Spontaneous resolution and recurrence of a Chiari I malformation and associated syringomyelia. Case report. J Neurosurg 92:207–210

239. Sullivan LP, Stears JC, Ringel SP (1988) Resolution of syringomyelia and Chiari I malformation by ventriculoatrial shunting in a patient with pseudotumor cerebri and a lumboperitoneal shunt. Neurosurgery 22:744–747

240. Tachibana S, Iida H, Yada K (1992) Significance of positive Queckenstedt test in patients with syringomyelia associated with Arnold-Chiari malformation. J Neurosurg 76:67–71

241. Taylor MJ, Boor R, Keenan NK, Rutka JT, Drake JM (1996) Brainstem auditory and visual evoked potentials in infants with myelomeningocele. Brain Dev 18:99–104

242. Teo C, Parker EC, Aureli S, Boop FA (1997) The Chiari II malformation: a surgical series. Pediatr Neurosurg 27:223–229

243. Terae S, Miyasaka K, Abe H, Abe S, Tashiro K (1994) Increased pulsatile movement of the hindbrain in syringomyelia associated with the Chiari malformation: cine-MRI with presaturation bolus tracking. Neuroradiology 36:125–129

244. Tew B, Laurence KM (1975) The effects of hydrocephalus on intelligence, visual perception and school attainment. Dev Med Child Neurol 17 [Suppl 35]:129–134

245. Tognetti F, Calbucci F (1993) Syringomyelia: syringosubarachnoid shunt versus posterior fossa decompression. Acta Neurochir (Wien) 123:196–197

246. Tokuno H, Hakuba A, Suzuki T, Nishimura S (1988) Operative treatment of Chiari malformation with syringomyelia. Acta Neurochir Suppl (Wien) 43:22–25

247. Tomlinson RJ Jr, Wolfe MW, Nadall JM, Bennett JT, MacEwen GD (1994) Syringomyelia and developmental scoliosis. J Pediatr Orthop 14:580–585

248. Tulipan N, Hernanz-Schulman M, Bruner JP (1998) Reduced hindbrain herniation after intrauterine mye-

249. Tulipan N, Hernanz-Schulman M, Lowe LH, Bruner JP (1999) Intrauterine myelomeningocele repair reverses preexisting hindbrain herniation. Pediatr Neurosurg 31:137–142

250. Vanaclocha V, Saiz-Sapena N, Garcia-Casasola MC (1997) Surgical technique for cranio-cervical decompression in syringomyelia associated with Chiari type I malformation. Acta Neurochir (Wien) 139:529–540

251. Van Calenbergh F, Van den Bergh R (1993) Syringoperitoneal shunting: results and problems in a consecutive series. Acta Neurochir (Wien) 123:203–205

252. Van Gilder JC, Menezes AH (1985) Craniovertebral junction anomalies. In: Wilkins RH, Rengecharry SS (eds) Neurosurgery, vol 3. Williams and Wilkins, New York, pp 2097–2101

253. Van Gilder JC, Menezes AH (1988) Craniovertebral anomalies and their treatment. In: Schmidek HH, Sweet WH (eds) Operative neurosurgical techniques. Indications, methods, and results, 2nd edn. Grune and Stratton, New York, pp 1281–1293

254. Van Velthoven V, Jost M, Siekmann R, Eggert HR (1993) Surgical strategies and results in syringomyelia. Acta Neurochir (Wien) 123:199–201

255. Vandertop WP, Asai A, Hoffman HJ, Drake JM, Humphreys RP, Rutka JT, Becker LE (1992) Surgical decompression for symptomatic Chiari II malformation in neonates with myelomeningocele. J Neurosurg 77:541–544

256. Veilleux M, Stevens JC (1987) Syringomyelia: electrophysiologic aspects. Muscle Nerve 10:449–458

257. Venes JL, Black KL, Latack JT (1986) Preoperative evaluation and surgical management of the Arnold-Chiari II malformation. J Neurosurg 64:363–370

258. Ventureyra ECG, Higgins MJ (1994) Syringomyelia and the Chiari type I malformation: new pathophysiological concepts. Crit Rev Neurosurg 4:275–285

259. Versari PP, Aliberti G, Talamonti G, Collice M (1993) Foraminal syringomyelia: suggestion for a grading system. Acta Neurochir (Wien) 125:97–104

260. Vickers TH (1961) Die experimentelle Erzeugung der Arnold-Chiari Missbildung durch Trypanblau. Beitr Pathol Anat 124:295–310

261. Wagner W, Peghini-Halbig L, Maeurer JC, Hüwel NM, Perneczky A (1995) Median nerve somatosensory evoked potentials in cervical syringomyelia: correlation of preoperative versus postoperative findings with upper limb somatosensory function. Neurosurgery 36:336–345

262. Warkany J, Wilson JG, Geiger JF (1958) Myeloschisis and myelomeningocele produced experimentally in the rat. J Comp Neurol 109:35–64

263. Welch K, Shillito J, Strand R, Fischer EG, Winston KR (1981) Chiari I malformation – an aquired disorder? J Neurosurg 55:604–609

264. West RJ, Williams B (1980) Radiographic studies of the ventricles in syringomyelia. Neuroradiology 20:5–16

265. Williams B (1977) Difficult labour as a cause of communicating syringomyelia. Lancet 2:51–53

266. Williams B (1978) A critical appraisal of posterior fossa surgery for communicating syringomyelia. Brain 101:223–250

267. Williams B (1993) Surgery for hindbrain related syringomyelia. Adv Tech Stand Neurosurg 20:107–164

268. Williams B (1997) Management schemes for syringomyelia: surgical indications and nonsurgical management. In: Anson JA, Benzel EC, Awad IA (eds) Syringomyelia and the Chiari malformations. American Association of Neurological Surgeons, Park Ridge, pp 125–143

269. Wolpert SM, Bhadelia RA, Bogdan AR, Cohen AR (1994) Chiari I malformations: assessment with phase-contrast velocity MR. AJNR Am J Neuroradiol 15:1299–1308

270. Yeager BA, Lusser MA (1992) Spontaneous resolution of idiopathic syringomyelia: MR features. J Comput Assist Tomogr 16:323–324

271. Zadeh HG, Sakha SA, Powell MP, Mehta MH (1995) Absent superficial abdominal reflexes in children with scoliosis. An early indicator of syringomyelia. J Bone Joint Surg Br 77:762–767

272. Zager EL, Ojemann RG, Poletti CE (1990) Acute presentations of syringomyelia. Report of three cases. J Neurosurg 72:133–138

273. Zerah M (1999) [Syringomyelia in children.] Neurochirurgie 45 [Suppl 1]:37–57

3.2
Rhombencephalic Malformations

Under this heading we wish to describe a number of malformations that show some overlap and are not always clearly defined in the literature. They consist of pathologies that combine malformations and dysplasias of vermis, cerebellar hemispheres, the fourth ventricle, and meninges of the posterior fossa. The most common of these is the Dandy-Walker malformation (DWM) described below. Some authors distinguish the so-called Dandy-Walker variant (DWV) from DWM to describe varying degrees of dysplasia of posterior fossa elements associated with an enlarged fourth ventricle. Finally, the Chiari IV malformation (CM IV) shares similarities with the DWM. Sometimes the so-called megacisterna magna (MCM) and arachnoid cysts of the posterior fossa are also mentioned under this heading [5].

3.2.1
Dandy-Walker Malformation

DWM is characterized by a grossly enlarged fourth ventricle and varying degrees of hypoplasia of the vermis; it occurs in approximately 3% of patients with hydrocephalus [15]. The posterior fossa is enlarged due to elevation of the tentorium, with upward displacement of torcula and lateral venous sinuses (Fig. 3.40). Dandy [9, 10] and Taggert and Walker [35] considered congenital obstruction of the foramina of Luschka and Magendie obligatory for the development of the mal-

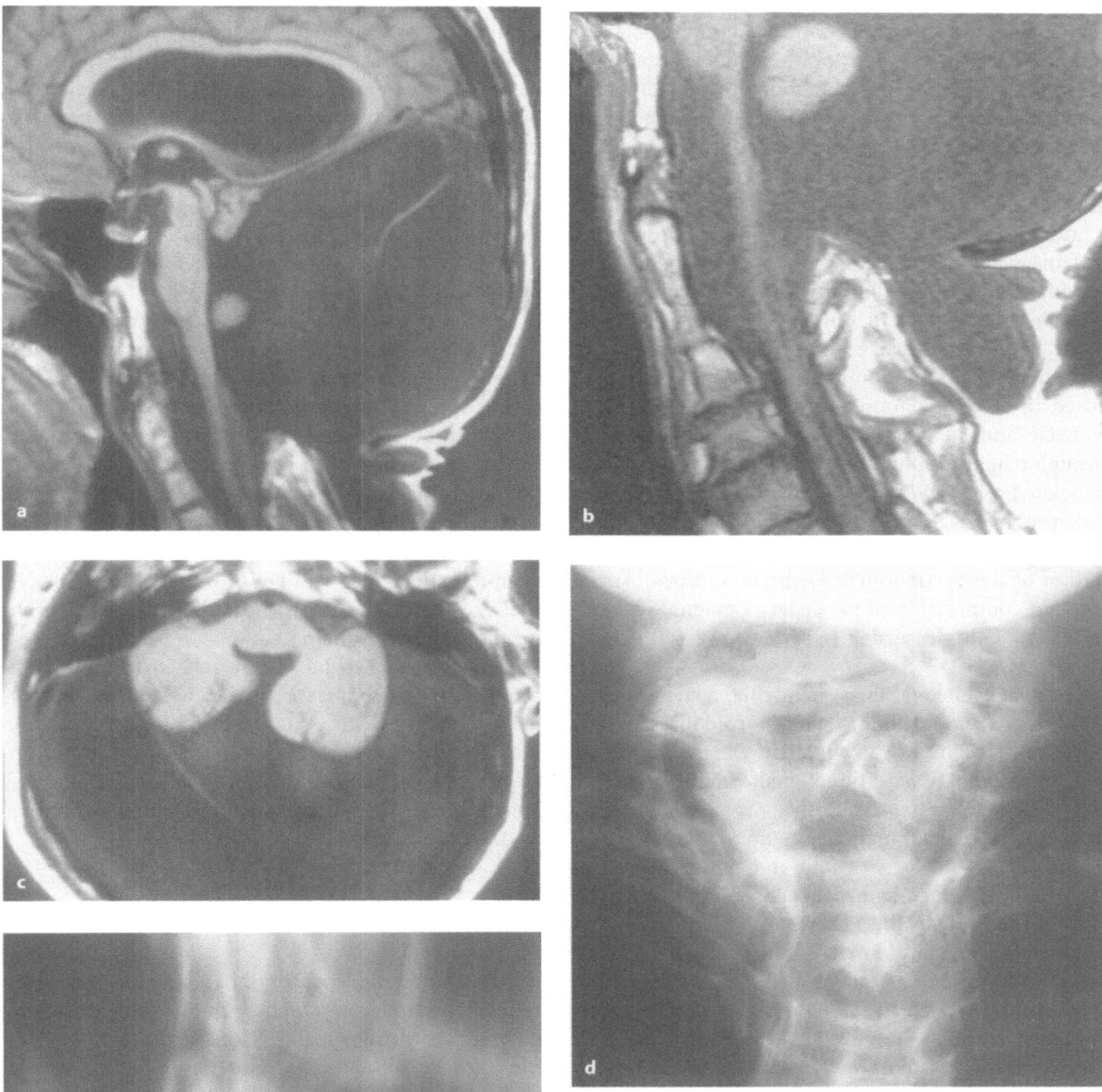

Fig. 3.40 a–e. This 48-year-old woman presented with a slight gait ataxia and urinary incontinence. The remainder of the neurological examination was normal. **a** The sagittal T1-weighted MRI displays a large Dandy-Walker cyst, with elevation of the tentorium and a marked enlargement of the posterior fossa. The vermis is aplastic. There is marked hydrocephalus. At the foramen magnum a meningocele can be seen. **b** A closer look at the craniocervical junction shows luxation of the C1/C2 joint, a Klippel-Feil syndrome C2/3, and a cervical syrinx. **c** The axial scan of the posterior fossa demonstrates aplasia of the vermis and hypoplastic cerebellar hemispheres. X-ray of the cervical spine (**d**) and a lateral tomography (**e**) show a cervical spina bifida and the C1/2 luxation. As neurological symptoms were rather mild, the patient was hesitant to undergo a neurosurgical intervention

formation which now bears their name. However, even though a significant proportion demonstrate obstruction of the fourth ventricle foramina and – possibly as a secondary phenomenon due to hydrocephalus – the aqueduct, not all patients with DWM develop obstructive hydrocephalus. According to Hirsch et al. [15], communication between the fourth ventricle and subarachnoid space is sufficient in utero but may become insufficient after delivery. Yet, a significant proportion of fetuses with DWM develop hydrocephalus. Approximately 80% of children with DWM had normal-sized ventricles at birth but 77.5% became hydrocephalic in the first year of life, most of them within 3 months [15]. As the foramen of Magendie is always closed in DWM, communication between the fourth ventricle and subarachnoid space presumably exists through patent foramina of Luschka. Syringomyelia is associated with DWM in approximately 1% of cases [30], provided CSF obstruction at the foramen magnum is present. This may occur with downward herniation of the cystic fourth ventricle and/or obstruction and compression of the cisterna magna. The embryology of this disorder is reviewed elsewhere [13, 30].

The cyst wall consists of ependyma, a layer of cerebellar tissue, and arachnoid. The choroid plexus of the fourth ventricle may be hypoplastic. Depending on the time of diagnosis, additional malformations of the central nervous system and other organ systems may be found [13]. Examinations in utero have demonstrated that up to 86% of fetuses demonstrate additional findings, such as hydrocephalus or cardiac defects [11, 26, 29]. In the Ecker et al. study [11] on 99 pregnancies with DWM or DWV, half of the pregnancies were terminated. Only 3 of the diagnosed 50 patients with DWM survived birth. One child had a normal physical examination at 6 weeks of age. With additional cardiovascular malformations in particular, DWM carries a grim prognosis [11, 20, 26, 29, 32].

Most patients with DWM become symptomatic within the first year of life [25, 32]. The predominant clinical problem for infants is obstructive hydrocephalus, which usually appears within 3 months of life [15]. Supratentorial shunts [36], cystoperitoneal shunts [6, 23, 32, 33], combined supratentorial and cystoperitoneal shunts [18, 25], and cyst wall fenestrations [22, 31, 39] have been performed. Cystoperitoneal shunting appears to be the safest and most effective treatment modality [4, 15] for infants. Miyamori et al. [23] even observed a descent of the confluens sinuum and normal development of the cerebellar hemispheres after successful cystoperitoneal shunt placement in a 1-month-old infant. However, cystoperitoneal shunting is not without risks. Lee et al. [21] reported a 42% complication rate with this technique. Hirsch et al. [15] mentioned a mortality rate of 12.5% after cysto-

peritoneal shunting. Supratentorial shunting, however, carries the risk of transtentorial cyst herniation due to aqueduct stenosis [4, 28, 40]. Cyst wall excision or fenestration was suggested by Walter Dandy in 1921 [9], but is reported by most authors to be a rather risky procedure with unacceptable complication rates [15, 38] and a total failure rate of up to 75% [13, 15]. Surviving children are likely to sustain significant neurodevelopmental delay, with psychomotor and cognitive deficits even after early and successful treatment of hydrocephalus [2, 26].

With a more delayed onset of symptoms in childhood (which may be observed in approximately 20% of patients born with DWM), cerebellar ataxia or signs of brainstem dysfunction become more significant clinical problems if hydrocephalus is delayed, arrested, or absent [22]. A few case reports in the literature describe patients with DWM and the onset of clinical symptoms in adulthood or even old age (Fig. 3.40) [8, 12, 17, 22, 27, 31, 38]. The majority of symptomatic adults with DWM were treated with cyst wall excision, rather than shunting, with good results for the majority of them.

CMIV appears to be closely related to DWM. The cerebellum is hypoplastic, while the fourth ventricle may be enlarged in a similar fashion as the Dandy-Walker cyst. However, the posterior fossa is not enlarged and the tentorium is not elevated (Fig. 3.41). Management follows the same guidelines as outlined for DWM.

3.2.2
Atresia of Foramina of Luschka and Magendie

In 1921, Dandy reported [9] of patients who had occlusion of the foramina of Luschka and Magendie with obstructive hydrocephalus. He concluded that, apart from postinflammatory obstruction of the fourth ventricle outlets, a congenital variant exists where these foramina failed to open. He considered this to be the hallmark of the malformation which was described as DWM in the previous paragraph. However, atresia of fourth ventricle outlets may occur without cerebellar dysplasia or hypoplasia. A number of case reports in the literature have appeared regarding patients with isolated obstruction of the fourth ventricle openings [1, 3, 7, 14, 16, 24, 34, 41]. In contrast to DWM, almost all of them were in the adult age group and presented with signs of hydrocephalus or a posterior fossa mass lesion, rather than the cerebellar symptoms expected for adult patients with DWM. Whether this malformation can be considered a variant of DWM is far from clear, as the embryological history still needs clarification. As in DWM, isolated obstruction of the fourth ventricle may lead to syringomyelia if the enlarged fourth ventricle obstructs the foramen magnum and

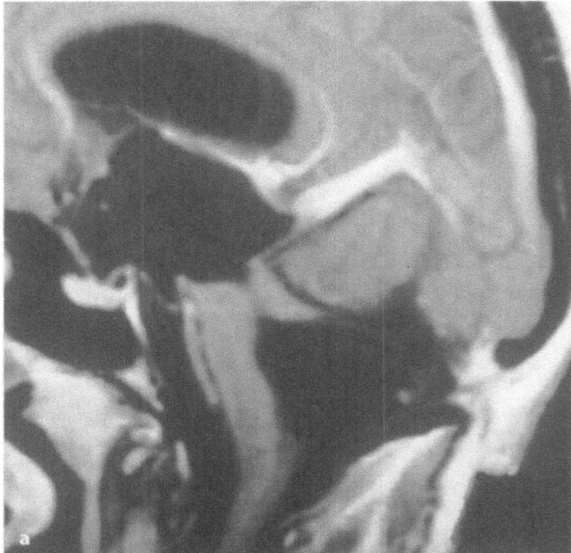

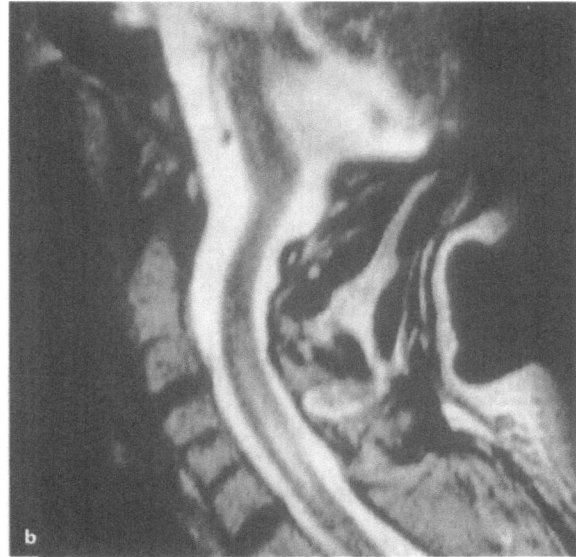

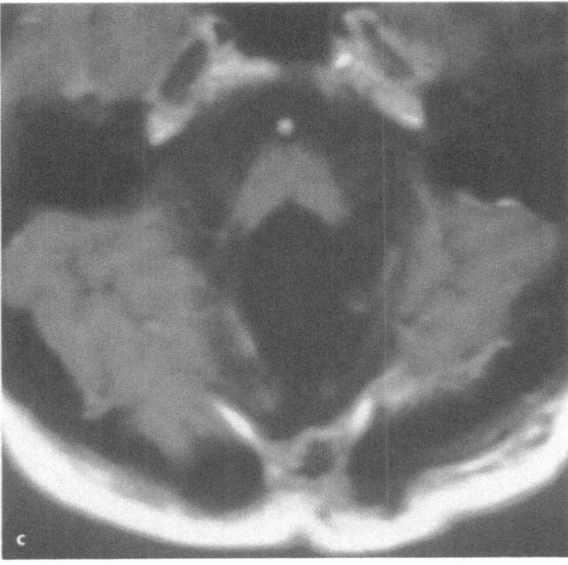

Fig. 3.41 a–c. This 32-year-old slightly retarded woman complained about progressive gait ataxia as the only new neurological symptom. a The sagittal T1-weighted MRI scan shows a
small posterior fossa, a bony defect corresponding to an occipital encephalocele which had been closed soon after birth, hydrocephalus, dysplasia of the midbrain, and aplasia of the cerebellum associated with a large Dandy-Walker cyst. b The T2-
weighted scan of the craniocervical junction demonstrates a
cervical syrinx and Klippel-Feil anomalies at the levels of C2/3
and C4–C6. c The axial T1-weighted image shows the complete
absence of the cerebellum in a small posterior fossa. Acknowl-
edging a certain overlap with DWM, we would classify this
configuration as a Chiari IV malformation. Currently the patient is followed clinically. If the patient's gait continues to deteriorate, a cystoperitoneal shunt will be recommended as the
least invasive form of treatment

causes CSF flow obstruction in this area [19, 37]. Acquired forms of fourth ventricular obstruction are related to arachnoiditis and meningitis and are described in the next chapter.

Recently, Suehiro et al. [34] reported of a patient
successfully treated by endoscopic third ventriculostomy. However, most patients had been treated by a direct approach to the fourth ventricle with fenestration
of the obstructed foramen of Magendie [3, 14, 24, 41]
rather than with shunts [1, 7]. Supratentorial ventriculoperitoneal or atrial shunts [1] are not recommended
anymore, unless there is evidence of additional significant arachnoid pathology, i.e., a history of meningitis.
Chai et al. [7] favor a fourth ventricle to cisternal
shunt over fenestration of the foramen of Magendie
and claim a lower rate of postoperative recurrences.
However, even in this series, a considerable shunt failure rate was observed. Furthermore, a foreign body
such as a shunt tube may aggravate problems of CSF
circulation, as it may induce arachnoid scarring.

Like most other authors, we favor a direct approach
to the pathology (Fig. 3.42). The patient is operated on
in the prone position, as described for CMI. The tonsils are gently retracted with microdissectors and a
thin translucent membrane becomes visible, which
obstructs the foramen of Magendie. The foramina of
Luschka are not inspected. It is sufficient to resect this
membrane to such a degree that wide communication
between the cisterna magna and fourth ventricle is obtained. If necessary, cerebellar tonsils may be shrunk
with bipolar coagulation to optimize communication
and CSF flow between the cisterna magna and fourth
ventricle. Depending on the size of the cisterna mag-

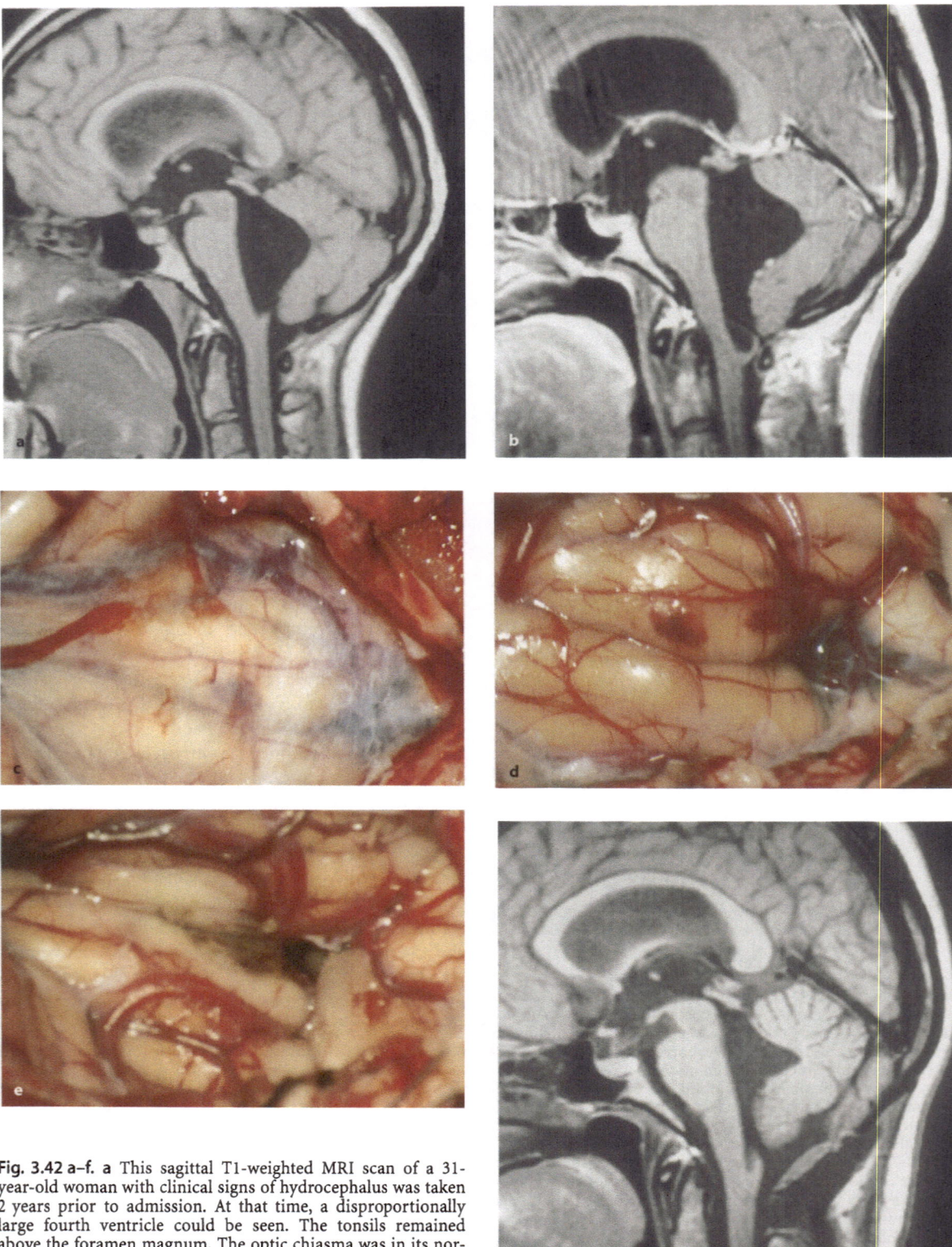

Fig. 3.42 a–f. a This sagittal T1-weighted MRI scan of a 31-year-old woman with clinical signs of hydrocephalus was taken 2 years prior to admission. At that time, a disproportionally large fourth ventricle could be seen. The tonsils remained above the foramen magnum. The optic chiasma was in its normal position (*arrow*). As clinical symptoms regressed spontaneously, no surgery was performed. **b** Two years later, the patient undergoes this MRI examination because signs of hydrocephalus reappeared. The fourth ventricle has enlarged further. Now the cerebellar tonsils reach below the foramen magnum level and the optic chiasma is pushed down and forward (*arrow*). An ophthalmologic examination disclosed papilledema.

na, we would insert a duraplasty or close the dura primarily. Provided no further arachnoid pathology is present, shunting of a ventricle supra- or infratentorially is not required. With more extensive arachnoid changes, however, shunting may still be necessary, even with a sufficient fourth ventricular outflow tract [3].

References

1. Aesch B, Goldenberg N, Maheut-Lourmiere J, Jan M (1991) [Hydrocephalus caused by obstruction of the foraminae of Luschka and Magendie in adults. Report of a case. Etiopathogenic discussion.] Neurochirurgie 37:269–272
2. Aletebi FA, Fung KF (1999) Neurodevelopmental outcome after antenatal diagnosis of posterior fossa abnormalities. J Ultrasound Med 18:683–689
3. Amacher AL, Page LK (1971) Hydrocephalus due to membranous obstruction of the fourth ventricle. J Neurosurg 35:672–676
4. Asai A, Hoffman HJ, Hendrick EB, Humphreys RP (1989) Dandy-Walker syndrome: experience at the Hospital for Sick Children, Toronto. Pediatr Neurosci 15:66–73
5. Calabro F, Arcuri T, Jinkins JR (2000) Blake's pouch cyst: an entity within the Dandy-Walker continuum. Neuroradiology 42:290–295
6. Carteri A, Gerosa M, Gaini SM, Villani R (1979) The dysraphic state of the posterior fossa. Clinical review of the Dandy-Walker syndrome and the so-called arachnoid cysts. J Neurosurg Sci 23:53–59
7. Chai WX (1995) Long-term results of fourth ventriculo-cisternostomy in complex versus simplex atresias of the fourth ventricle outlets. Acta Neurochir (Wien) 134:27–34
8. Cox TA (1979) Rebound nystagmus. An adult with Dandy-Walker syndrome. J Kans Med Soc 80:414–416
9. Dandy WE (1921) The diagnosis and treatment of hydrocephalus due to occlusions of the foramina of Magendie and Luschka. Surg Gynecol Obstet 32:112–124
10. Dandy WE, Blackfan KD (1914) Internal hydrocephalus. An experimental, clinical and pathological study. Am J Dis Child 8:406–482
11. Ecker JL, Shipp TD, Bromley B, Benacerraf B (2000) The sonographic diagnosis of Dandy-Walker and Dandy-Walker variant: associated findings and outcomes. Prenat Diagn 20:328–332
12. Engelhard HH, Meyer JR (1995) Adult-onset presentation of Dandy-Walker variant in siblings. Surg Neurol 44:43–47
13. French BN (1990) Midline fusion defects and defects of formation. In: Youmans JR (ed) Neurological surgery, 3rd edn. Saunders, Philadelphia, pp 1141–1149
14. Hashish H, Guenot M, Mertens P, Sindou M (1999) [Chronic hydrocephalus in an adult due to congenital membranous occlusion of the apertura mediana ventriculi quartii (Foramen of Magendie). Report of two cases and review of the literature.] Neurochirurgie 45:232–236
15. Hirsch JF, Pierre-Kahn A, Renier D, Sainte-Rose C, Hoppe-Hirsch E (1984) The Dandy-Walker malformation. A review of 40 cases. J Neurosurg 61:515–522
16. Holland HC, Graham WL (1958) Congenital atresia of the foramen of Luschka and Magendie with hydrocephalus. J Neurosurg 15:688–694
17. Ishimitsu H, Namba S, Nakasone S (1979) [An adult case of a Dandy-Walker syndrome.] No To Shinkei 31:583–589
18. James HE, Kaiser G, Schut L, Bruce DA (1979) Problems of diagnosis and treatment in the Dandy-Walker syndrome. Child's Brain 5:24–30
19. Kojima N, Tamaki N, Matsumoto S (1988) [Clinical evaluation of an isolated fourth ventricle.] No To Shinkei 40:679–687
20. Kolble N, Wisser J, Kurmanavicius J, Bolthauser E, Stallmach T, Huch A, Huch R (2000) Dandy-walker malformation: prenatal diagnosis and outcome. Prenat Diagn 20:318–327
21. Lee M, Leahu D, Weiner HL, Abbott R, Wisoff JH, Epstein FJ (1995) Complications of fourth-ventricular shunts. Pediatr Neurosurg 22:309–313; discussion 314
22. Lipton HL, Preziosi TJ, Moses H (1978) Adult onset of the Dandy-Walker syndrome. Arch Neurol 35:672–674
23. Miyamori T, Okabe T, Hasegawa T, Takinami K, Matsumoto T (1999) Dandy-Walker syndrome successfully treated with cystoperitoneal shunting – case report. Neurol Med Chir (Tokyo) 39:766–768
24. Osaka Y, Shin H, Sugawa N, Yoshino E, Horikawa Y, Yamaki T, Ueda S (1995) [Disproportionately large, communicating fourth ventricle due to membranous obstruction of Magendie's foramen.] No Shinkei Geka 23:429–433
25. Osenbach RK, Menezes AH (1992) Diagnosis and management of the Dandy-Walker malformation: 30 years of experience. Pediatr Neurosurg 18:179–189
26. Pascual-Castroviejo I, Velez A, Pascual-Pascual SI, Roche MC, Villarejo F (1991) Dandy-Walker malformation: analysis of 38 cases. Child's Nerv Syst 7:88–97
27. Peterson DI, Stirling K, Pena AM (1983) Dandy-Walker syndrome without hydrocephalus in an adult. Bull Clin Neurosci 48:115–121
28. Rosenfeld DL, Lis E, DeMarco K (1995) Transtentorial herniation of the fourth ventricle. Pediatr Radiol 25:436–439
29. Russ PD, Pretorius DH, Johnson MJ (1989) Dandy-Walker syndrome: a review of fifteen cases evaluated by prenatal sonography. Am J Obstet Gynecol 161:401–406

c The intraoperative view of the craniocervical junction after dura opening reveals normal arachnoid with no evidence of previous meningitis. d After arachnoid opening, a thin translucent membrane containing small blood vessels can be seen to obstruct the foramen of Magendie which lies at the level of C1. e After transecting this membrane the fourth ventricle is open. A duraplasty with a galea graft was inserted. f The postoperative MRI after 1 week shows a marked reduction of ventricular sizes – especially of the fourth ventricle – and a normal position of the optic chiasma (arrow). A minor subfascial CSF collection disappeared within a few weeks spontaneously and was no longer present at subsequent follow-up studies. The patient left hospital without any neurological symptoms

30. Sarnat HB (1991) Embryology and dysgenesis of the posterior fossa. In : Batzdorf U (ed) Syringomyelia. Current concepts in diagnosi#s and treatment. Williams and Wilkins, Baltimore, pp 19–23

31. Sato K, Kubota T, Nakamura Y (1996) Adult onset of the Dandy-Walker syndrome. Br J Neurosurg 10:109–112

32. Sawaya R, McLaurin RL (1981) Dandy-Walker syndrome. Clinical analysis of 23 cases. J Neurosurg 55:89–98

33. Shuto T, Sekido K, Ohtsubo Y, Saida A, Yamamoto I (1999) [Dandy-Walker syndrome associated with occipital meningocele and spinal lipoma – case report.] Neurol Med Chir (Tokyo) 39:544–547

34. Suehiro T, Inamura T, Natori Y, Sasaki M, Fukui M (2000) Successful neuroendoscopic third ventriculostomy for hydrocephalus and syringomyelia associated with fourth ventricle outlet obstruction. Case report. J Neurosurg 93:326–329

35. Taggart JK Jr, Walker AE (1942) Congenital atresia of the foramens of Luschka and Magendie. Arch Neurol Psychiatry 48:583–612

36. Tal Y, Freigang B, Dunn HG, Durity FA, Moyes PD (1980) Dandy-Walker syndrome: analysis of 21 cases. Dev Med Child Neurol 22:189–201

37. Toriyama T, Kawauchi M, Koike J, Harada T, Murata A, Kyoshima K (1991) [A case of disproportionately large communicating fourth ventricle combined with syringomyelia and Chiari malformation.] No Shinkei Geka 19:167–172

38. Unsgaard G, Sand T, Stovring J, Ringkjob R (1987) Adult manifestation of the Dandy-Walker syndrome. Report of two cases with review of the literature. Neurochirurgia 30:21–24

39. Villavicencio AT, Wellons JC III, George TM (1998) Avoiding complicated shunt systems by open fenestration of symptomatic fourth ventricular cysts associated with hydrocephalus. Pediatr Neurosurg 29:314–319

40. Wolfson BJ, Faerber EN, Truex RC Jr (1987) The keyhole: a sign of herniation of a trapped fourth ventricle and other posterior fossa cysts. AJNR Am J Neuroradiol 8:473–477

41. Yoshioka S, Matsukado Y, Uemura S, Nagahiro S, Ootsuka T, Yadomi C (1985) [Hydrocephalus due to membranous obstruction of the fourth ventricle aperture.] No Shinkei Geka 13:1135–1139

3.3
Foramen Magnum Arachnoiditis

The first surgical attempt to treat foramen magnum arachnoiditis (FMA) is attributed to Thurel [2] in 1935. Although several authors list FMA as a possible cause of syringomyelia [1, 6, 9, 10], the publication of Appleby et al. in 1969 [3] has remained the only study exclusively devoted to this subject. This may reflect the decrease in occurrence of syringomyelia due to FMA as antibiotics and improved hygiene have reduced the incidence of meningitis – tuberculous meningitis, in particular. However, it may also indicate uncertainty as to the treatment strategy or generally poor results for these patients. Appleby et al. [3] recommended restricting surgical attempts to shunting of the associated hydrocephalus.

We have encountered 21 patients with FMA and syringomyelia (Table 3.12). Of these 21 patients, 4 did not undergo surgery: 3 because of a stable clinical situation, and 1 patient refused surgery. All 17 operated patients presented with progressive neurological symptoms.

3.3.1
Clinical Presentation

Patients presented at an average age of 38±12 years with a mean history of 64±80 months. In 10 patients, the cause of arachnoiditis could be identified: meningitis in 5 patients, birth trauma or other traumatic incidents in 4 patients (Figs. 3.43, 3.44), subarachnoid hemorrhage in 1 patient, and a combination of subarachnoid hemorrhage and multiple operations in another patient. The average time interval between the presumed causal event and the development of FMA and syringomyelia symptoms was almost 10 years (115±117 months, range 8 months to 36 years). Interestingly, this time interval is almost identical compared with patients having syringomyelia related to spinal trauma or other causes of spinal arachnoid scarring [8].

The most common neurological symptom which the patients with FMA noticed first was progressive motor weakness of one upper limb (48%). Sensory disturbances or headaches were each reported in 20% of patients as the first symptom. Problems of gait, swallowing, or hydrocephalus were each encountered by 4% of patients as the first clinical problem. In contrast, patients with CMI and syringomyelia are more likely to report headaches and sensory disturbances as the first complaint, with problems of gait or motor power appearing later in the clinical course (Chi-square test: $P=0.0016$).

At presentation in our hospitals, patients with FMA complained mainly of progressive motor weakness (40%), gait problems (24%), or occipital pain (24%). Patients with CMI, however, predominantly complain of occipital headaches (30%), whereas motor weakness is less often the predominant problem (15%) (Chi-square test: $P=0.0038$). Patients with FMA presented with a significantly lower Karnofsky score compared with patients having CMI and syringomyelia (65±14 and 73±14, respectively; t-test: $P=0.0008$).

Table 3.12. Overview of patients with syringomyelia and foramen magnum arachnoiditis

No.	History (months)	Int. (months)	Grade	Associations and causes	Add. find.	Surgery	Outcome
1	12	–	2	Foramen magnum stenosis	–	Decompress arachnolysis	Improved
2	48	36	2	Cryptococcal meningitis	Hydro.	Decompress. arachnolysis	Clinical recurrence
2	3					Syringoperit. shunt	Stable
3	36	–	2	–	–	Decompress. arachnolysis	Stable
4	24	–	2	Hemorrhage, chronic infl.	–	Decompress. arachnolysis	Improved
5	20	192	2	Meningitis	–	Decompress. arachnolysis	Clinical recurrence
5	51					Syringoperit. shunt	Clinical recurrence
5	7					Decompress. arachnolysis	Improved
6	12	108	2	Head trauma, spinal trauma C4	–	Decompress. arachnolysis	Clinical recurrence
6	3				Hydro.	Ventriculoperitoneal shunt	Clinical recurrence
6	6					Decompress. arachnolysis	Improved
7	60	–	2	–	–	Syringosub. shunt	Clinical recurrence
7	24					Decompress. arachnolysis	Improved
8	120	–	2	Meningitis, chronic otitis media	Arach cyst	Decompress. arachnolysis	Improved
9	60	–	2	–	–	Decompress. arachnolysis	Stable
10	84	96	2	Meningitis	Hydro	Decompress. arachnolysis	Clinical recurrence, died 4 years postop
11	36	–	2	–	–	Decompress. arachnolysis	Improved
12	60	–	2	–	Arach. cyst	Perit. shunt of arachnoid cyst	Clinical recurrence
13	348	–	2	–	–	Decompress. arachnolysis	Clinical recurrence
14	18	–	2	Foramen magnum stenosis	–	Decompress. arachnolysis	Stable
15	1	–	–	–	Hydro.	No surgery	Stable
16	60	60	2	AVM – hemorrhage, multiple surgeries	Hydro.	Decompress. arachnolysis	Clinical recurrence
17	228	120	2	Birth trauma	Hydro. arach. cyst	Decompress. arachnolysis	Improved
18	156	36	–	Meningitis	–	No surgery recom.	Stable
19	6	–	–	Platybasia	–	No surgery recom.	Stable
20	72	60	–	Birth trauma	–	Surgery recom.	Progressive
21	84	432	1	Birth trauma	–	Decompress. arachnolysis	Stable

Int., interval until symptoms of syringomyelia developed; Add. find., additional findings; Decompress., decompression of foramen magnum; Hydro., hydrocephalus; Syringoperit., syringoperitoneal; Infl., inflammation; Syringosub., syringosubarachnoidal; Arach. cyst, arachnoidal cyst; Perit., peritoneal; postop., postoperatively; Recom., recommended

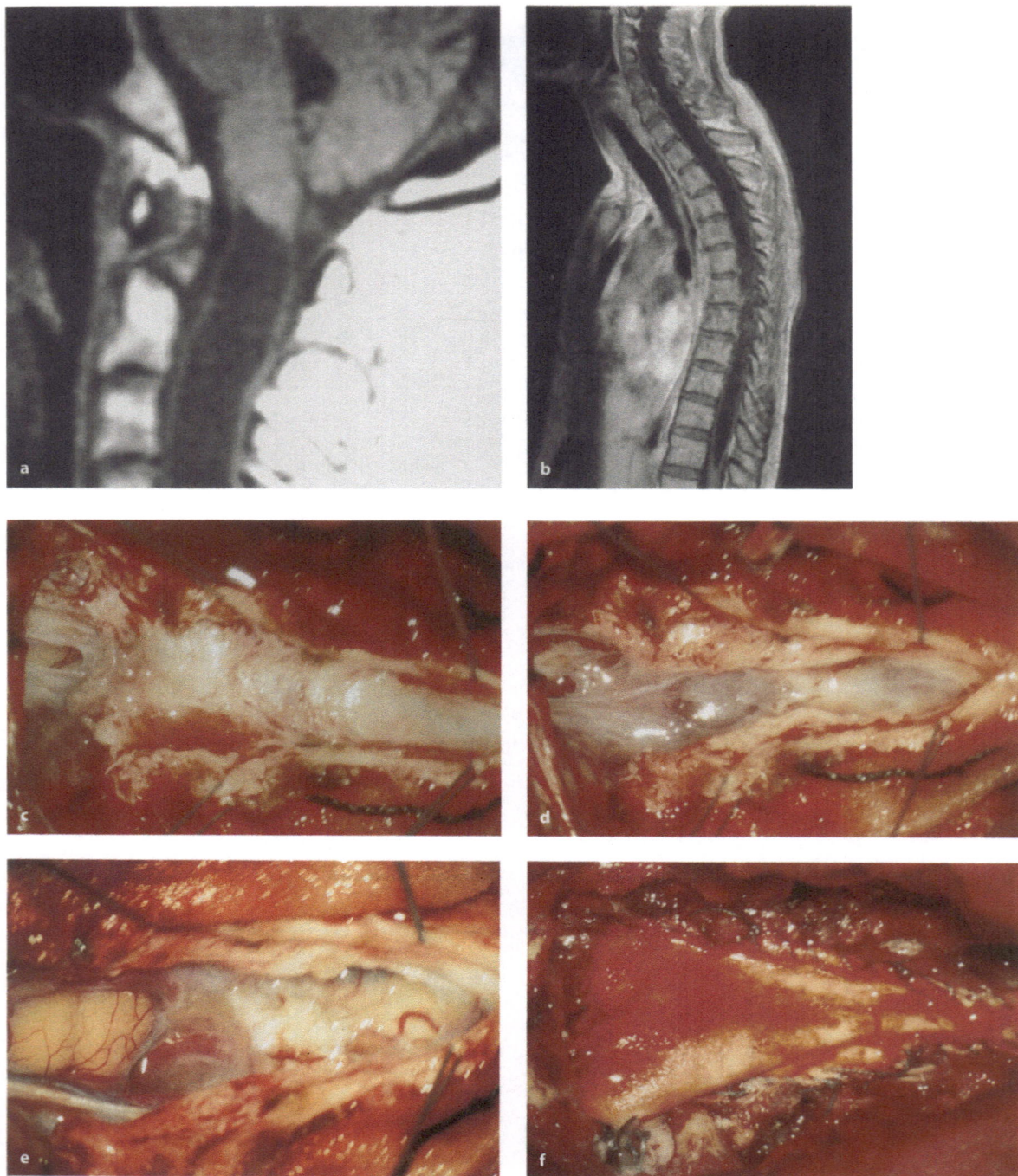

Fig. 3.43 a–g. The T1-weighted MRI scans of this 44-year-old woman display a large syrinx extending from the foramen magnum (**a**) down to Th11 (**b**). Comparing the cyst morphology on both ends of the cyst, the rather irregular shape at the upper pole suggests that obstruction of CSF flow may be situated at the foramen magnum. There is no Chiari malformation. The patient gave a history of birth trauma and complained about progressive gait ataxia and motor weakness of her hand muscles for the past 2 years. There was no history of meningitis. Surgery was recommended under the presumptive diagnosis of foramen magnum arachnoiditis. **c** After dura opening, dense arachnoid adhesions became visible, causing a complete block of CSF flow at the foramen magnum. **d** After partial resection of the arachnoid scar, some blood vessels on the spinal cord surface and cerebellar cortex became visible. **e** This view under higher magnification shows the final stage of dissection. A small layer of scarring was left on the spinal cord as it did not interfere with CSF flow. The fourth ventricle is open and the left PICA is visible. **f** A large synthetic duraplasty (Neuropatch) has been inserted. **g** Postoperative MRI after 1 week shows a significant decrease of the syrinx. Neurological symptoms remained unchanged

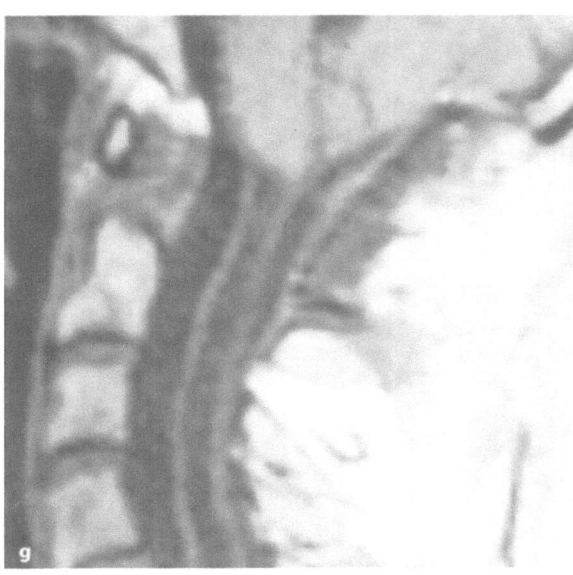

Fig. 3.43 g

3.3.2
Neuroradiology

Five patients in this group demonstrated radiological evidence of hydrocephalus. In two of these, the hydrocephalus was related to meningitis; in one patient each, it was related to trauma or previous surgery, while no obvious cause was detected in the remaining patient. An arachnoid cyst in the posterior fossa was seen in three patients – again related to meningitis or trauma in one patient each, with no apparent cause in the third patient. Hydrocephalus and posterior fossa arachnoid cysts associated with a syrinx indicate a rather widespread problem of CSF circulation that may go beyond the area of the foramen magnum. Likewise, a history of previous operations at the foramen magnum or meningitis indicates that thick arachnoid adhesions may be encountered.

In the absence of hydrocephalus or an arachnoid cyst, the arachnoid pathology at this level may be difficult to diagnose. When examining standard MRI scans in a patient with suspected FMA, one should look for compression, displacement, or other types of distorted MRI images of the cord, brainstem, or cerebellum, such as bulging of the upper cervical cord and medulla or displacement of the medulla on axial scans due to arachnoid scarring. The severity of the arachnoid pathology, however, cannot be determined preoperatively.

The method of choice to demonstrate FMA is cardiac-gated MRI, which demonstrates obstruction of CSF flow at the foramen magnum as indirect evidence for arachnoid pathology. This imaging modality allows visualization of CSF flow. This study was diagnostic in each of the patients presented here since it was first employed in 1990. Standard MRI may provide indirect signs of arachnoiditis, such as irregular margins of central nervous structures or adhesions between dura mater and cerebellum or spinal cord.

3.3.3
Surgical Management

In patients with an associated hydrocephalus, the hydrocephalus should be treated first. If the patient continues to deteriorate, the function of the ventricular shunt should be checked before an operation at the foramen magnum is considered. Once hydrocephalus has been ruled out and CSF flow obstruction at the foramen magnum has been demonstrated, the strategy of treatment becomes obvious: exploration of the foramen magnum with the objective to establish free CSF passage. It is very difficult to provide a reasonably accurate prognosis as to the postoperative outcome even when the operation succeeds and normal flow of CSF is obtained. Therefore, we recommend surgery only for those patients in whom the clinical situation has clearly deteriorated. Seventeen patients of our series underwent exploration of the foramen magnum. Figures 3.43 and 3.44 provide illustrative examples. The surgical technique is similar to those described under Sects. 3.1.4.2 and 3.1.6.

After a midline incision and detachment of the neck muscles from the occipital bone, a small occipital craniectomy including the foramen magnum was performed. In the majority of cases, a laminectomy of C1 was done as well. The dura was incised in a Y-shape, the arachnoid was inspected, and arachnoid scarring classified intraoperatively as described in paragraph 3.1.4.2.

Obstruction of CSF pathways could be found in every patient undergoing surgery at the foramen magnum. The arachnoid scarring was so severe that, in all but one patient, no CSF flow could be observed after dura opening. CSF flow could only be observed after opening and sharp dissection of the arachnoid toward the foramen of Magendie, the cerebellopontine cisterns, and the spinal canal. The foramen of Magendie was obstructed in each of these patients and opened. The size of the tonsils was reduced by bipolar coagulation or subpial suction [5] if necessary to visualize the foramen. If the PICA was embedded in thick arachnoid adhesions, no attempt was made to dissect it free. Likewise, no dissection was carried out laterally toward perforating arteries or caudal cranial nerves. The only objective of surgery was to provide free CSF pathways.

Any operation trying to improve a problem related to arachnoid scarring may create new arachnoid scar

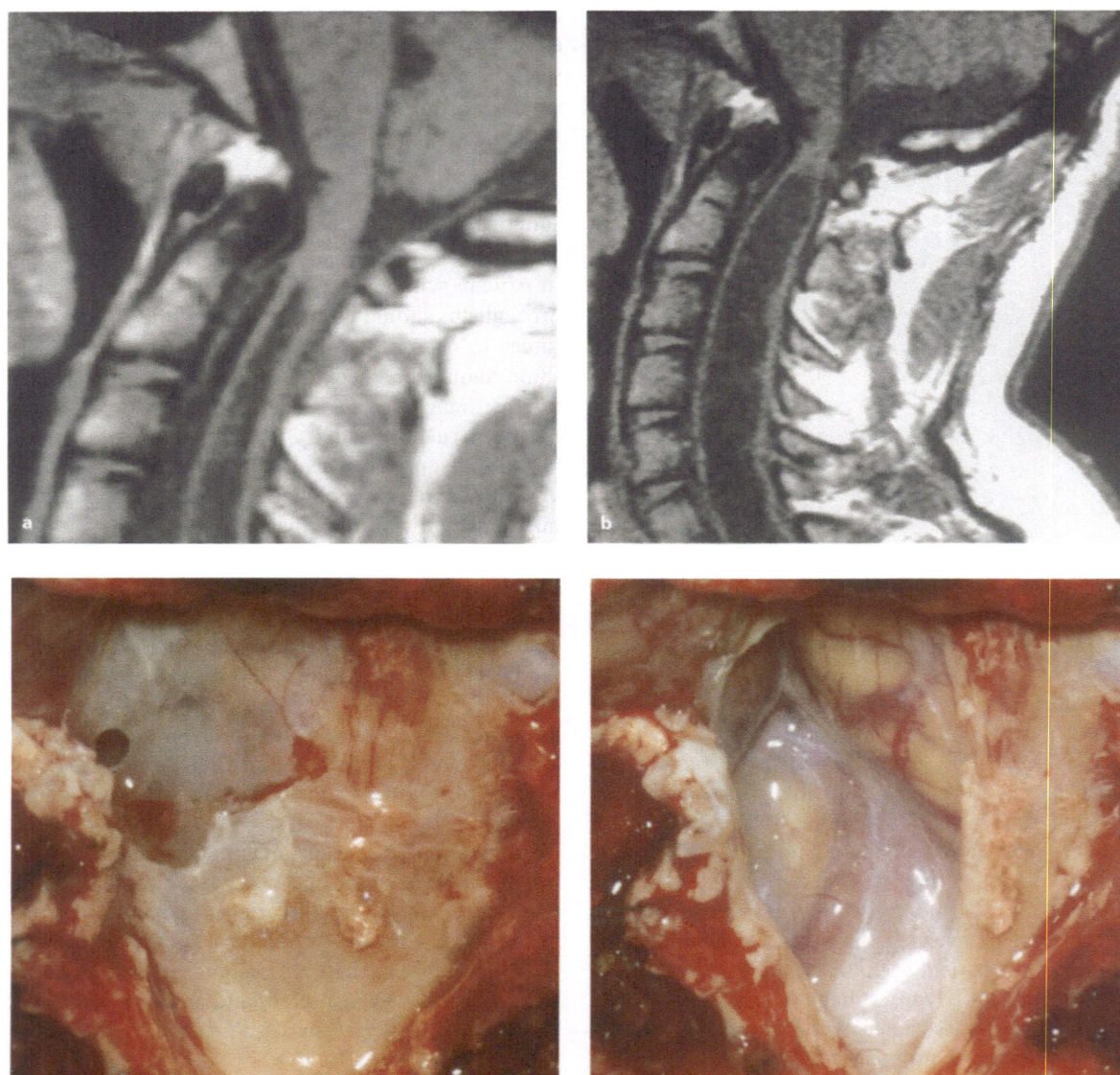

Fig. 3.44 a–f. This 29-year-old man also gave a history of birth trauma. Symptoms began 19 years ago with progressive weakness of his left arm. He underwent orthopedic surgery for scoliosis 4 years ago. Then syringomyelia and hydrocephalus were discovered and a ventriculoperitoneal and syringosubarachnoid shunt were placed. On admission, the patient had a plegic left arm, marked weakness of his right arm with atrophy of small hand muscles, dysesthesias in his right arm, gait ataxia, and sensory deficits on the left side of his body since implantation of the syringosubarachnoid shunt. There were no clinical signs of hydrocephalus. **a** This T1-weighted MRI scan shows the upper pole of a syrinx, no Chiari malformation. **b** The parasagittal scan reveals an additional arachnoid cyst in the posterior fossa. The diagnosis of foramen magnum arachnoiditis was made and surgery recommended. **c** In the semi-sitting position, the dura was opened and severe arachnoid scarring became immediately apparent. **d** After partial resection of the outer layer of this scar, the spinal cord, left PICA, and both tonsils became visible. Please note the twisted and slightly turned position of these structures: the cord is turned to the right and the fourth ventricle displaced to the left side of the midline. **e** After further arachnoid dissection, the foramen of Magendie could be opened; the right tonsil was coagulated to gain access to the arachnoid cyst for fenestration. Free CSF passage to both cerebellopontine cisterns and toward the spinal canal were present. Therefore, no further dissection was undertaken and a duraplasty inserted. **f** The postoperative MRI scan 6 months later shows a decrease of the syrinx, but also a rather shallow cisterna magna which could indicate that adhesions have formed between cerebellar tonsils and duraplasty. So far, the clinical situation is stable with improvement of dysesthesias and no further progression of neurological deficits

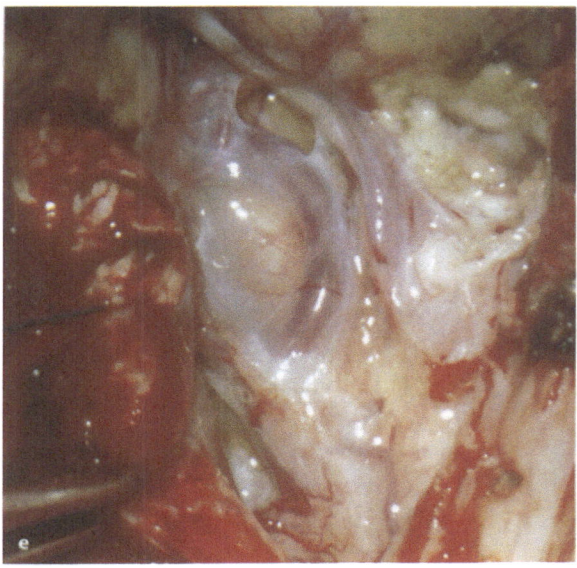
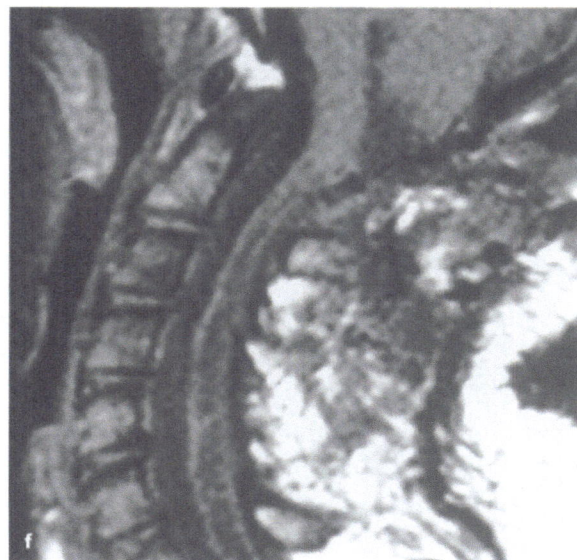

Fig. 3.44 e, f

formation: the less the extent of dissection and the less contamination of the surgical field with blood, the better the chance for a long-lasting free CSF passage. Presumably for this reason, the postoperative results of foramen magnum operations by Appleby et al. [3] were not very successful, so that they recommended limiting surgical therapy to ventricular shunting.

After providing a free CSF pathway from the fourth ventricle and the cerebellopontine cisterns toward the spinal canal, a large cisterna magna was created with a spacious dura graft.

Shunting of the syrinx will not influence the mechanism that caused the syrinx. It will also not influence those symptoms which may be directly related to the arachnoiditis itself. Therefore, shunting of the syrinx should be performed only in those instances where the CSF flow obstruction cannot be corrected, i.e., patients with extensive arachnoid pathology after meningitis, etc.

3.3.5
Postoperative Outcome

We encountered a complication rate of 19% with CSF leaks as the predominant problem (14%). Preliminary swallowing problems were observed in 5% of these patients. After opening of the foramen magnum, arachnolysis, and insertion of a dura graft, improvement was observed during the first postoperative year in sensory disturbances, dysesthesias, and pain, whereas motor weakness, gait, sphincter functions, and swallowing problems tended to remain unaltered. Considering the severe preoperative motor deficits in these patients, this lack of postoperative improvement is re-

flected in an unchanged Karnofsky score during the first postoperative year. As patients with FMA demonstrate a similar arachnoid pathology as patients with CMI and arachnoid scarring grade 2, we compared these two groups. In FMA, postoperative results are less satisfactory. In CMI with grade 2 arachnoid scarring, improvement was seen in sensory disturbances, pain, motor power, and bladder function, whereas dysesthesias, gait, and swallowing function remained unchanged (Table 3.13).

Four patients required multiple operations: one patient stabilized after foramen magnum surgery and syringoperitoneal shunting, one patient finally improved after two foramen magnum procedures and a syringoperitoneal shunt, another patient improved after two foramen magnum procedures and a ventriculoperitoneal shunt, one last patient underwent a foramen magnum procedure after syringosubarachnoid shunting and improved. In terms of clinical recurrence rates, the overall figure for patients with FMA and syringomyelia after a foramen magnum procedure was 57% within 5 years. This figure was significantly worse than patients having CMI and grade 1 or grade 2 arachnoiditis (17% and 41%, respectively; log-rank test: $P=0.0255$) (Fig. 3.45).

Compared with patients having CMI and various degrees of associated arachnoid changes, results for patients with syringomyelia and FMA are considerably worse [1, 3, 9]. The optimal clinical result for patients with FMA is stabilization of a previously progressive course. Even this can only be achieved in approximately half of the patients with a single operation at the foramen magnum. Two major reasons may account for this outcome. First, the rather severe arach-

Table 3.13. Preoperative and postoperative clinical symptoms for FMA and CMI

Group	Preop.	Postop.	3 months	6 months	1 year	P
Sensory deficits						
FMA	2.9±0.5	3.3±0.6	3.4±0.8	3.4±0.8	3.3±0.8	n.s.
CMI + arach.	3.4±1.2	3.6±1.2	3.6±1.2	3.6±1.2	3.6±1.2	
Dysesthesias						
FMA	4.2±0.8	4.3±0.8	4.3±0.8	4.3±0.8	4.4±0.8	n.s
CMI + arach.	3.9±0.9	4.0±0.9	4.1±0.8	4.0±1.0	3.9±1.0	
Pain						
FMA	3.5±1.0	3.9±0.8	4.0±0.8	4.0±0.8	3.8±0.9	$P<0.01$
CMI + arach.	4.0±0.9	4.2±0.4	4.6±0.5	4.6±0.5	4.6±0.5	
Motor power						
FMA	2.9±1.3	2.9±1.4	3.1±1.4	3.0±1.5	2.9±1.6	$P<0.05$
CMI + arach.	3.6±1.2	3.6±1.2	3.8±1.2	3.8±1.2	3.8±1.2	
Gait ataxia						
FMA	3.4±1.6	3.5±1.6	3.7±1.3	3.5±1.4	3.4±1.6	n.s.
CMI + arach.	3.6±1.0	3.6±1.0	3.6±0.9	3.6±0.9	3.6±1.0	
Bladder function						
FMA	4.3±1.0	4.2±1.0	4.2±1.0	4.2±1.0	4.3±1.0	n.s.
CMI + arach.	4.1±1.5	4.4±0.8	4.4±0.8	4.4±0.8	4.4±0.8	
Bowel function						
FMA	4.8±0.6	4.8±0.6	4.8±0.6	4.8±0.6	4.8±0.6	n.s.
CMI + arach.	4.6±0.7	4.5±0.8	4.6±0.7	4.6±0.7	4.6±0.7	
Swallowing function						
FMA	4.8±0.6	4.9±0.4	4.9±0.4	4.9±0.4	4.9±0.4	n.s.
CMI + arach.	4.7±0.7	4.6±0.7	4.7±0.5	4.8±0.4	4.8±0.4	
Karnofsky score						
FMA	65±14	67±14	70±14	69±16	66±20	n.s.
CMI + arach.	69±16	71±16	74±14	74±14	73±15	

FMA, foramen magnum arachnoiditis; CMI + arach., Chiari I malformation and arachnoiditis grade 2; *P*, *P*-value comparing postoperative results for both groups after 1 year; n.s., not significant

noid pathology in this group of patients may preclude a better postoperative result as the objective of surgery – free CSF pathways at the foramen magnum – cannot be fully achieved in many instances. Often the surgeon has to compromise to avoid undue risks. Second, unlike patients with CMI who generally improve postoperatively due to brainstem decompression rather than regression of syringomyelia [4, 7, 9], brainstem compression does not play a role in FMA.

References

1. Abe T, Okuda Y, Nagashima H, Isojima A, Tani S (1995) [Surgical treatment of syringomyelia.] Rinsho Shinkeigaku 35:1406–1408
2. Alajouanine T, Hornet T, Thurel R, Andre R. (1935) Le feutrage arachnoidien posterieur dans la syringomyelie (sa place dann sla pathologie des leptomeninges). Rev Neurol (Paris) 64:91–98

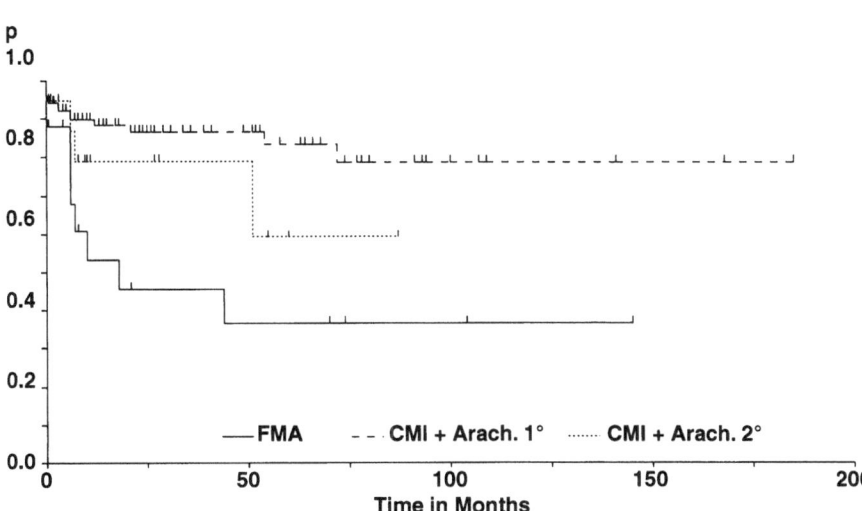

Fig. 3.45. Kaplan-Meier analysis of clinical recurrences comparing patients with foramen magnum arachnoiditis (FMA) and Chiari I malformation with grade 1 (CMI + Arach. 1°) or grade 2 (CMI + Arach. 2°) arachnoid scarring (log-rank test: $P=0.0255$)

3. Appleby A, Bradley WG, Foster JB, Hankinson J, Hudgson P (1969) Syringomyelia due to chronic arachnoiditis at the foramen magnum. J Neurol Sci 8:451–464

4. Bindal AK, Dunsker SB, Tew JM Jr (1995) Chiari I malformation: classification and management. Neurosurgery 37:1069–1074

5. Halamandaris GG, Batzdorf U (1989) Adult Chiari malformation. Contemp Neurosurg 11:1–6

6. Hurth M, Parker F (1999) [History, controversy and pathogenesis.] Neurochirurgie 45 [Suppl 1]:138–157

7. Klekamp J, Batzdorf U, Samii M, Bothe HW (1996) The surgical treatment of Chiari I malformation. Acta Neurochir (Wien) 138:788–801

8. Klekamp J, Batzdorf U, Samii M, Bothe HW (1997) Treatment of syringomyelia associated with arachnoid scarring caused by arachnoiditis or trauma. J Neurosurg 86:233–240

9. Parker F, Aghakhani N, Tadie M (1999) [Non-traumatic arachnoiditis and syringomyelia. A series of 32 cases]. Neurochirurgie 45 [Suppl 1]:67–83

10. Williams B (1993) Surgery for hindbrain related syringomyelia. Adv Tech Stand Neurosurg 20:107–164

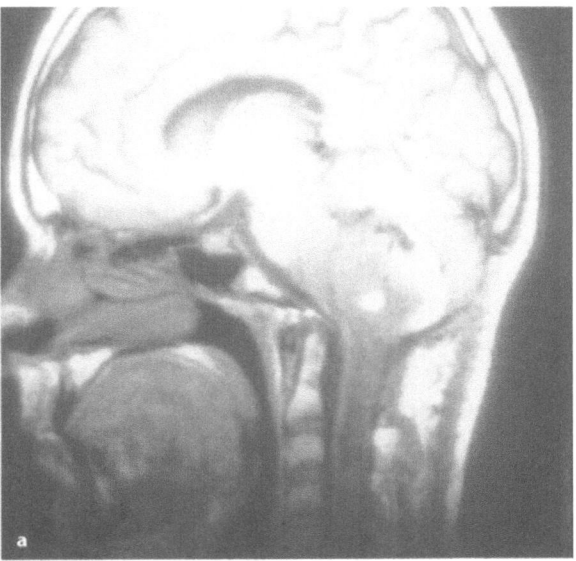

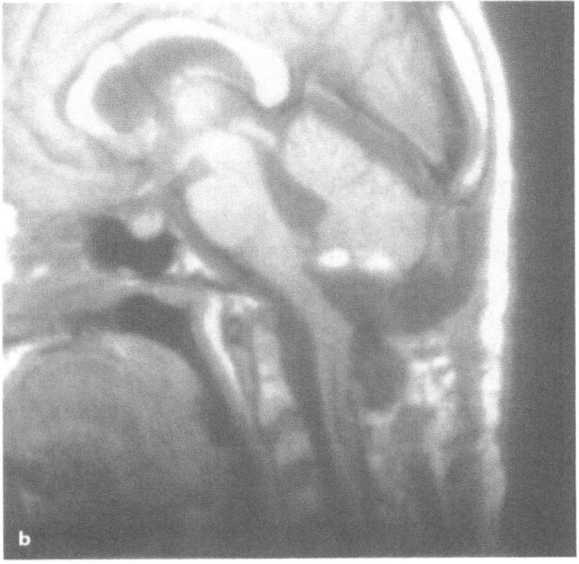

Fig. 3.46a, b. This 17-year-old boy presented with a 13-month history of headache, vertigo, and progressive visual loss. A CT scan disclosed a tumor of the posterior fossa in the midline with obstructive hydrocephalus. A preliminary diagnosis of a meningioma was made and a ventriculoperitoneal shunt was inserted 11 months before admission to our department. On admission, the patient presented with cerebellar ataxia and nystagmus. No motor weakness or sensory deficit could be detected. The progressive visual loss had resolved completely with ventriculoperitoneal shunting. **a** A T1-weighted MRI scan without gadolinium demonstrated a large meningioma in the posterior fossa in the midline, which had pushed the cerebellar tonsils into the foramen magnum. A small intratumoral hemorrhage is visible. The upper level of a syringomyelic cavity can be detected at C2. The lower limit of the syrinx was not visualized. Through a midline suboccipital approach, the tumor was removed completely. Arachnoid adhesions at the foramen magnum had to be dissected before the tumor could be resected. A dural graft was inserted to enlarge the cisterna magna. The histological diagnosis was hemangioblastic meningioma. **b** The postoperative MRI scan confirmed complete removal of the tumor, a patent cisterna magna, and a collapse of the syrinx. On follow-up examination after 1 month, the neurological state was identical to the preoperative state

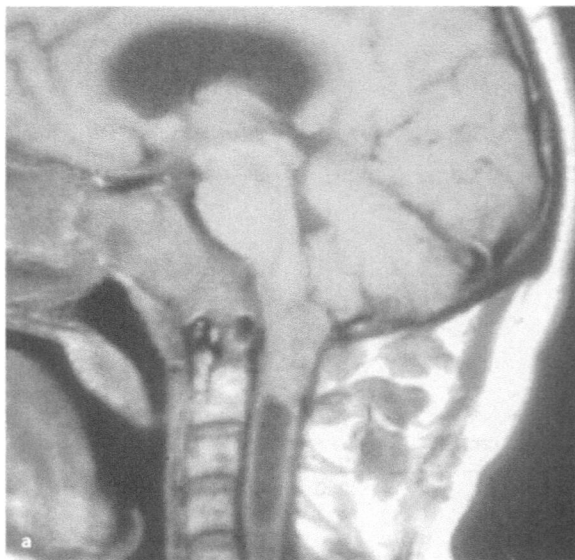

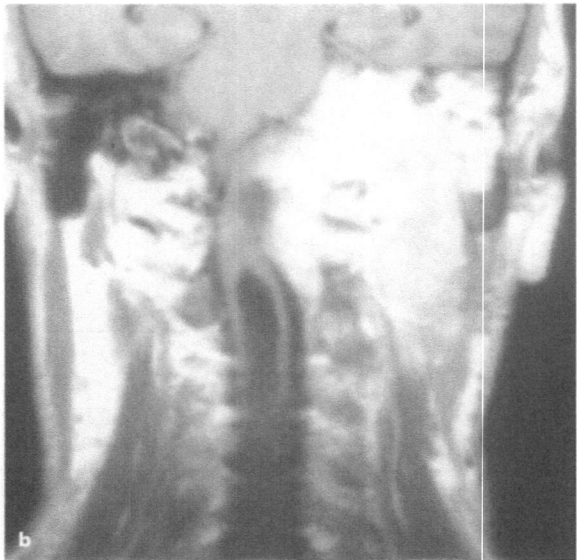

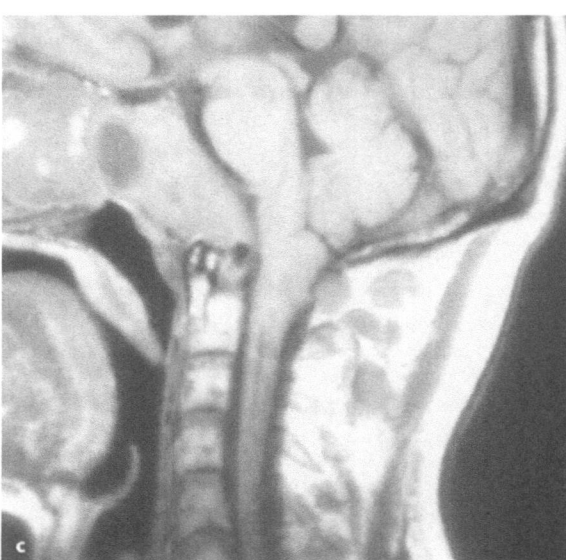

Fig. 3.47 a–c. This 48-year-old man presented with a 34-year history of a synovialoma of the skull base. He was operated on six times before presenting at our institution. The last operation with a partial removal of the tumor had been performed 2 years earlier. On admission, he presented with pain in his left shoulder and dysesthesias in his left hand, which he could provoke by coughing or sneezing. He had lost function of cranial nerves III, V, VII, and IX–XII on the left side. The remainder of the neurological examination was normal. **a** A T1-weighted MRI scan without gadolinium demonstrated obstruction of the cisterna magna by tumor and a syrinx between C2 and C4. **b** The coronal scan after gadolinium revealed a large tumor which replaced almost the entire skull base on the left side, crossing the midline in the posterior fossa and obliterating the cisterna magna. There was no evidence of obstructive hydrocephalus. A partial tumor removal was achieved via an extended lateral suboccipital approach. Most of the tumor in the paravertebral, retromandibular, and craniocervical region could be removed. Arachnoid scarring toward the foramen magnum was found and dissected to achieve free CSF passage. **c** The postoperative MRI scan after 1 year showed residual tumor in the cisterna magna but a decrease in syrinx caliber, due to the improvement of CSF flow attributable to arachnoid dissection. At 2 years postoperatively, the residual tumor was unchanged and the syrinx had disappeared. He complained about incomplete facial, accessory, and recurring nerve palsies on the left side, and slight dysesthesias, all of which were no longer aggravated by coughing or sneezing

3.4
Intracranial Tumors

The association of intracranial tumors with syringomyelia is an absolute rarity [20]. Apart from arachnoid cysts [1, 3, 5, 8, 13], solid tumors [2, 6, 9, 10, 11, 15, 18, 19] of the posterior fossa have been observed to cause herniation of cerebellar tonsils and syringomyelia. Five patients were reported as autopsy findings [4, 7, 17]. Even a few patients with supratentorial tumors have been described [12, 14, 15, 16].

Intracranial space-occupying lesions may cause CMI and produce syringomyelia. As syringomyelia

takes some time to develop, it is not surprising that slow-growing tumors such as meningiomas were the most common among these. Most, but not all patients, showed signs of obstructive hydrocephalus. Kumar et al. [11] reported a cerebellar astrocytoma with exophytic growth along the posterior aspect of the medulla oblongata down to C2 without causing hydrocephalus. This 16-year-old boy showed signs of upper extremity weakness and a sensory loss from C2 to T10. Symptoms improved with subtotal removal and radiotherapy.

One patient had signs of a dissociated sensory disturbance in her upper limbs which improved after re-

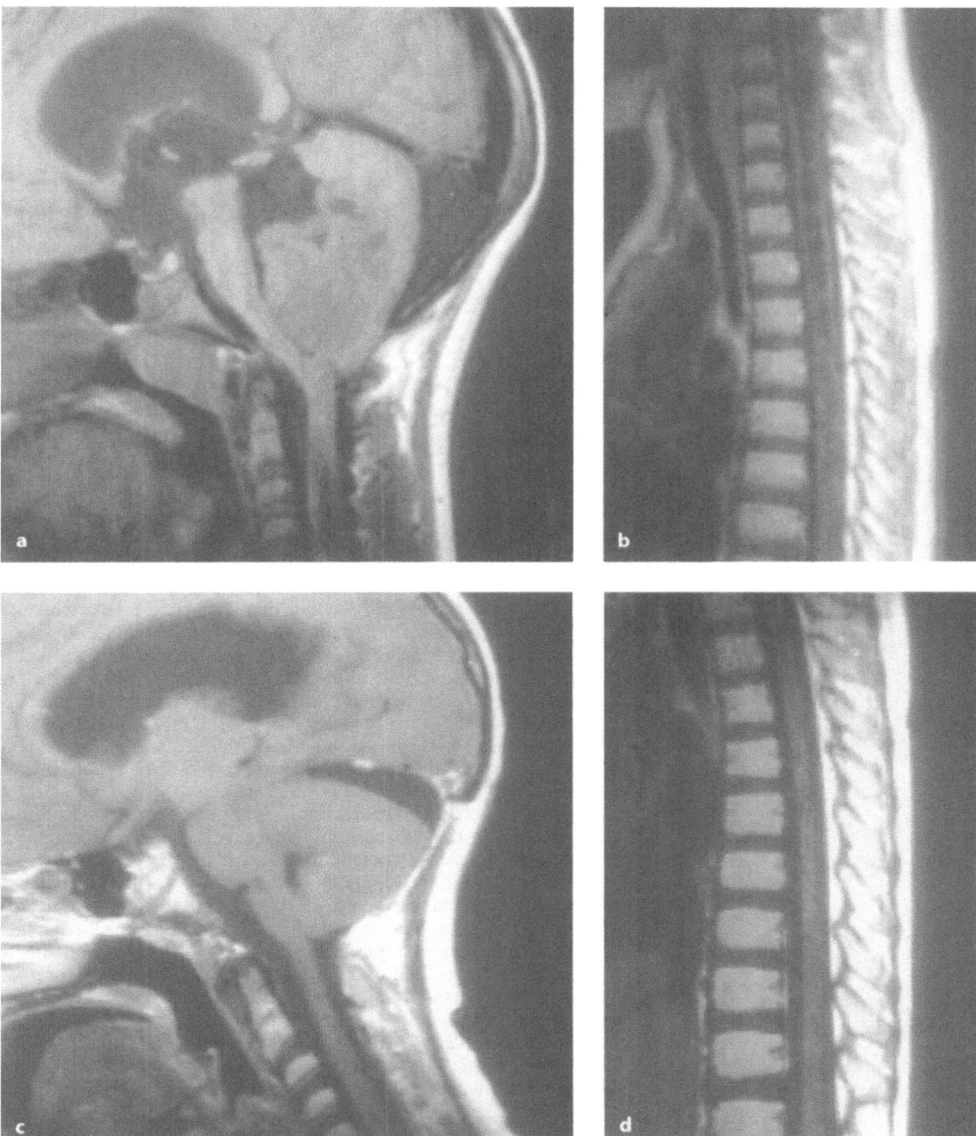

Fig. 3.48 a–d. This 8-year-old girl presented with a 4-month history of hydrocephalus with headache, meningism, cerebellar ataxia, dysarthria, and vomiting. On admission, there were no additional neurological deficits to be detected. **a** A T1-weighted MRI scan without gadolinium disclosed a large tumor of the fourth ventricle with obstructive hydrocephalus and impaction of the cerebellar tonsils into the foramen magnum. **b** A syrinx was demonstrated between C2 and Th8. A provisional diagnosis of a medulloblastoma was made. The patient was operated on via a midline suboccipital approach and total tumor re-

moval could be achieved. No arachnoid changes were detected at the fourth ventricle or foramen magnum. The histological examination confirmed the diagnosis of medulloblastoma. **c** The postoperative MRI scan with gadolinium showed no residual tumor and complete disappearance of the syrinx (**d**). The child made a slow recovery from operation over a period of 3 months. Unfortunately, due to the chemotherapy regimen, she developed severe aplastic anemia leading to staphylococcal and candida septicemia. She eventually died 7 months after the operation

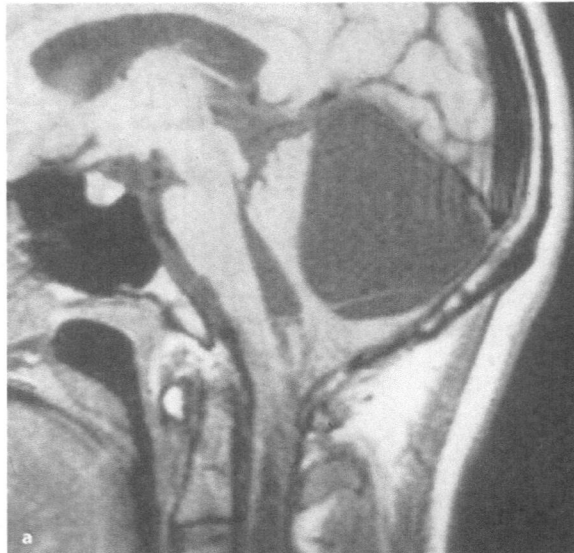
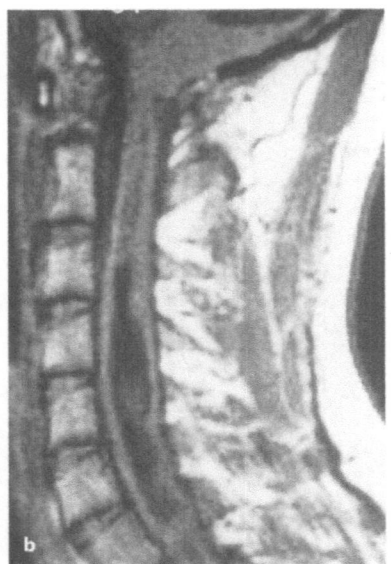
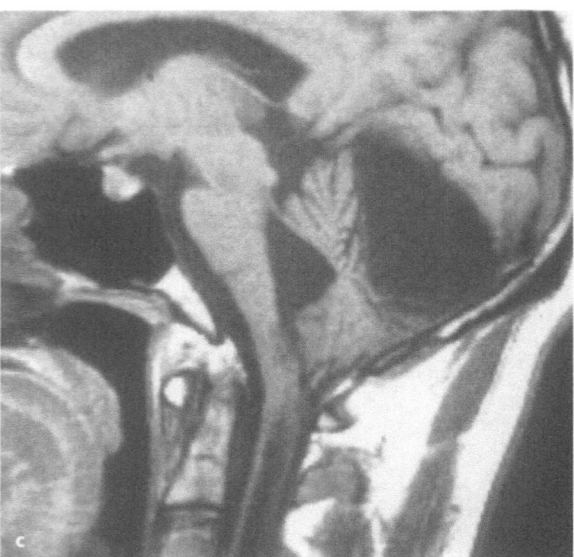

Fig. 3.49 a–c. This 26-year-old man reported a 5-year history of occipital pain. On examination, he had hemihypesthesia on his right side excluding his face, gait ataxia, and moderate weakness of his right upper limb. He could provoke dysesthesias in his neck by bending his head forward. **a, b** The T1-weighted MRI scans revealed a large arachnoid cyst in the posterior fossa on the left side, Chiari I malformation, and a syrinx which extended from C2 to the conus medullaris. There was no evidence of hydrocephalus. Cardiac-gated MRI demonstrated pulsations within the arachnoid cyst but no apparent communication to the subarachnoid space. At the foramen magnum, CSF flow was obstructed. The patient underwent cystoperitoneal shunting. Postoperatively, the patient was left unchanged. **c** The shunt led to a substantial decrease of the cyst volume, decompression of vermis and 4th ventricle, but free CSF passage at the foramen magnum was not achieved – presumably due to additional arachnoid scarring at that level. Therefore, foramen magnum decompression was recommended. For a number of years the patient was hesitant towards a second operation. Due to his progressive neurological symptoms, he finally decided to undergo this surgery at another hospital 4 years after the cystoperitoneal shunt. Since then, his neurological situation is stable

moval of the meningioma [10], whereas the other syrinx cavities were asymptomatic [2, 6, 19]. The syrinx collapsed or disappeared with removal of the tumor. There is no necessity for additional shunts of the syrinx similar to the strategy for CMI.

Of a series of more than 3000 posterior fossa tumors operated on in our department, we observed four patients with tonsillar herniation and syringomyelia; their neuroradiological features and postoperative results are presented in Figs. 3.46 to 3.49. All the cases listed in the literature and the four patients described here showed an obstruction of the foramen magnum, either because the tumor obstructed the foramen magnum itself or pushed the cerebellar tonsils down into it [18]. Arachnoid adhesions at the out-

flow foramina of the fourth ventricle, which are often encountered in patients with CMI, were present in two of our patients.

In each patient, establishment of open subarachnoid space at the foramen magnum with at least a partial tumor removal led to shrinkage or even complete disappearance of the syrinx with concomitant clinical improvement. The cystoperitoneal shunt (Fig. 3.49), however, was not sufficient to improve CSF passage, so that the syrinx was left unchanged and an additional foramen magnum procedure was required in this patient. In conclusion, no additional measures need to be taken to treat the syrinx once the tumor causing the CSF flow obstruction at the foramen magnum has been removed.

References

1. Banna M (1988) Syringomyelia in association with posterior fossa cysts. AJNR Am J Neuroradiol 9:867–873
2. Budrewicz S, Paradowski B, Podemskij R, Betlej M (1994) [Multiple intracranial meningiomas in a patient with asymptomatic syringomyelia.] Neurol Neurochir Pol 28:251–256
3. Cano G, Andersen M, Kutschbach P, Borden J, Saris S (1993) Hydromyelia associated with a posterior fossa cyst. Surg Neurol 40:512–515
4. Castellano F, Ruggiero G (1953) Meningiomas of the posterior fossa. Acta Radiol 104:1–157
5. Firsching R, Sanker P (1993) MRI follow-up in syringomyelia. Observations from twelve cases. Acta Neurochir (Wien) 123:206–207
6. Fukui K, Kito A, Iguchi I (1993) Asymptomatic syringomyelia associated with cerebellopontine angle meningioma – case report. Neurol Med Chir (Tokyo) 33:833–835
7. Hinokuma K, Ohama E, Oyanagi K, Kakita A, Kawai K, Ikuta F (1992) Syringomyelia. A neuropathological study of 18 autopsy cases. Acta Pathol Japonica 42:25–34
8. Jain R, Sawlani V, Phadke R, Kumar R (2000) Retrocerebellar arachnoid cyst with syringomyelia: a case report. Neurol India 48:81–83
9. Klekamp J, Samii M, Tatagiba M, Sepehrnia A (1995) Syringomyelia in association with tumours of the posterior fossa: pathophysiological considerations, based on observations on three related cases. Acta Neurochir (Wien) 137:38–43
10. Kosary IZ, Braham J, Shaked I, Tadmor R (1969) Cervical syringomyelia associated with occipital meningeoma. Neurology 19:1127–1130
11. Kumar C, Panagapoulos K, Kalbag RM, McAllister V (1987) Cerebellar astrocytoma presenting as a syringomyelic syndrome. Surg Neurol 27:187–190
12. Lee M, Rezai AR, Wisoff JH (1995) Acquired Chiari-I malformation and hydromyelia secondary to a giant craniopharyngioma. Pediatr Neurosurg 22:251–254
13. Modrego Pardo PJ, Lopez del Val J, Morales Asin F (1990) [Syringomyelia, posterior fossa cyst and acute respiratory distress.] Neurologia 5:336–337
14. Morioka T, Shono T, Nishio S, Yoshida K, Hasuo K, Fukui M (1995) Acquired Chiari I malformation and syringomyelia associated with bilateral chronic subdural hematoma. Case report. J Neurosurg 83:556–558
15. Sasaki J, Miura S, Onishi H (1995) [Syringomyelia associated with tentorial meningioma.] No To Shinkei 47:795–798
16. Sheehan JM, Jane JA (2000) Resolution of tonsillar herniation after supratentorial tumor resection: case report and review of the literature. Neurosurgery 47:233–235
17. Stein BM, Leeds NE, Taveras JM, Pool JL (1963) Meningiomas of the foramen magnum. J Neurosurg 20:740–751
18. Tachibana S, Harada K, Abe T, Yamada H, Yokota A (1995) Syringomyelia secondary to tonsillar herniation caused by posterior fossa tumors. Surg Neurol 43:470–477
19. Urasaki E, Soejima T, Yokota A, Matsuoka S (1989) [Association of asymptomatic syringomyelia with tentorial meningioma.] No Shinkei Geka 17:985–989
20. Williams B (1993) Surgery for hindbrain related syringomyelia. Adv Tech Stand Neurosurg 20:107–164

4 Syringomyelia Associated with Diseases of the Spinal Canal

This chapter will describe the management of patients with disorders of the spinal canal that have caused a syrinx. A major problem in this group may be the exact localization of this underlying pathology. Tumors can be easily visualized with gadolinium-enhanced MRI. All other entities described below may offer diagnostic problems, so that counseling of the patient, indication for surgery, and planning the surgical strategy may be quite difficult. Nevertheless, it is our firm belief that idiopathic syringomyelia does not exist. In each patient, it is possible to identify the cause of syrinx formation. Therefore, every effort should be made to demonstrate the underlying disorder.

Basically, the evaluation and treatment of these patients follow the same guidelines as outlined for patients with craniocervical disorders. Once a tumor has been excluded, clinical and neuroradiological evaluations have to be performed to demonstrate the exact extent and morphology of the syrinx and the presence of pathologies that may interfere with CSF circulation and/or spinal cord mobility, i.e., a tethered cord. Treatment should primarily aim at this underlying pathology. This chapter will describe how patients with syringomyelia related to spinal diseases should be approached in terms of diagnosis and management.

4.1
Syringomyelia Related to Spinal Arachnoid Scarring

The pathophysiology of syringomyelia related to trauma or arachnoiditis is still incompletely understood. Hematomyelia [8, 19, 65, 92, 104, 179, 185] related to spinal cord trauma and spinal cord ischemia [8, 31, 52, 107, 135, 139] due to arachnoiditis are generally believed to cause syringomyelia in these instances. However, hematomyelia and cord ischemia will lead to instant neurological problems, i.e., myelomalacia, and not to a slowly progressing syrinx after years of delay. Furthermore, the development of a syrinx after mild spinal trauma [92, 147] or a small area of arachnoiditis cannot be explained by either ischemia or hematomyelia of the spinal cord.

The relevance of arachnoid changes for changes of CSF flow, spinal cord mobility, and the development of syringomyelia in these instances is not widely re-

cognized. Shunting of the syrinx to either the subarachnoid, pleural, or peritoneal space is still widely accepted as the treatment of choice for patients with syringomyelia due to trauma or arachnoiditis [4, 121, 134, 165, 178, 188].

It has been known for a long time that spinal arachnoiditis or arachnoid scarring may be associated with syringomyelia [2, 3, 16, 21, 29, 33, 47, 66, 73, 124, 126, 133, 142, 143, 156, 194]. Many authors, for instance, report on arachnoid adhesions at the level of the spinal injury in patients with posttraumatic syringomyelia [19, 31, 46, 53, 104, 117, 143, 144, 156, 178]. However, the relevance of arachnoid scarring for neurological symptoms related to spinal cord tethering and syringomyelia has only recently become more appreciated.

Arachnoid scarring may be caused by a variety of mechanisms. Inflammatory reactions of the arachnoid due to bacterial, fungal, or viral infections [38, 85], chemical substances such as contrast media [34, 69, 162] or breakdown products of blood after subarachnoid hemorrhages [89, 119], or due to mechanical irritation related to trauma, degenerative diseases of the spine, scoliosis, kyphotic deformities, or instabilities [122] can lead to arachnoid scarring in a focal, circumscribed area of the spinal canal [25, 27, 28, 37, 41, 46, 47, 50, 54, 58, 67, 71, 88, 98, 100, 106, 146, 149, 162]. Another important cause of arachnoid scarring is intradural surgery. Any surgical intervention in the spinal subarachnoid space may lead to disturbances of CSF flow and even spinal cord tethering at the site of surgery. Depending on the cause of arachnoid pathology, the scarring may be limited to a very circumscribed area of just a few millimeters or may extend over several spinal segments. The most severe forms of spinal arachnoiditis are reported after tuberculous meningitis [38, 52, 59, 116, 139, 171].

Even with a carefully documented patient history, the cause of spinal arachnoid scarring cannot be clarified in each individual patient. The most likely explanation in such patients may still be posttraumatic arachnoid scarring, even though the patient does not recall such an incident. Minor accidents may cause focal arachnoid scarring due to small tears or hemorrhages from little blood vessels inside the arachnoid layer without any neurological symptoms at the time of trauma [190].

Table 4.1. Patient data for spinal arachnoid scarring and syringomyelia *Interval* time span between trauma or – if known – the inflammatory process leading to arachnoid scarring – and the development of symptomatic syringomyelia

	Posttraumatic scarring	Postinflammatory scarring
n	68	86
Male:Female	2.9:1	1:1.1
Age	45+13 years	44+15 years
History	51+70 months	48+75 months
Interval	107+106 months	109+136 months
Follow up	29+38 months	26+31 months

For the purpose of this book, we suggest the terms posttraumatic syringomyelia (PTS) for patients with spinal arachnoid scarring and a history of spinal trauma at that level and postinflammatory syringomyelia (PIS) for patients with spinal arachnoid scarring but no such history.

4.1.1
Clinical Presentation

Our series of patients with spinal arachnoid pathologies consists of 154 patients. In 68 patients, arachnoid scarring resulted from trauma, whereas 86 patients developed scarring as a result of an inflammatory reaction. Except for differences in sex distribution, there was no statistical difference between both groups of patients in terms of age, history, or follow-up (Table 4.1).

4.1.1.1
Posttraumatic Syringomyelia

Posttraumatic syringomyelia requires a traumatic lesion of the arachnoid. It does not necessitate spinal cord trauma. Tethering of the spinal cord and CSF flow obstruction due to arachnoid scarring or spinal canal stenosis [122, 123, 136] may then cause progressive syringomyelia. However, severe forms of spinal trauma will lead to a combination of soft tissue, bony, leptomeningeal and spinal cord lesions in various combinations. If spinal cord tissue is damaged severely, a necrotic area may result in a defect inside the spinal cord, i.e., myelomalacia. As a general rule, the extent of myelomalacia is restricted to the spinal level of the cord injury and does not progress (Fig. 4.1). PTS, however, begins at the level of the injury and may progress from there in either direction (Fig. 4.2). Clinically, myelomalacia is almost always associated with instant symptoms related to the extent of spinal cord damage but without further clinical progression.

In syringomyelia, progressive clinical symptoms start to develop after an interval of typically several years (Table 4.1). The neurological distribution of these new symptoms are related to the spinal representation of the syrinx. Especially after severe spinal cord trauma, myelomalacia and syringomyelia may coexist [56] (Fig. 4.2). Therefore, the term posttraumatic cystic myelopathy was introduced which may be separated into a stationary, i.e., myelomalacia, and a progressive, i.e., syringomyelia, form.

The first description of a posttraumatic cystic lesion of the spinal cord was given by Bastian [20] in 1867. In 1898, Cushing [36] described two patients with hematomyelia and supposed that residual symptoms of these patients were related to cyst formation after resorption of the hematoma. Lloyd [97] postulated as early as 1894 a pathophysiological relationship between posttraumatic arachnoid scarring and cyst formation. Collier [35] explained posttraumatic arachnopathy on the basis of small hemorrhages into the arachnoid or the subarachnoid space in 1916.

The incidence of PTS is not precisely known. About 2% of patients with spinal cord trauma will develop new neurological symptoms with each ongoing year for a number of possible reasons, such as spinal instability, spinal cord compression, or syringomyelia [122, 123, 145]. Before the era of MRI, the incidence of PTS was assumed according to clinical and autopsy data somewhere between 1.25% and 8% [14, 17, 46, 62,

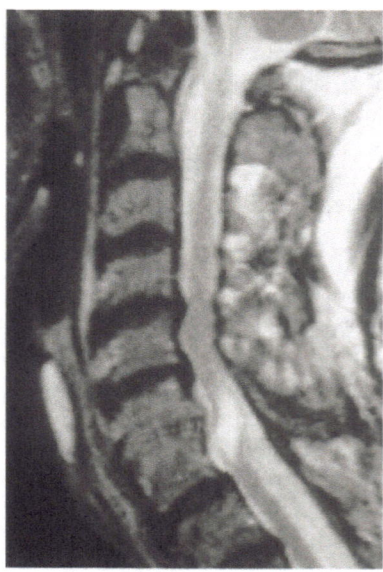

Fig. 4.1. This T2-weighted sagittal MRI scan of a 59-year-old man shows a myelomalacia at C6/7 due to an operated traumatic disc prolapse at this level 9 years ago. Fortunately, the patient recovered from an incomplete spinal cord lesion. At the time of this scan he complained about dysesthesias in both arms. There were no signs of cervical myelopathy. No surgery was recommended

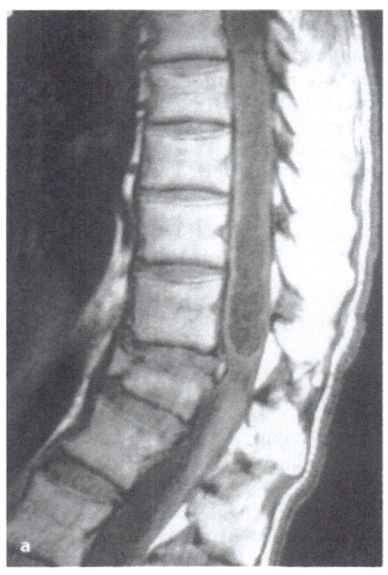 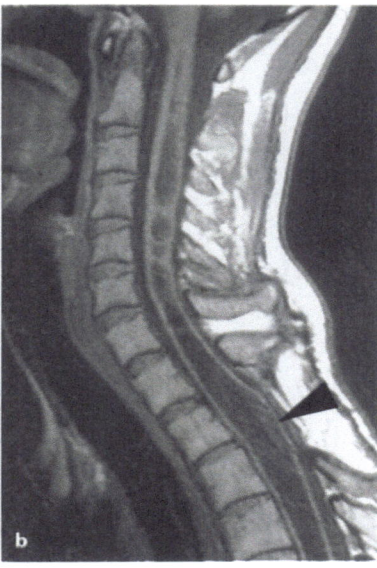

Fig. 4.2 a, b. These T1-weighted MRI scans of a 24-year-old woman were performed 16 years after a complete spinal cord lesion at Th12. **a** There is evidence of a small myelomalacic cyst at this level and kyphotic angulation due to the Th12 fracture. A syrinx extends from Th11 to C3. At Th2 a syringoperitoneal shunt had been placed at another institution with no effect on syrinx size (*arrow*) (**b**). There were no progressive symptoms reported. Therefore, no surgery was recommended

135, 141, 177, 181]. With routine MRI examinations of patients with spinal cord trauma, Backe et al. [12] gave a figure of 51% for patients with posttraumatic spinal cord cysts after an average interval of 1.6 years. Similar figures were given by several other authors [24, 122, 145, 154]. However, no distinction was made between syringomyelia and myelomalacia, and patients with spinal trauma without affection of the spinal cord did not enter these studies.

There is no clear-cut relationship between spinal level of the trauma and the likelihood for PTS to develop [12]. Several studies described syringomyelia to be more common after thoracic injuries [18, 70, 123, 147, 172, 177, 189], whereas others found syringomyelia more often associated with a cervical trauma [46, 129, 154, 192]. Discrepancies between older and more recent studies on this point may be explained by a reduced mortality rate of patients after cervical injuries.

We have seen 68 patients with PTS at an average age of 45±13 years. Males predominated by a factor of 2.9:1. Thirty-six percent developed a syrinx after a cervical trauma, 53% after thoracic, and 11% after conus

medullaris injuries. Compared with postinflammatory arachnoid scarring, there was a significantly higher percentage of patients with cervical scarring and fewer thoracic cases (Table 4.2).

Seventeen patients were not operated on as they did not demonstrate progressive neurological symptoms (Figs. 4.2 to 4.4). The remaining 51 patients underwent 76 operations. The mean interval between trauma and development of symptomatic syringomyelia was extremely variable [7, 17, 46, 50, 70, 84, 91, 94, 123, 135, 141, 147, 148, 154, 177, 184, 189]. For one patient, it took 38 years before the first clinical signs of a posttraumatic syrinx were observed. Another patient showed signs of progressive neurological deterioration 2 weeks after the injury. Typically, several years (mean 9 years and 9 months) elapsed before a syrinx became symptomatic (Table 4.1). Some authors described a shorter interval after complete spinal cord injuries [99, 129] whereas others denied such a correlation [177]. After clinical symptoms of syringomyelia had started, it took another 51±70 months until patients presented to us.

A complete spinal cord injury preceded the syrinx in 24% of cases, an incomplete lesion in 40%, while 36% developed PTS without an initial cord injury. This distribution is similar to the observations by Barnett and Jousse [17] who described PTS to occur more often after incomplete than complete lesions, whereas other authors made the opposite observation [46]. Most authors, however, could not find a correlation between severity of trauma and occurrence of PTS [70, 129, 147]. Posttraumatic arachnopathy is the key for the development of a syrinx and not the amount of cord damage due to the initial trauma. Several authors noted that a syrinx may develop even without an initi-

Table 4.2. Spinal level of arachnoid scarring for patients with postinflammatory and posttraumatic syringomyelia

Spinal level	Postinflammatory scarring	Posttraumatic scarring
Cervical	16%	36%
Thoracic	72%	53%
Conus medullaris	12%	11%

Chi-square-test: *P*=0.0055

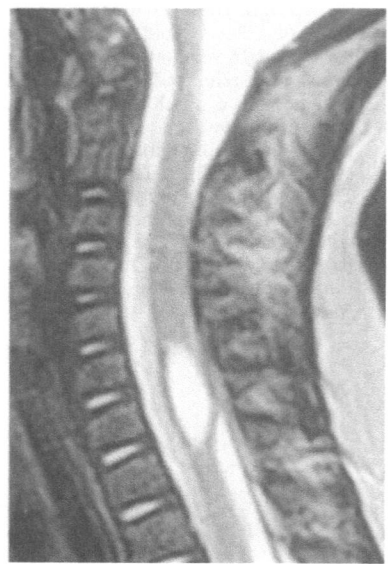

Fig. 4.3. This T2-weighted MRI scan of a 3-year-old girl shows a posttraumatic syrinx at the C7/Th1 related to birth trauma. Since birth the girl has suffered from delayed motoric development in her legs but has continued to improve her neurological function ever since. Repeated MRI scans showed no progression of the syrinx. The patient is followed clinically for three years since this scan was taken. Surgery will be recommended if progressive neurological symptoms develop

Fig. 4.4 a, b. The T1-weighted MRI scans of this 53-year-old woman demonstrate a posttraumatic syrinx after a vertebral body fracture at L1 (*arrow*) 24 years ago. The patient acquired an incomplete conus lesion with slight urinary dysfunctions and sensory deficits. Otherwise, her neurological examination is normal with no progression. The syrinx extends from Th12 (**a**) to the foramen magnum (**b**)

▼

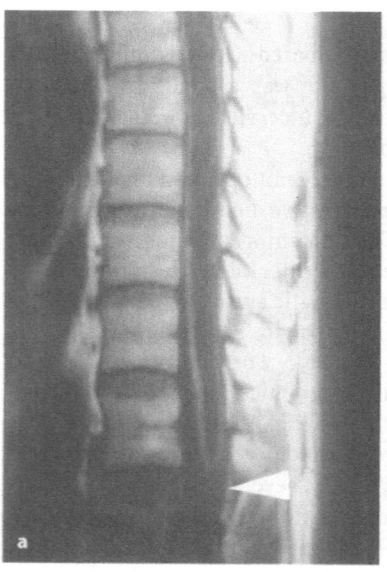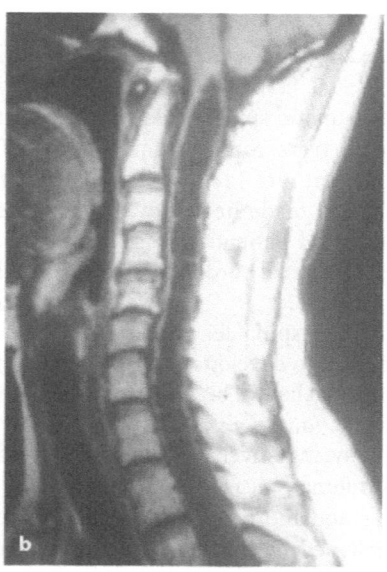

al cord injury [81, 92]. A leptomeningeal hemorrhage may be sufficient to cause scarring and syringomyelia [190]. It has been suggested that bulging of the yellow ligament toward the spinal cord may lead to such leptomeningeal injuries [190].

PTS started in most instances with progressive motor weakness (30% of patients) or pain (28% of patients). Gait problems (12%) and dysesthesias (16%) were encountered less often [123]. Sensory problems (9%), sphincter disturbances (2%), swallowing problems (1%) [177], or cardiorespiratory dysfunctions (1%) [5, 103] were rare initial presentations.

Fifty-one patients demonstrated clinical signs of neurological progression [6, 17, 68, 129, 135, 138, 165, 177, 178]. The major complaint at the time of surgery was local pain or pain radiating into dermatomes representing the spinal levels of the syrinx for 36% of patients and gait problems for 23%. Dysesthesias (18%) and motor weakness (15%) were less often considered to be the main clinical problem. Sensory deficits (4%), sphincter disturbances (1%), swallowing problems (1%), or cardiorespiratory dysfunctions (1%) rarely predominated the clinical picture. In the literature, pain and sensory deficits are usually considered to be the most common symptoms, whereas motor weakness tends to develop at a later stage (Table 4.3) [7, 17, 99, 104, 123, 129, 135, 148, 177, 189].

Table 4.3. Clinical symptoms of patients with posttraumatic and postinflammatory arachnoid scarring and syringomyelia

Symptom		Posttraumatic syringomyelia		Postinflammatory syringomyelia	
Pain		89%		63%	
Sensory disturbance		100%		74%	
Dysesthesias		78%		47%	
Gait ataxia	Unable to walk	100%	44%	74%	26%
Motor weakness		78%		53%	
Sphincter disturbance	Catheter dependent	56%	11%	37%	16%
Cardiorespiratory disturbance		3%		3%	
Swallowing disturbance		11%		1%	

4.1.1.2
Postinflammatory Syringomyelia

For 86 patients, spinal arachnoid pathology could not be related to a particular traumatic incident (Fig. 4.5). The underlying process that had caused this inflammatory reaction could be identified in 34 patients: nine patients provided a history of meningitis, three patients had suffered from spondylodiscitis or spinal abscess formation, 17 patients had undergone intradural surgical procedures, three peridural anesthesia, and two patients had suffered a subarachnoid hemorrhage. For 52 patients, however, the cause of arachnoid scarring remained obscure, i.e., 60% of patients developed symptomatic syringomyelia without any preceding clinical problem. One may speculate whether minor traumatic accidents, which the patient did not recall, might have been responsible. As even a minor trauma may cause arachnoid scarring and symptoms of PTS usually appear after several years, this seems to be the most likely explanation. Nagai et al. [108] even described a family with two siblings suffering from spinal arachnoiditis and syringomyelia.

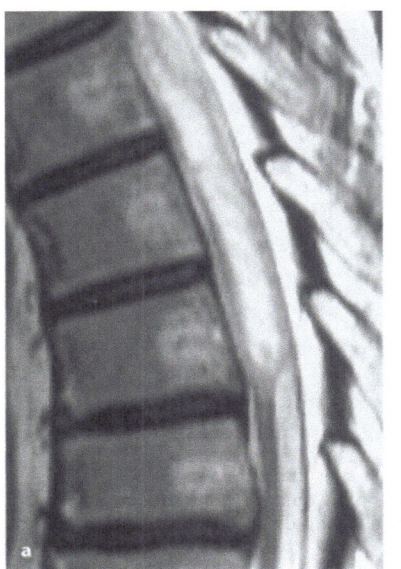 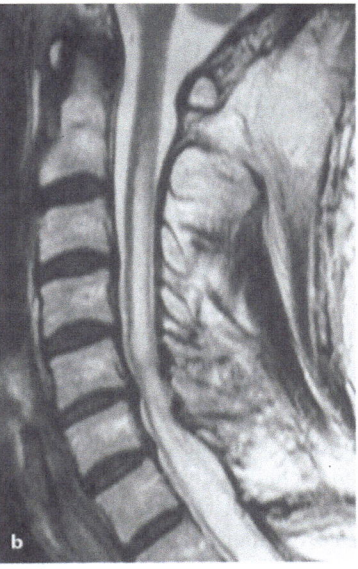 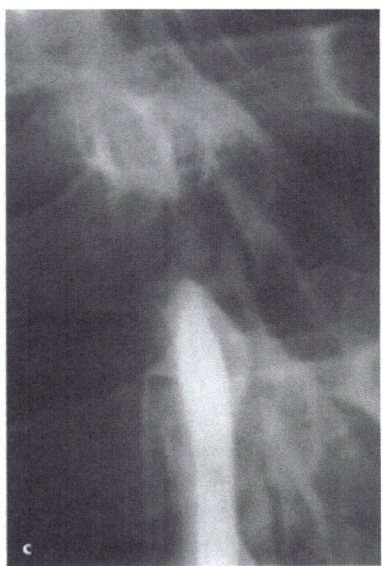

Fig. 4.5 a–c. This patient with postinflammatory syringomyelia between C2 and Th5 demonstrates the different syrinx morphology at the site of the scarring compared to the opposite end of the syrinx in T2-weighted MRI scans. **a** The arachnoid scarring is located at the lower pole of the syrinx. Here, the spinal cord abruptly changes its diameter due to some compressive effect of the arachnoid scar. The posterior surface of the spinal cord appears to be in direct contact with the dura suggesting fixation of the cord in an arachnoid scar. **b** At the upper pole of the syrinx there is a gradual decrease in syrinx and spinal cord diameter. **c** With ascending myelography, a subtotal block of contrast passage was determined at Th5/6. Due to progressive gait ataxia surgery was indicated

Forty-two patients underwent 65 operations, whereas 44 patients were not operated on as they did not demonstrate clinical signs of neurological progression. For 16%, the arachnoid pathology was located in the cervical spine, for 72% in the thoracic area, and for 12% arachnoid scarring was situated at the level of the conus medullaris. Compared with posttraumatic arachnoid scarring, this distribution was significantly different in favor of thoracic postinflammatory scarring (Chi-square-test: $P=0.0055$).

The average interval between inflammatory reaction and onset of symptoms related to syringomyelia was just over 9 years and similar to observations for posttraumatic patients. In one patient, it took 50 years for the syrinx to develop and to produce clinical manifestations [59]. Once symptoms had appeared, it took another 4 years on average before the diagnosis was made and the patient was sent to a neurosurgeon.

The most common symptoms at the beginning of clinical manifestations of syringomyelia were gait ataxia (28%), back pain radiating to dermatomes of the syrinx (23%), dysesthesias (21%), and motor weakness (16%). Forty-two patients demonstrated clinical progression of neurological symptoms [6, 15, 17, 59, 68, 106, 119, 138, 165] so that surgery was indicated. During such a progressive course, however, the clinical picture only changed in terms of severity of particular symptoms. At the time of surgery, patients still reported those symptoms as their major complaint with which syringomyelia had started to be clinically noticed.

Apart from the fact that a significant number of patients with PTS develop syringomyelia on top of a complete or incomplete spinal cord lesion with instant neurological symptoms, the clinical course of patients with PIS or PTS is not very different. The worse preoperative neurological status of posttraumatic patients (preoperative Karnofsky score 54±19 and 69±18, respectively; t-test: $P < 0.0001$) is related to the severity of spinal cord trauma and not to different dynamics of syrinx progression (Table 4.3) [47, 80, 83, 98, 165].

4.1.2
Neuroradiology

Once a Chiari malformation, other pathologies at the foramen magnum or a tumor have been excluded, the entire spinal canal should be carefully examined for signs of CSF flow obstruction or spinal cord tethering. In posttraumatic patients, the level of CSF flow obstruction will be at the site of the trauma with a combination of arachnoid scarring, spinal stenosis related to kyphotic angulations or fracture dislocations [14, 17, 31, 46, 57, 87, 91, 104, 105, 114, 115, 117, 122, 123, 132, 144, 178, 189]. The diagnostic difficulties to distinguish

myelomalacia and syringomyelia have already been mentioned.

In patients without a history of trauma, a number of medullary lesions may be mistaken for syringomyelia, such as cystic intramedullary tumors, glioependymal cysts of the conus medullaris, medullary changes associated with arteriovenous fistulas, or hematomyelia. A cystic intramedullary tumor will usually take up some contrast in the wall of the cyst. The cyst fluid tends to have a higher protein content than a syrinx and gives a less hypodense signal in a T1-weighted MRI image (Fig. 4.6). Finally, flow phenomena are detected less regularly in a cystic tumor than a syrinx [101, 168, 169]. Depending on the time delay after the hemorrhage, hematomyelia may disclose different signal intensities on T1- and T2-weighted images. Hematomyelia may occur after trauma or due to a spontaneous intramedullary hemorrhage from an intramedullary tumor or arteriovenous malformation (Fig. 4.7). Traumatic hematomyelia does not provide diagnostic difficulties as the clinical history will provide the necessary information. Spontaneous hemorrhages of an intramedullary tumor require a certain amount of vascularization of the tumor (Fig. 4.7). Therefore, enhancement of the tumor after gadolinium application can be ex-

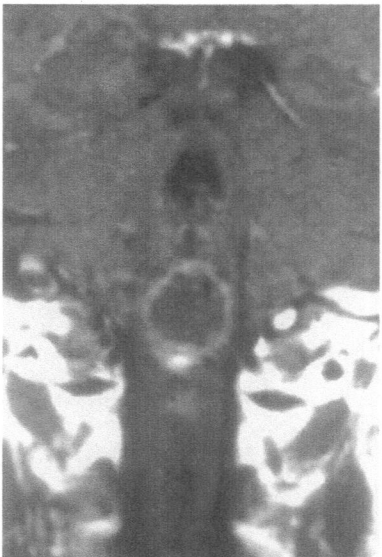

Fig. 4.6. This 37-year-old woman with neurofibromatosis type II presented with swallowing disturbances and gait ataxia due to sensory problems on the left side. The coronal T1-weighted MRI shows a round hypodense lesion of the medulla oblongata at the foramen magnum. The margin of this lesion enhances with contrast. The lesion was operated and the histological diagnosis was pilocytic astrocytoma. The patient did not acquire new deficits from surgery and recovered in terms of gait and swallowing over a period of 3 months. She is free of local recurrence for 10 years but had to undergo further surgeries for other tumors since then

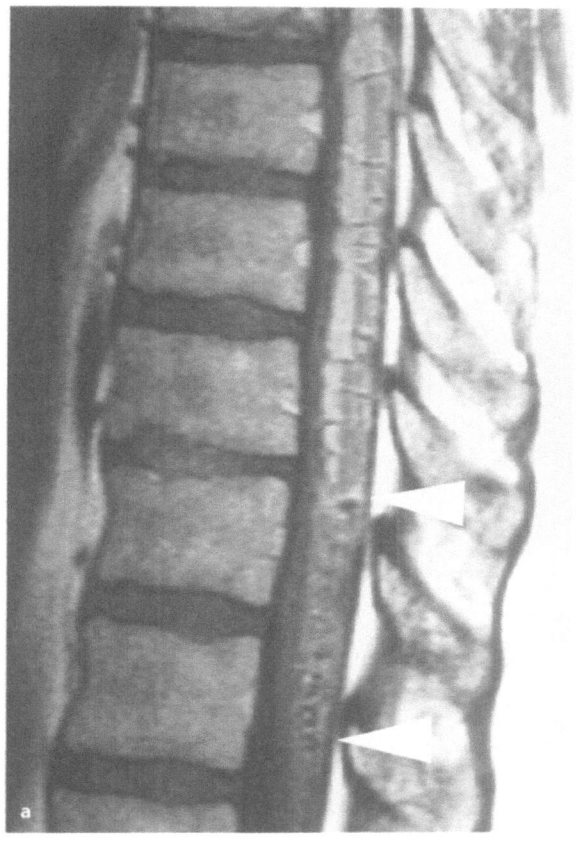

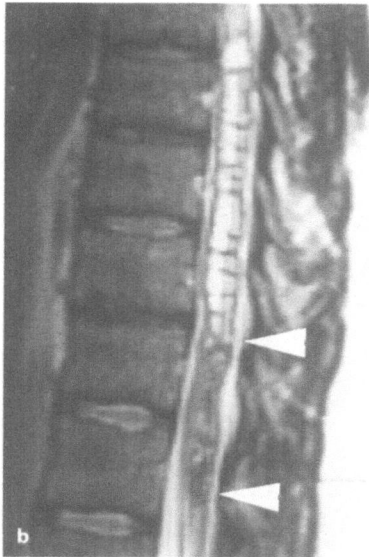

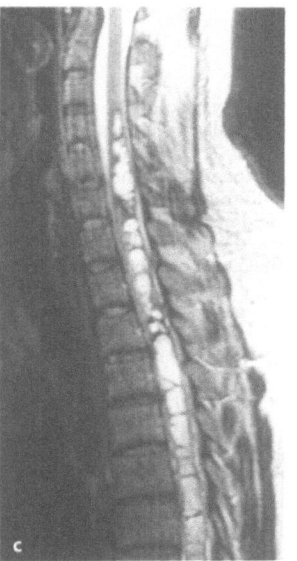

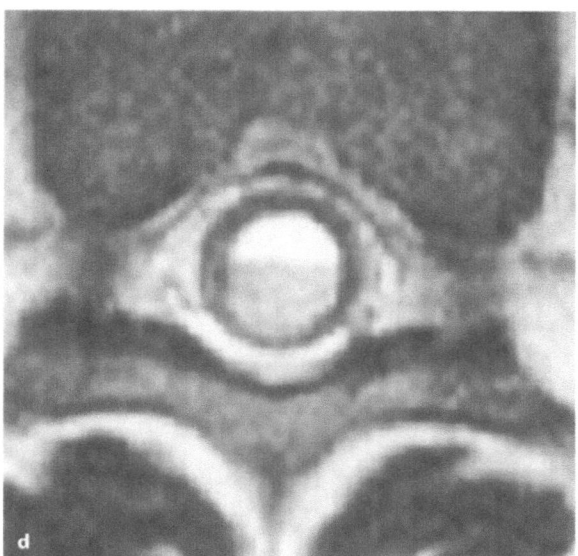

Fig. 4.7 a–d. This 36-year-old man presented with a history of acute onset of paraparesis and sphincter problems. The sagittal T1- (**a**) and T2-weighted (**b**, **c**) MRI scans show an intramedullary astrocytoma at the level of Th11/12 (*arrows*) in combination with a spinal arteriovenous malformation and a septated syrinx extending up to C4. The acute exacerbation of symptoms was caused by an intramedullary hemorrhage, i.e. hematomyelia. The cervical part of this syrinx reveals patches of hemosiderin in its wall (**c**). The axial T2-weighted image displays the sedimented blood in the dependent part of the cyst (**d**)

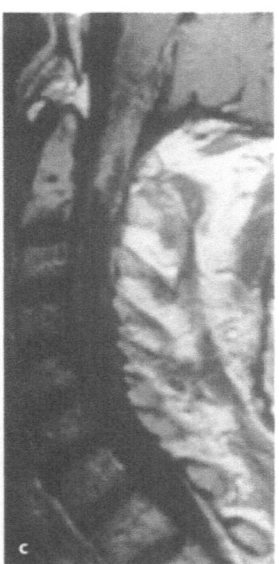

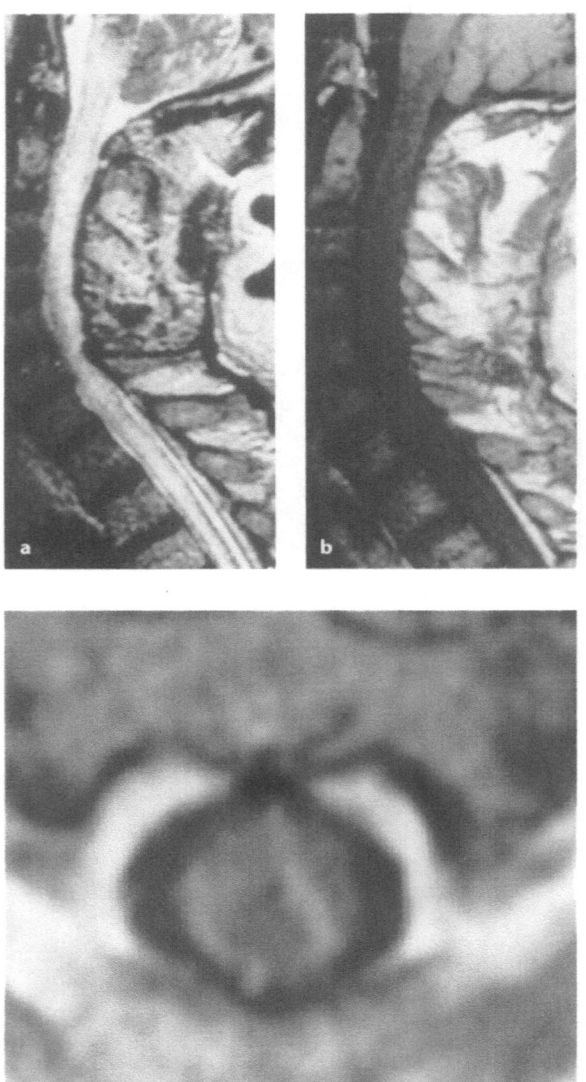

Fig. 4.8 a–d. The MRI scans of this 60-year-old man with acute progressive tetraparesis show the medullary changes associated with a dural arteriovenous fistula. **a** There is marked spinal cord edema with a CSF like signal intensity of the cord in the T2-weighted image in the cervicothoracic cord up to the medulla oblongata. **b** The T1-weighted scan without gadolinium shows the corresponding finding. **c, d** After gadolinium administration, a patchy and delayed uptake can be seen at the border of the pathology almost suggesting a cystic tumor in the sagittal and axial plane. These features represent the Foix-Alajouanine syndrome

pected. Figures 4.8 and 4.9 provide examples for rare cystic lesions of the spinal cord related to dural arteriovenous fistulas and glioependymal conus cysts, respectively. If no trauma occurred and very slow contrast enhancement is seen at the margin of the lesion on MRI, an arteriovenous malformation should be suspected (Fig. 4.8). A glioependymal cyst does not take up contrast in the cyst wall. Radiologically, it may be impossible to differentiate such a cyst from a syrinx. Missing signs of CSF flow obstructions and no ascension of the cyst in serial examinations may be the only clues for the differential diagnosis (Fig. 4.9).

Another group of patients presents with small slit-like cysts of the thoracic cord and unspecific back pain (Figs. 4.10, 4.11). Whether these are just widenings of the central canal with no pathological significance or the early stage of a syrinx can hardly be decided with a single examination. Whenever in doubt as to the nature of a cystic process in the spinal cord, repeated examinations of the area may disclose its dynamics and help in the differential diagnosis.

Once the diagnosis of syringomyelia has been made and a tumor excluded, the site of the CSF flow obstruction has to be determined. In posttraumatic patients, most syringomyelia cysts develop rostral to the arachnoid pathology (Table 4.4). Holmes [72] already noticed this in his famous lecture in 1915. In patients with a syrinx above and below the area of scarring,

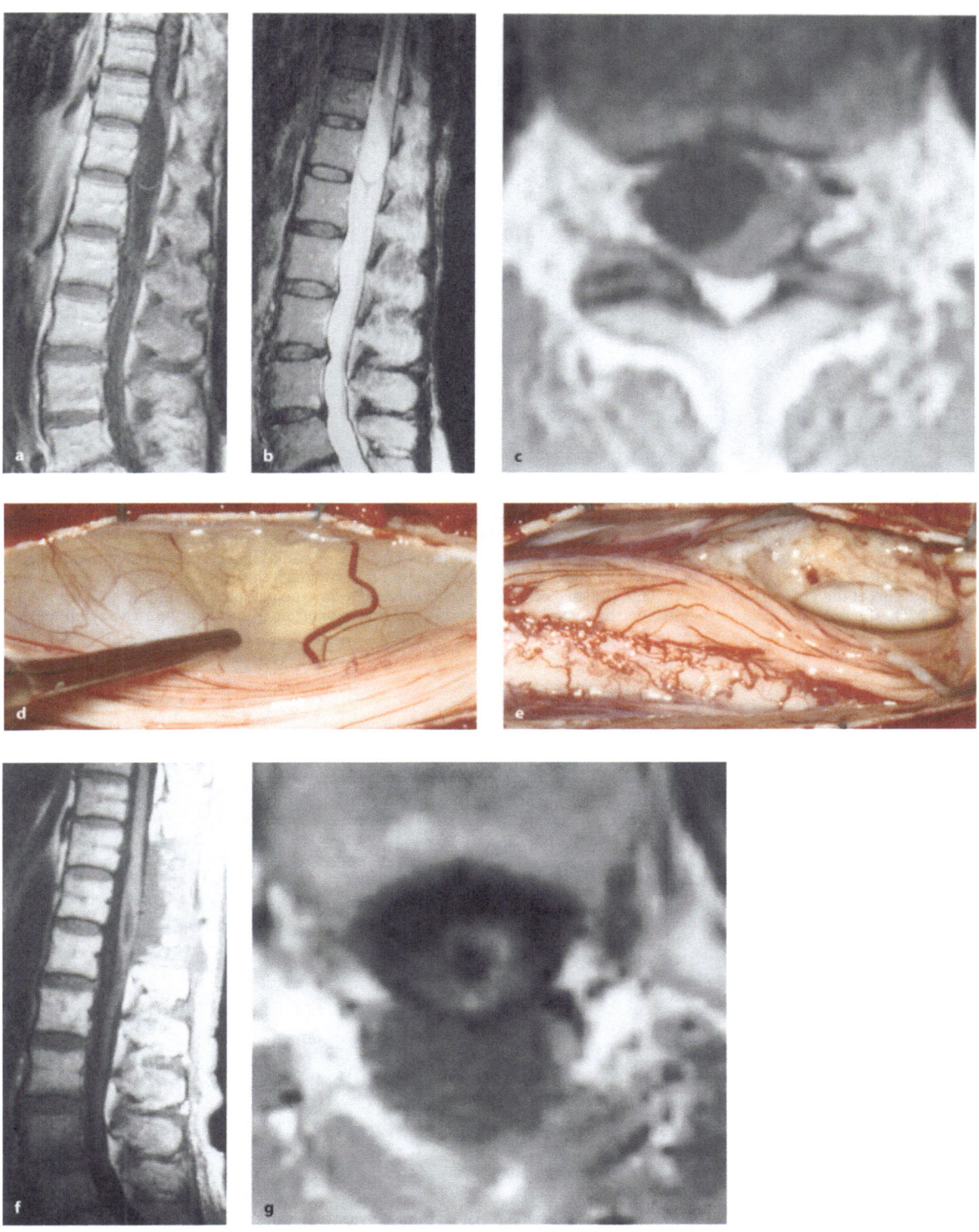

Fig. 4.9 a–g. This 66-year-old woman demonstrated motor deficits of her L4 and L5 nerve roots on the right side. Sensory disturbances, sphincter problems or pain were not reported. **a** The T1-weighted MRI scan shows a cystic process in the ventral part of the conus medullaris at the Th11/12 level. **b** The T2-weighted image clearly demonstrates the intramedullary loca- tion of this cyst. **c** The axial T1-weighted image demonstrates the eccentric position of this lesion on the right side. **d** This intraoperative view displays the translucent wall of a glioependy- mal cyst. **e** The cyst was fenestrated and part of the wall ex- cised. Postoperatively, motor weakness improved and the cord started to reestablish its normal morphology (**f, g**)

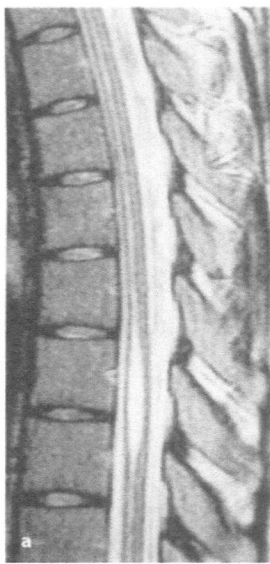
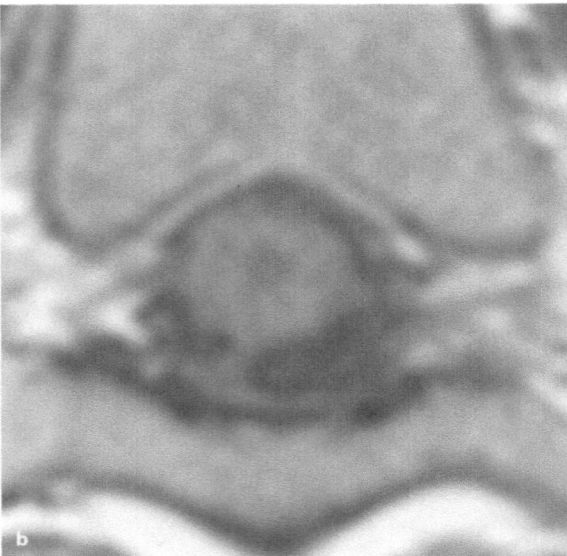
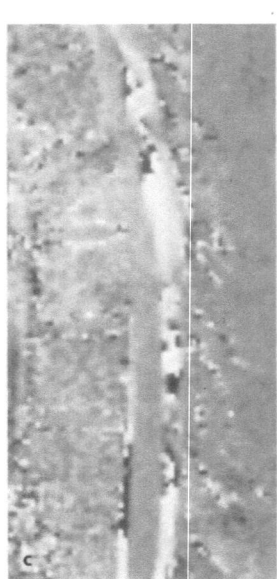

Fig. 4.10 a–c. This 22-year-old woman complained about uncharacteristic back pain provoked by physical activities. Her neurological examination was normal except for some hypesthesia on her trunk which was inconsistent on repetitive testings. **a** The T2-weighted MRI scan shows a small centrally located syrinx at the Th6/7 level consistent with a dilated central canal. **b** The T2-weighted axial scan illustrates the central position of this cyst. Neither phase contrast cine-MRI (**c**) nor ascending myelography were able to establish an area of CSF flow obstruction. Only repeated MRI examinations over the next months or even years and a clinical control may provide further information to distinguish this slit-like dilatation of the central canal, which may have no pathological significance, from a true syrinx that may expand and produce progressive symptoms

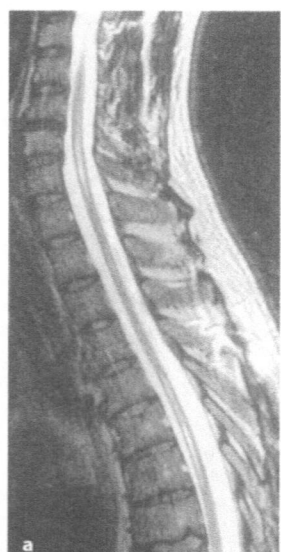
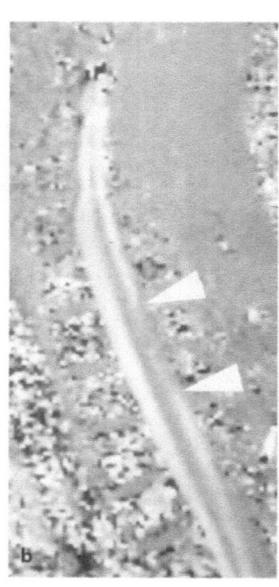
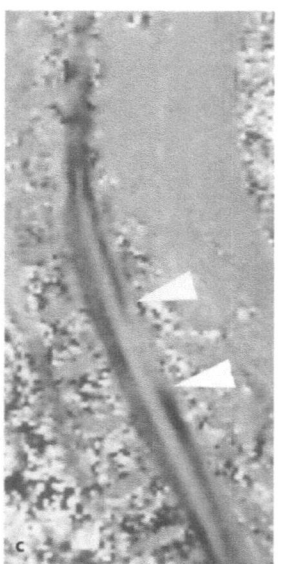

Fig. 4.11 a–c. This 45-year-old man complained about slight neck pain radiating to his left shoulder. The neurological examination disclosed no further signs or symptoms. **a** The T2-weighted MRI scan demonstrated two slit-like dilatations of the central canal area between C6 and C7 and between Th4 and Th7. The systolic (**b**) and diastolic (**c**) phase of the phase contrast cine-MRI display a missing flow signal in the posterior subarachnoid space (*arrows*) indicating an area of CSF flow disturbance at Th1/2. The patient is followed clinically. If neurological symptoms appear surgery at this level will be recommended

Table 4.4. Orientation of the syrinx in relation to spinal level of arachnoid scarring

Orientation	Posttraumatic syringomyelia	Postinflammatory syringomyelia
Rostral	38%	40%
Caudal	21%	24%
Both	41%	36%
Syringobulbia	8%	5%

the rostral part usually is more extensive and of greater caliber [17, 26, 44, 46, 105, 135, 145, 192].

Compared with PTS, patients with postinflammatory scarring and syringomyelia share the same relationship between spinal level of scarring and orientation of the syrinx: in the majority of patients, the lower part of the cyst is the site of the arachnoid pathology [3].

Another clue, where to look for an area of CSF flow obstruction can be obtained from a carefully taken clinical history and a study of the shape of the cyst. As a general rule, a syrinx starts to develop at the spinal level of the arachnopathy and extends from there rostrally and/or caudally. Therefore, it can be assumed that the caliber of the syrinx will be largest in the area close to the scarring and gradually subside towards the opposite end of the cyst. Consequently, it can be expected that the first clinical signs of a patient with a postinflammatory syrinx will be related to the spinal level of or close to the area of the arachnopathy [43, 46, 80, 88]. With further progress of syrinx and clinical signs, radiological extent and neurological symptoms then may start to affect additional spinal segments in an ascending or descending manner, depending which direction the syrinx has taken. Serial examinations, thus, may disclose the spinal level of scarring. With a syrinx extending rostrally, the arachnopathy will be found at the caudal end of the cyst and vice versa.

Radiological signs of a locally restricted, focal area of arachnoid scarring may be difficult to detect on standard MRI scans. Arachnoid scarring may lead to adhesions of the spinal cord to the dura (Figs. 4.5, 4.12), abrupt changes in spinal cord caliber (Figs. 4.5, 4.13), or signal irregularities of the spinal cord contour (Figs. 4.14, 4.15). In a patient with two separate syrinx cavities, the arachnoid pathology will most likely be found at the spinal level between both cavities (Figs. 4.11, 4.16). T2-weighted MRI images are the preferred method to detect these radiological signs.

Additionally, dynamic imaging with phase contrast cine-MRI can be employed to search for an area of CSF flow obstruction as an indirect indicator of a focal area of arachnoid pathology (Fig. 4.11). Such images will also demonstrate flow phenomena inside the syrinx itself [11, 49, 79, 150, 151, 152, 168, 169], which even tend to be more profound than the surrounding subarachnoid space [30] (Fig. 4.17). The fastest flow velo-

Fig. 4.12 a–c. This 40-year-old woman presented with left leg pain and sensory disturbances related to surgery on a lipoma of her left thigh. Her diagnostic examinations included this T2-weighted MRI scan displaying a small syrinx at Th10 and Th11 and posterior displacement of the conus medullaris suggesting arachnoid scarring at Th11/12 (**a**). Phase contrast cine-MRI demonstrated a corresponding CSF flow obstruction at that level in the systolic (**b**) and diastolic phase (**c**). As this lesion is currently not symptomatic the patient is observed clinically

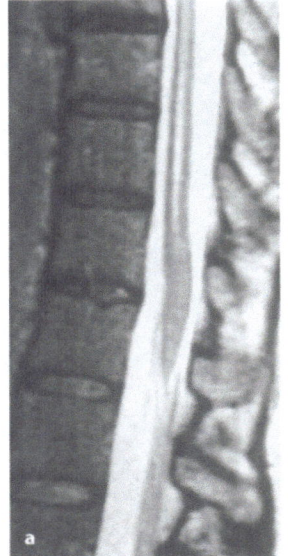 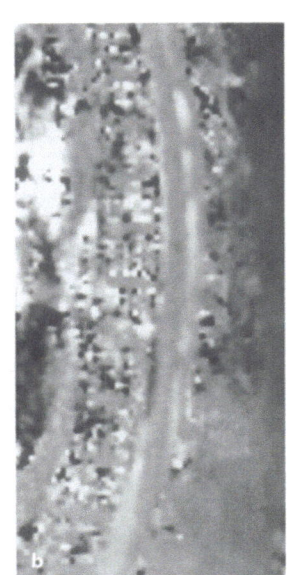 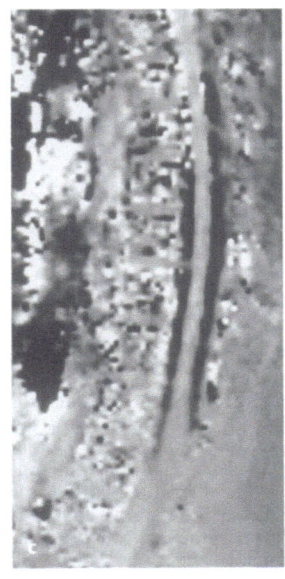

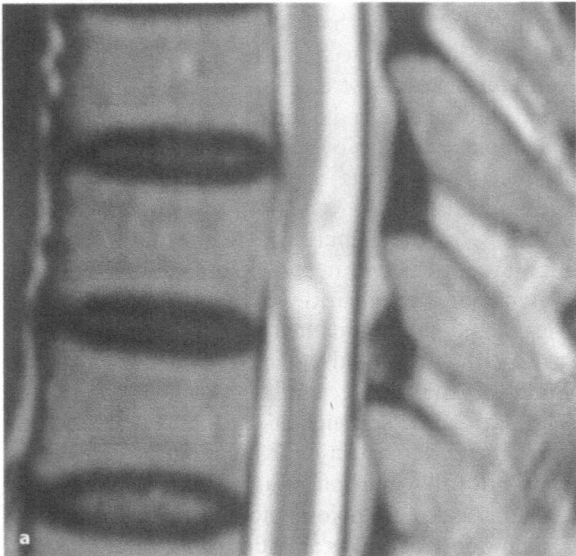

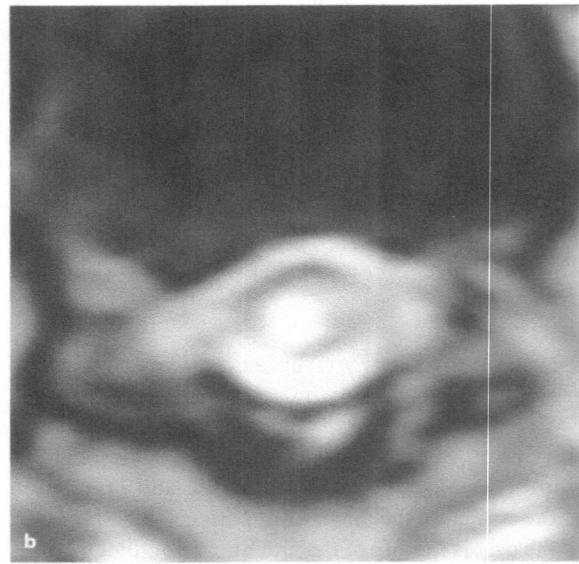

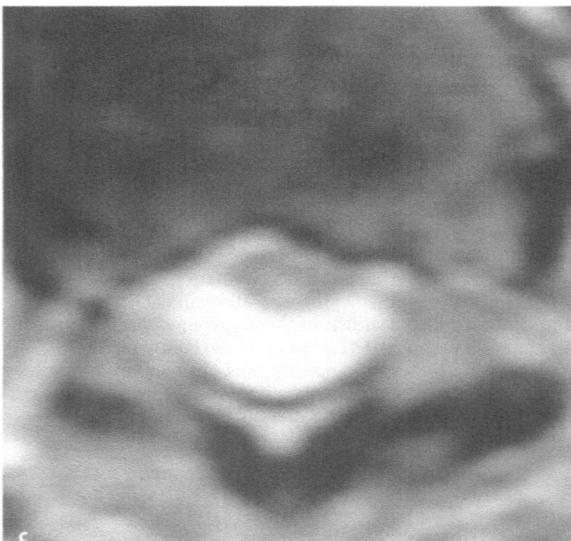

Fig. 4.13 a–c. This 69-year-old man complained about progressive gait ataxia and a sensory level at Th10. **a** The T2-weighted MRI scan show a syrinx at the level of Th8/9 and compression of the spinal cord from posterior at Th8. **b** The axial scan at Th9 displays the syrinx. **c** At Th8 the compression of the cord becomes evident. At surgery, arachnoid scarring forming a pouch was discovered at this level. CSF flow was established and the syrinx collapsed. The patient is well 2 years after surgery with improved gait

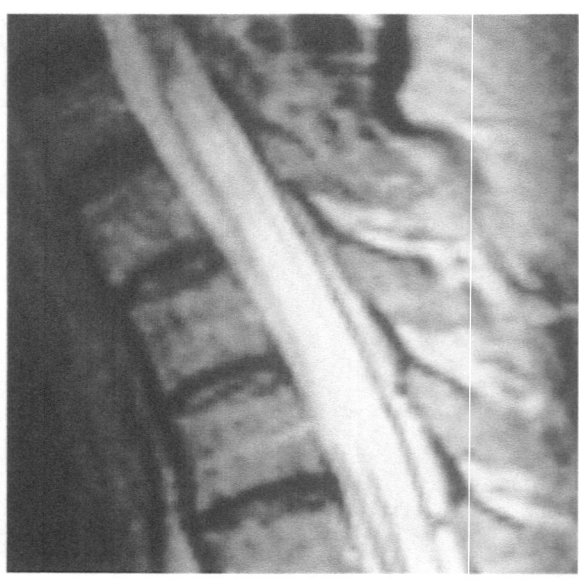

Fig. 4.14. This T2-weighted MRI scan of a 58-year-old man with gait ataxia, a sensory level at Th7 and dysesthesias of his trunk displays a syrinx between Th3 and Th6. At Th6 the caliber of the spinal cord changes abruptly. The posterior margin of the cord is ill defined at Th5 and Th6 compared to the other spinal levels. At surgery, an arachnoid scar acting like a constrictive band was found at Th6. After dissection of this scar and establishment of a free CSF passage the syrinx collapsed completely. Postoperatively, the syrinx remained collapsed until the last follow up visit 4 years later. However, the patient still complains about very irritating dysesthesias

cities inside the syrinx will be detected close to the area of scarring, whereas no flow or a significant flow reduction will be detected at this level in the subarachnoid space.

Such flow studies may not only disclose the area of underlying pathology in a patient with a syrinx. They also may be of prognostic significance [30]. Tobimatsu et al. [169] found a good correlation between syrinx flow velocities and clinical signs of progression. It may also help to distinguish between myelomalacia and syringomyelia in posttraumatic cases. A myelomalacia will not demonstrate profound flow phenomena in contrast to a posttraumatic syrinx [101].

As flow velocities and patterns in the subarachnoid space vary considerably according to the spinal level [45, 48, 96, 140, 168] considerable experience is required not to misinterpret such flow studies. In the cervical canal the major flow is observed ventrally, whereas in the thoracic canal the dorsal part of the subarachnoid space harbors most of the flow [60, 61]. While the influence of cisternal action on CSF flow diminishes in a caudal direction, the respiratory influence on CSF flow due to thoracic pressure changes is the major motor of CSF flow in the thoracic area [48, 61, 131, 137, 150, 164].

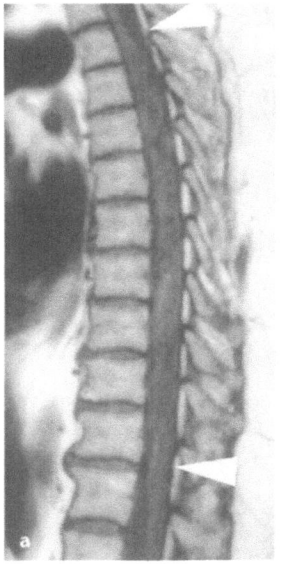
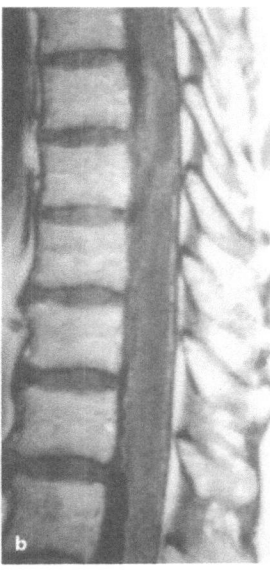

Fig. 4.15 a,b. These T1-weighted MRI scans without gadolinium demonstrate typical features of a syrinx after spinal meningitis in a 43-year-old woman. She had suffered a meningoencephalitis with spastic paraparesis 4 years earlier and made a partial recovery. Her major complaints now were back pain radiating into both legs and increased spasticity. The scan shows a syrinx between Th2 and Th10 (*arrows*) and irregular margins of the spinal cord of variable signal intensity. We advised against surgery in this patient and recommended conservative treatment

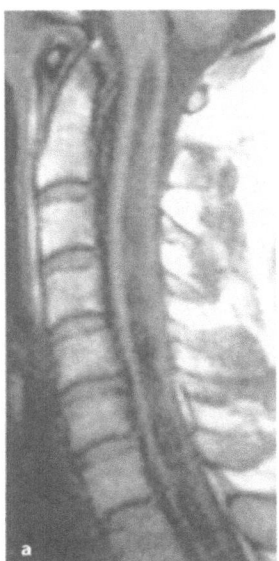
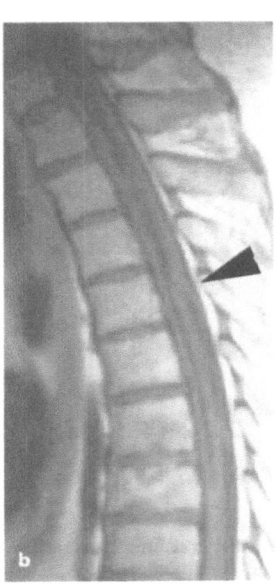
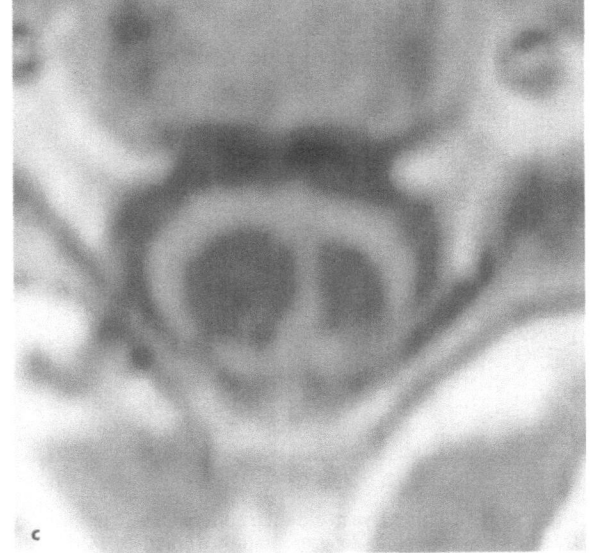

Fig. 4.16 a–e. This 49-year-old man complained about gait ataxia and a sensory disturbances in his left arm for the past 10 years without progression. The T1-weighted MRI scans display a syrinx between C1 and Th6 (**a**, **b**). At the level of Th4 (*arrow*) a sudden change in caliber is apparent (**b**). The axial scan at C5 (**c**) shows a vertically septated syrinx cavity (continued on next page)

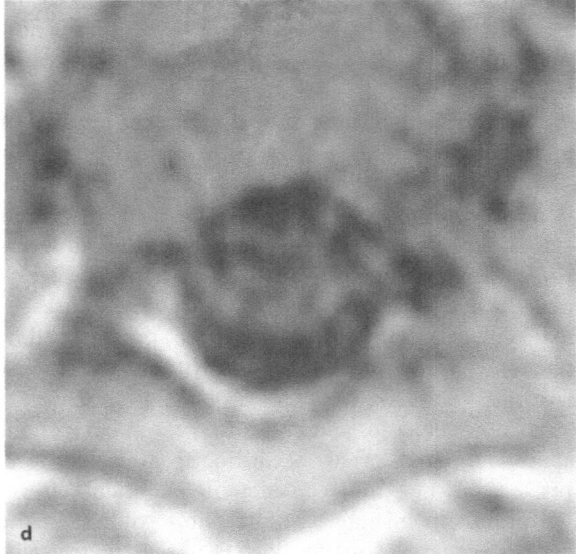

Fig. 4.16 d, e. d At Th4, the spinal cord margins become blurred suggesting arachnoid scarring at this level. **e** At Th5, the cord displays an irregular shape suggesting arachnoid adhesions pulling the left side of the cord posteriorly. Currently, the patient is still observed clinically. As soon as progression of his symptoms occurs surgery will be recommended at the Th4/5 level

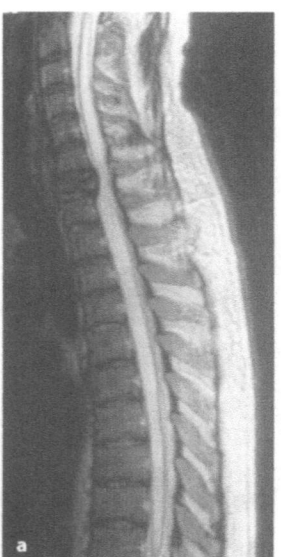
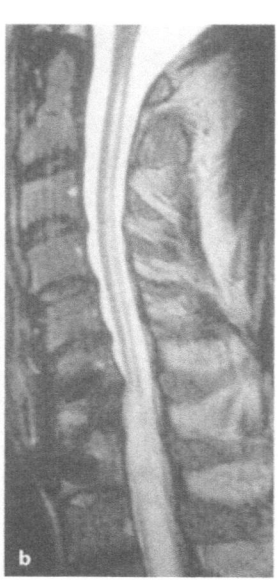
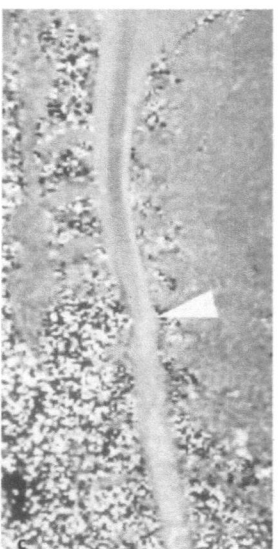
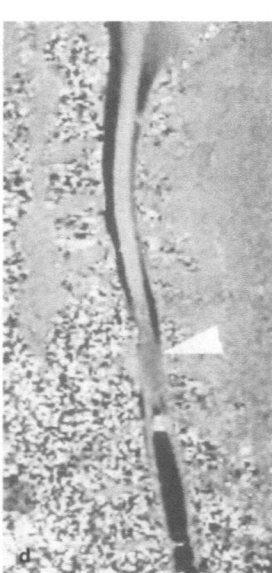

Fig. 4.17 a–d. This 37-year-old man suffered a C7 compression fracture 19 years prior to presentation with these MRI scans. For the past 8 years he had experienced dysesthesias in his left arm and trunk. Now progressive sensory disturbances, motor weakness of his left hand and gait ataxia developed. **a** This T2-weighted MRI shows the syrinx between foramen magnum and Th12 and the old fracture at C7. **b** Under higher magnification the sudden change of spinal cord caliber at C7 becomes visible. Due to the arachnoid pathology at C7 the cord margins become less defined at this level. The systolic (**c**) and diastolic phase (**d**) of the phase contrast cine-MRI demonstrate the level of CSF flow obstruction (*arrow*) and profound fluid movements inside the caudal part of the syrinx. After surgery at C7 his neurological symptoms improved. The syrinx was slightly reduced in caliber 2 weeks postoperatively

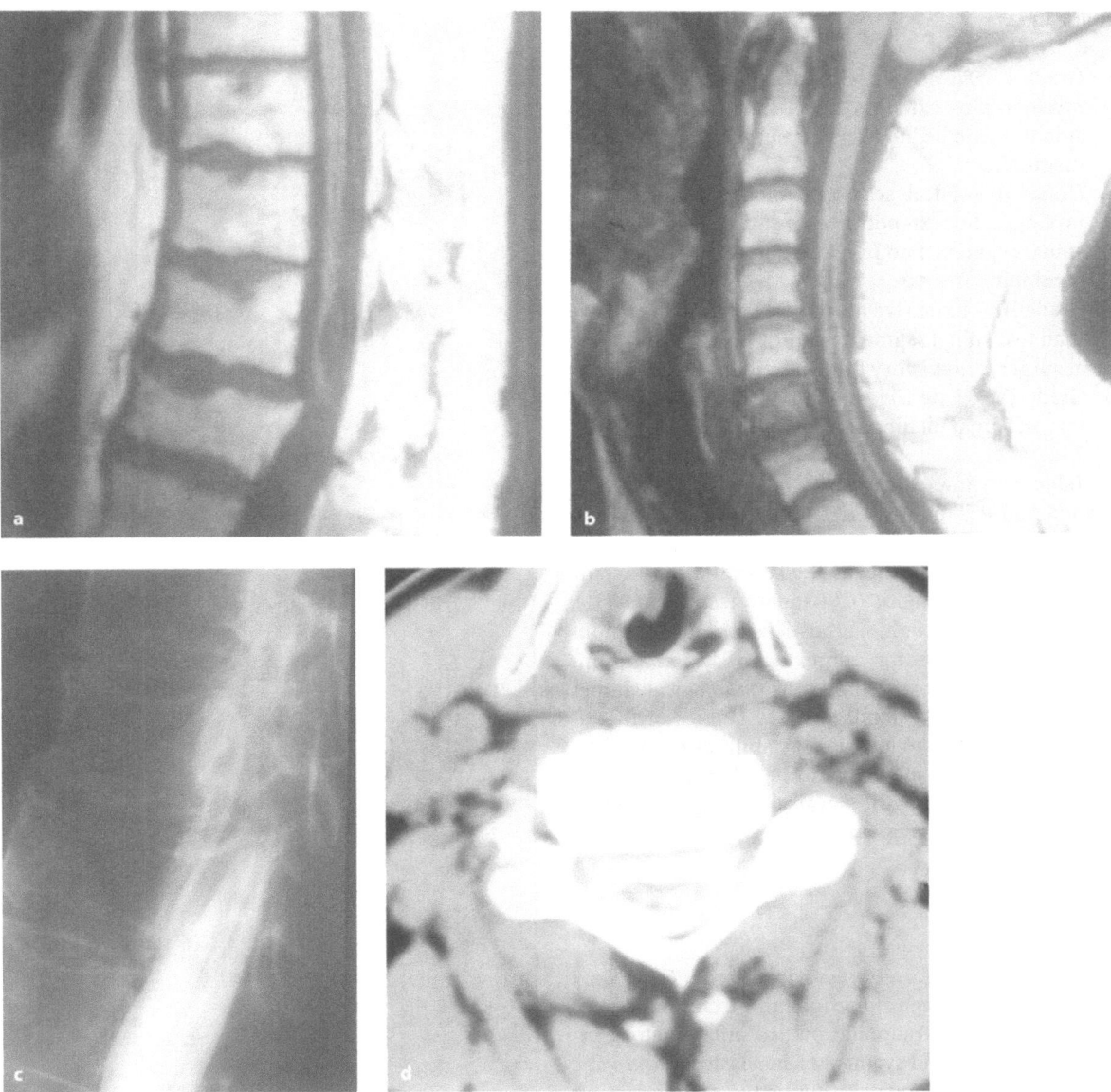

Fig. 4.18 a–d. a This T1-weighted MRI scan shows an old fracture at Th12 with myelomalacia at Th11. **b** A syrinx extends up to the level of C4. **c** Myelography demonstrated an almost complete block of contrast at Th12. **d** The postmyelographic CT at C6 shows an atrophic cord with contrast in the syrinx. This 55-year-old man was operated at Th12 because of increasing gait problems. Postoperatively, his gait was left unchanged. However there was no further progression until his last follow up visit 4 years later

If phase contrast cine-MRI imaging is not available or MRI cannot be used at all, for instance in patients after spinal instrumentation, myelography and postmyelographic CT can be used to localize CSF flow obstructions. In posttraumatic patients, a complete or incomplete block of contrast can almost always be demonstrated at the level of the injury, i.e., the level of arachnoid scarring (Fig. 4.18). In postinflammatory cases, the arachnoid scar and, thus, the area of flow obstruction may be limited to either the anterior or posterior part of the subarachnoid space. In such an instance, the pathology may be very difficult to prove with this method as the contrast material may pass the pathological area without delay along the opposite side of the subarachnoid space [47, 187]. Sometimes, the postmyelographic CT may then demonstrate signs of arachnoid pathology such as arachnoid septations or changes of spinal cord contour [144] and can also be used to demonstrate the syrinx itself as water soluble contrast will accumulate in the cyst [10].

The extent of arachnoid scarring was graded in the following way:

► Grade I – Focal scar without block of contrast on myelography extending over no more than two spinal segments; no previous surgery; no history of meningitis
► Grade II – Focal scar with block of contrast on myelography extending over no more than two spinal segments; no previous surgery; no history of meningitis
► Grade III – Extensive arachnoid scarring over more than two spinal segments and/or previous intradural surgery; no history of meningitis
► Grade IV – Extensive arachnoid scarring with history of spinal meningitis

Table 4.5 shows the severity of arachnoid scarring for PIS and PTS in our series. PIS was associated with a significantly worse grade of arachnoid scarring than in posttraumatic patients as the latter did not include patients with meningitis (Chi-square-test: $P < 0.0001$). Apart from a thorough diagnostic work-up to demonstrate the exact position and extent of syrinx and underlying arachnoid scarring, neuroradiological studies should also include standard X-ray studies of the affected spinal levels to look for instabilities or kyphotic angulations which may have to be taken into consideration for planning the surgical strategy appropriately [122, 123, 141] (Fig. 4.19).

4.1.3
Neurophysiology

Similar to syringomyelia associated with CMI, only few data exist on neurophysiological examinations in patients with posttraumatic or postinflammatory arachnoid scarring and syringomyelia. Basically, the same principles as in CMI may be applied to diagnostic and intraoperative monitoring of evoked potentials in this patient group (see Fig. 3.13). The incidence of patients with complete waveform absence is higher. Therefore, the options to monitor and survey the positioning and monitoring processes are reduced in patients with spinal arachnoid scarring. However, all detected waveforms are regarded as essential to be preserved at sur-

Table 4.5. Grade of arachnoid scarring for patients with posttraumatic and postinflammatory syringomyelia

	Grade I	Grade II	Grade III	Grade IV
Posttraumatic	31%	32%	37%	–
Postinflammatory	38%	16%	30%	16%
Total	35%	23%	34%	8%

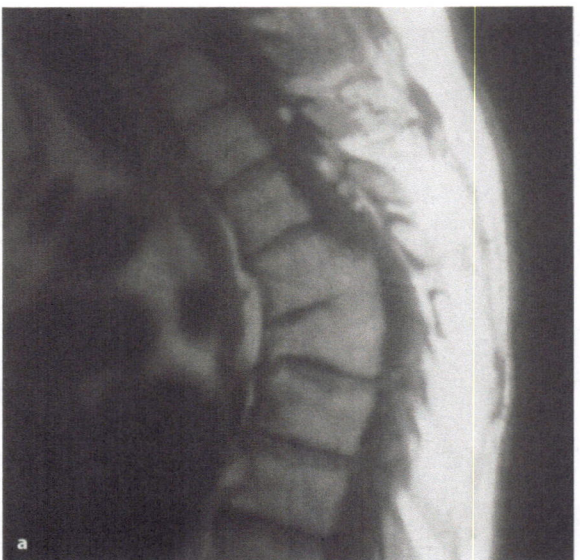
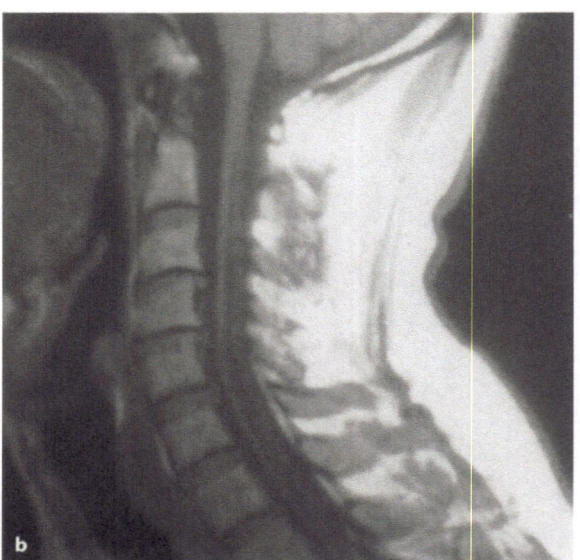

Fig. 4.19 a–b. a This T1-weighted MRI scan demonstrates a fracture at Th5 with a posttraumatic syrinx. The syrinx extends to C2 (**b**). After the motor cycle accident, he made an almost full recovery except for a peroneus lesion on the left side. Twenty-one years later, this now 40-year-old patient had lost his ability to walk completely and complained about progressive weakness of his right arm and hand. In this patient, it was decided that causal treatment would have to involve major surgery combining orthopedic realignment of the spine and arachnoid dissection at Th5. The risks to loose the remaining neurological functions in such an operation were considered too high by the patient so that a syringoperitoneal shunt was inserted at Th1. The patient experienced some improvement of his motor power for about a year and declined further surgery

gery. We agree with the hypothesis of a few other investigators that stable or slightly improved SSEPs are usually correlated with good or excellent clinical outcome [180].

Tibial-SEP were found to be the most sensitive modality to predict the presence of syringomyelia as this method obtained pathological results in the majority of patients [75, 111, 159]. However, no correlation was found between these SSEP changes and clinical symptoms or length of history [75, 112]. Obviously, arachnoid scarring and tethering of the cord will also cause SSEP changes [77], so that pathological values have to be attributed to both phenomena: syringomyelia and cord tethering [77].

Some authors studied EMG changes [40, 135], motor evoked potentials [113] and tried to quantify thermhypesthesia using warmth-induced sensory potentials [170]. Even though pathological values were detected in patients with syringomyelia, no prognostic significance could be deduced from these studies.

4.1.4
Surgical Management

The first surgical attempt to treat a syrinx was published by Abbe and Coley [1] in 1892. They exposed the spinal cord in a patient with spinal arachnoiditis and punctured the intramedullary cyst. Postoperatively, the neurological condition of the patient was unchanged. Treatment of posttraumatic and postinflammatory arachnoid scarring and syringomyelia should concentrate on the underlying disorder of CSF flow and spinal cord mobility: arachnoid scarring. The management of patients with additional bony compression of spinal cord and subarachnoid space [147] is discussed below under 4.1.4.2.

The first publication of a surgical procedure to treat spinal arachnoiditis dates back to 1909 and was published by Victor Horsley [74]. He reported on 21 patients with arachnoid dissection to free the spinal cord out of scar tissue. The dura was left open. He made no comments on syringomyelia in this series. Similar smaller series were published by Brouwer [29], Kikuchi [86], and Batten [21]. The first series with arachnoid dissection and spinal decompression to treat syringomyelia was published by Adelstein [2] in 1938. He reported on three patients with syringomyelia and arachnoiditis where he observed a collapse of the syrinx after dura opening and arachnoid dissection. He also left the dura open.

The aim of surgery should be to obtain a free CSF passage in the area of arachnoid scarring and to untether and decompress the spinal cord. Progressive symptoms may be related to:

▶ CSF flow obstruction and syringomyelia

Table 4.6. Operations for patients with posttraumatic and postinflammatory arachnoid scarring and syringomyelia

	Posttraumatic syringomyelia	Postinflammatory syringomyelia
Decompression	35	35
– Dura graft	29	23
– Plus shunt	2	5
– Dura open	4	6
– Plus shunt	–	1
Syrinx shunts	34	28
– Peritoneal	20	16
– Pleural	10	2
– Subarachnoidal	4	10
Fusion	6	1
Untethering	–	1
Thalamic stimulator	1	–

▶ tethering of the cord due to arachnoid scarring
▶ compression of the spinal cord by arachnoid pathologies
▶ compression of the spinal cord by spinal stenosis or kyphotic angulations
▶ spinal instability

All these mechanisms can be involved in the process of myelopathy and the development of syringomyelia [25, 32, 43, 80, 94, 104, 119, 123, 128, 129, 132, 155].

Fifty-one patients with PTS underwent 76 surgical procedures, while 42 patients with PIS underwent 65 procedures (Table 4.6). Except for seven spinal fusions for concomitant degenerative diseases or spinal instabilities and one thalamic stimulator for treatment of pain, all other operations aimed to treat the syrinx.

For several years now, decompression of the subarachnoid space and arachnoid dissection are performed as the first surgical option. No syrinx shunt has been implanted within the last 6 years.

4.1.4.1
Arachnolysis and Decompression of the Spinal Canal

Figures 4.20, 4.21, and 4.22 give examples of postinflammatory and posttraumatic syringomyelia and different grades of arachnoid scarring. The operation is performed in the prone position, except for cervical cases which are operated in the semi-sitting position. The head is fixed in the Mayfield clamp in neutral position. Median- and tibial-SSEP are employed for neu-

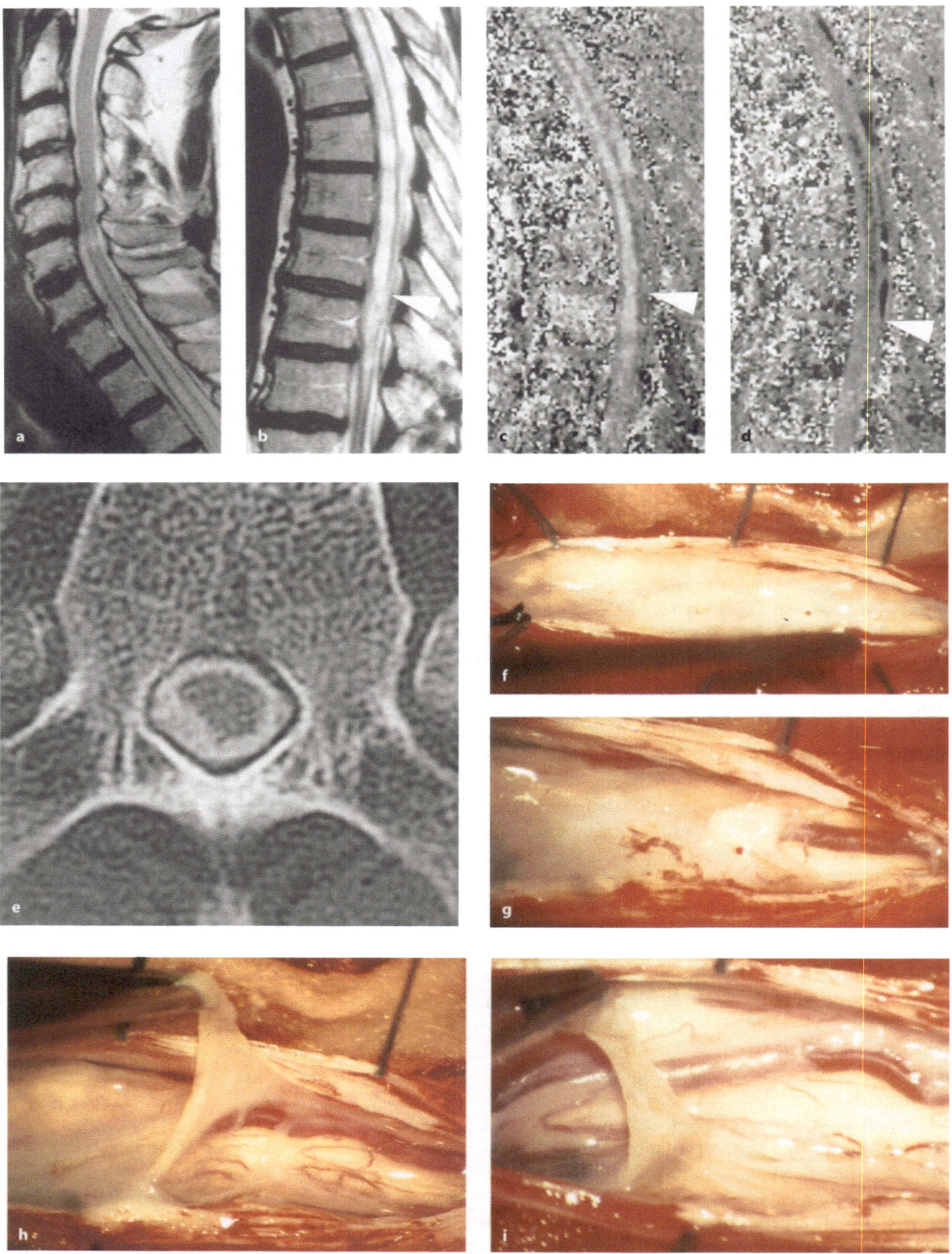

Fig. 4.20 a–i

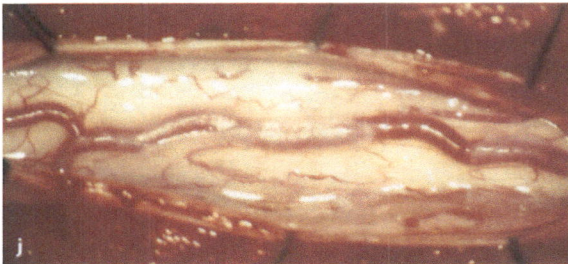
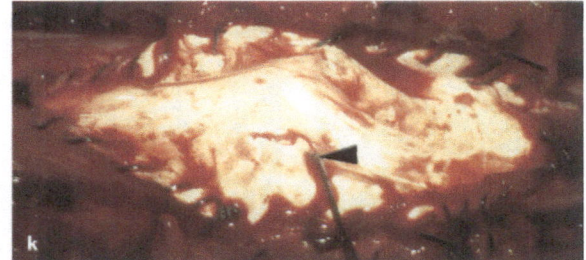
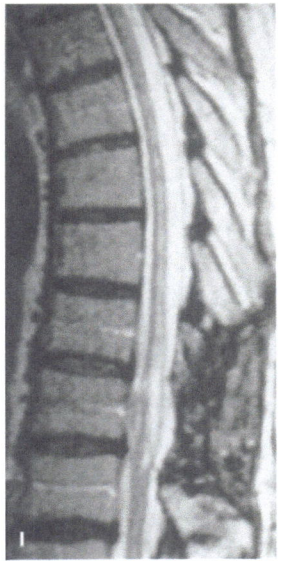
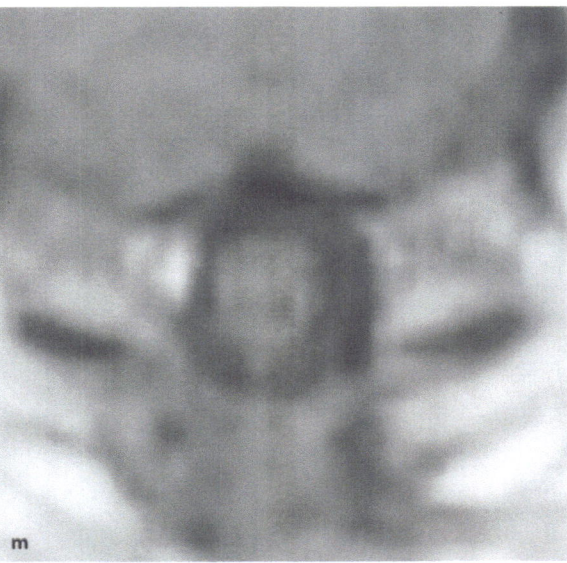

Fig. 4.20 a–m. This 61-year-old patient underwent myodil myelography 35 years ago after a whiplash injury of his cervical spine. Eight years later he started to develop sensory changes in his left leg. At presentation, he had a progressive paraparesis and pain provoked by movements of his trunk radiating into the Th8 and Th9 dermatomes on the right side. **a** The T2-weighted MRI scan shows the upper limit of the syrinx at C7 and an old spinal cord contusion at C6 due to the former accident. **b** The T2-weighted MRI scan of the thoracic spine shows an area of arachnoid scarring at the lower end of the syrinx at Th8/9 (*arrow*). The systolic (**c**) and diastolic phase contrast cine-MRI (**d**) show a corresponding CSF flow obstruction at that level (*arrow*). **e** The postmyelographic CT at Th8/9 demonstrates compression of the spinal cord on the right side due to an arachnoid pouch as a result of the myodil myelography 35 years earlier. **f** The intraoperative view after dura opening shows thickened arachnoid obscuring the underlying spinal cord from view. At either end of the dura opening, the arachnoid is translucent indicating the limited extent of this ar-achnopathy. **g** The arachnoid is opened at the lower part first starting below the scarring. **h** With sharp dissection, the scar is resected limiting the dissection to the posterior aspect of the spinal canal. **i** Under higher magnification, the last piece of scarring which is removed can be seen. Please note that some arachnoid scarring is left in place on the cord surface to avoid injury to the pia or spinal cord vessels. Nevertheless, untether-ing of the cord was achieved. **j** The final view displays a free CSF passage in this area. **k** A Gore-Tex duraplasty is inserted and lifted off the cord surface with a tenting suture (*arrow*). **l** The postoperative T2-weighted MRI scan 3 months later shows a free CSF passage at the level of surgery and a considerable de-crease of the syrinx size. **k** The axial T1-weighted scan at Th8/9 demonstrates the now normal shaped spinal cord surrounded by CSF with no adhesion to the overlying dura graft. The pa-tient experienced improvement of his preoperative symptoms. The pain provoked by movement of his trunk has disappeared completely

rophysiological monitoring. After a midline incision, vertebral laminae are exposed according to the extent of arachnoid pathology. The fascia is incised on either side of the spinous process and muscles are detached with subperiosteal dissection. The laminectomy is re-stricted to a width of 15 mm to avoid damage of inter-vertebral joints. The yellow ligament is resected and the dura mater becomes visible. As contamination of the CSF with blood may cause inflammatory reactions of the arachnoid, great care is taken to achieve good hemostasis [71, 158, 190]. For this purpose, the entire surgical field is covered by cotton strips which keep soft tissues moist, facilitate hemostasis, and soak up any minor bleeding.

With ultrasound, the intradural situation can now be examined: the syrinx can be visualized. Pulsations of syrinx fluid and CSF may become visible. Some-times, arachnoid septations can be seen. Most impor-tantly, the safest spot for opening of the dura can be chosen using this technique. Arachnoid scarring may

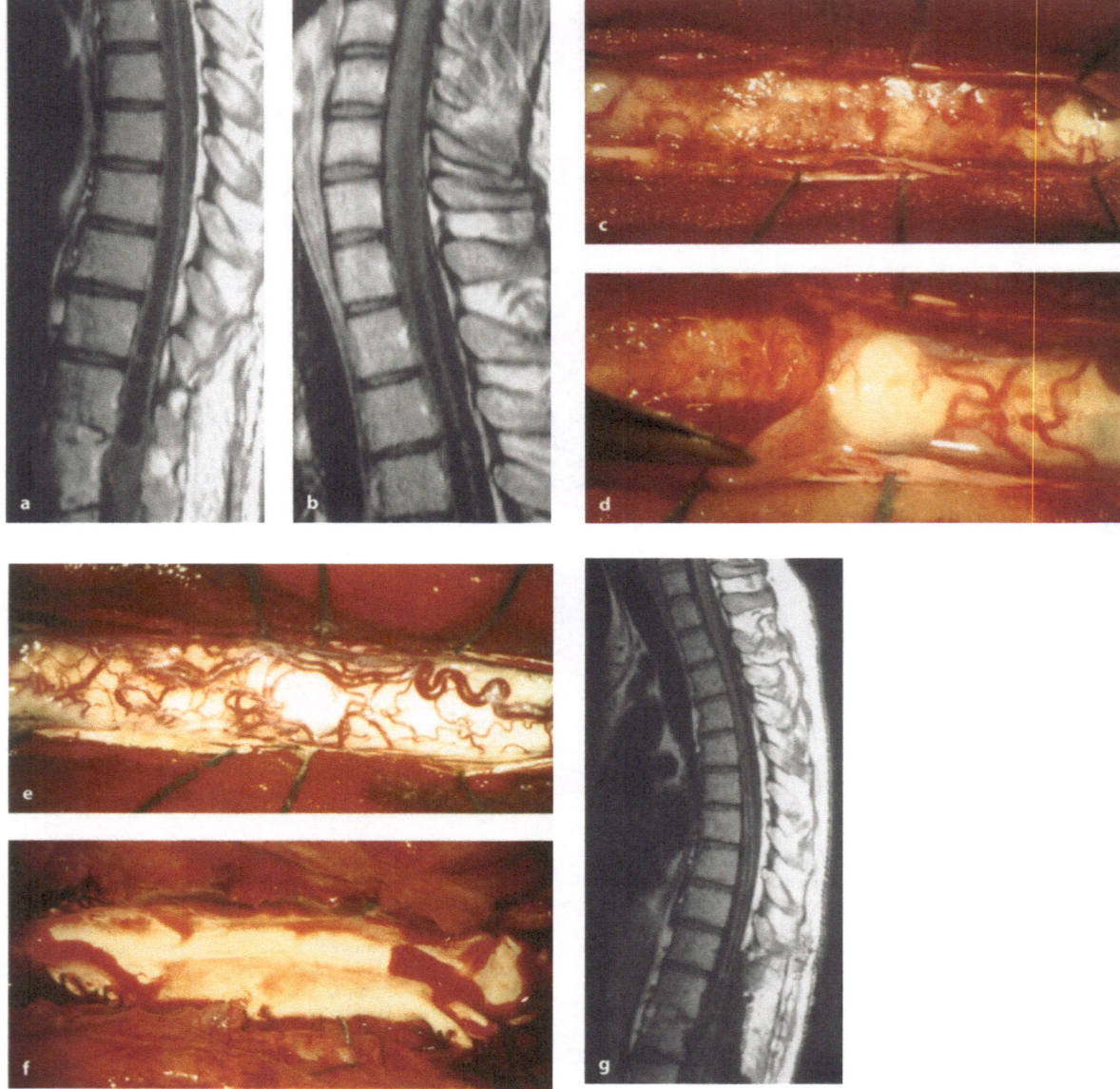

Fig. 4.21 a–g. a, b The T1-weighted MRI scans of this 26-year-old man with a fracture at Th12 and an incomplete cord lesion after a climbing accident 8 years ago show a posttraumatic syrinx between Th11 and C5. Due to increasing gait problems and sensory disturbances on the left side up to C5, surgery was recommended. **c** After dura opening the arachnoid scarring and the translucent, normal appearing arachnoid at both ends of the opening are visible. **d** The scarring is gradually resected starting at the lower end of the exposure using sharp dissection. **e** At the end of the microsurgical dissection, the cord appears collapsed. A small area representing the site of the spinal cord contusion is visible in the center of the picture. Untethering of the cord was not possible due to the anterior extension of the scarring. **f** A large Gore-Tex duraplasty is inserted. **g** Two weeks later, the T1-weighted MRI scan shows a marked decrease of syrinx caliber and an enlarged subarachnoid space at the level of surgery. Signal irregularities of the ventral spinal cord surface reveal the anterior part of the arachnopathy which prevented untethering in this case. The slight epidural CSF collection disappeared subsequently. The patient's gait stabilized while his sensory disturbances improved

cause adherence of the cord to the overlying dura. With ultrasound, such an area can be avoided for the initial dura incision. Once the outer and inner layer of the dura have been incised in the midline under the microscope, the dura is held under gentle tension on either side by retracting sutures. As the underlying arachnoid is thickened and often densely adherent to the cord surface, further opening of the dura should be attempted, preserving the arachnoid layer. In this way, any injury to nervous tissue or small vessels can

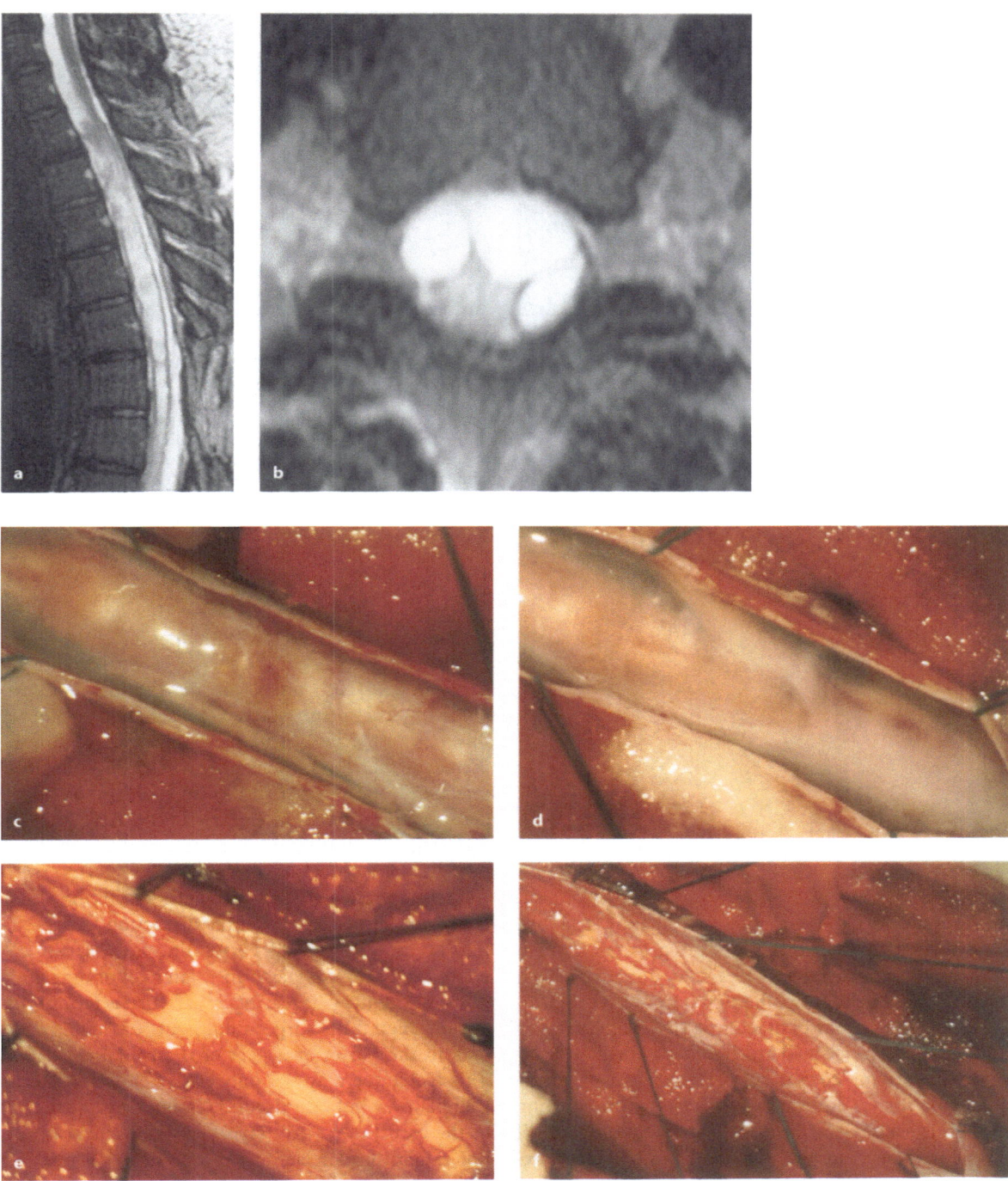

Fig. 4.22 a–i. a This T2-weighted MRI scan demonstrates a syrinx due to an extensive arachnopathy caused by subarachnoid hemorrhage 2 years earlier. The syrinx extends from Th3 to Th12. At Th7, an endoscopic exploration of the spinal canal had been performed in another hospital without clinical benefit. **b** This axial scan at Th2 demonstrates the multiple septations of the subarachnoid space by a series of arachnoid webs anterior of the cord. The major CSF flow obstruction was thought to be situated between Th1 and Th3. Due to rapidly progressive gait ataxia of this patient surgery was offered despite the large extension of this arachnoid pathology. **c** The intraoperative view after dura opening reveals the milky appearance of the arachnoid throughout the exposure. **d** Layer by layer of arachnoid webs could be removed. This view displays the situation midway through the resection. **e** The final result is apparent in this magnified view. Please note that no attempts were undertaken to dissect arachnoid scars laterally or anteriorly. **f** This overview displays the situation before closure. CSF was entering the surgical field from either end (continued on next page).

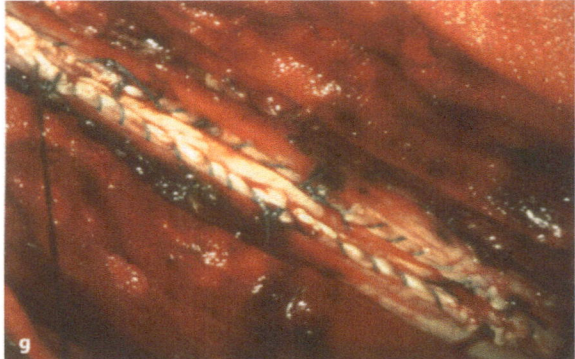

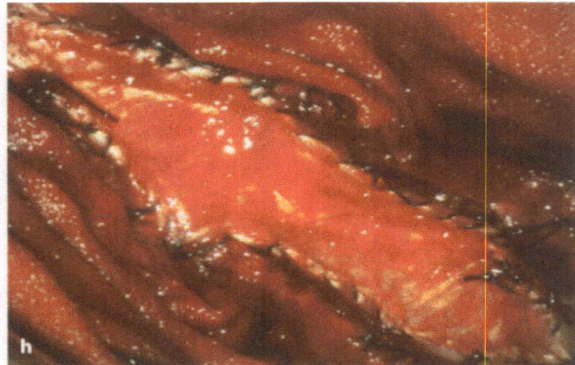

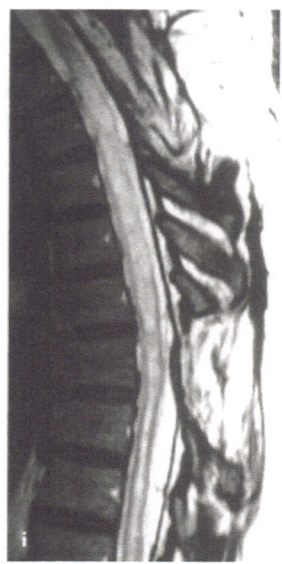

Fig. 4.22 g–i. g At the time of this operation, fascia lata was still used for duraplasty. This view shows the duraplasty before tenting sutures were applied. h After anchoring the duraplasty along the suture line to neighboring soft tissue, the duraplasty is lifted up and no longer contacts the spinal cord surface. Postoperatively, the patient kept his ability to walk with no further clinical progression. i The T2-weighted MRI scan 4 years later shows extension of the syrinx now up to Th2. The posterior subarachnoid space still appears patent at the level of surgery

be easily avoided (Figs. 4.20g, 4.21c, 4.22d). The arachnoid itself may contain perforating arteries which may bleed considerably. Once the dura has been opened, the arachnoid pathology becomes visible. In most instances, areas of arachnoid scarring can easily be depicted, as thickened arachnoid obscures the view to the underlying cord tissue. If the exposure is adequate, the rostral and caudal end of the dura opening should reveal a normal, translucent arachnoid layer. If this is not the case, the dura opening has to be extended. In order to obtain a sufficient CSF passage, the operation has to extend into the unaffected subarachnoid space on either side of the CSF obstruction.

With a microdissector, arachnoid and dura can be separated from each other without any problem in areas without arachnoid scarring, i.e., at either end of the exposure. In the area of scarring, sharp dissection with microscissors may be required to achieve this. Starting at the rostral and caudal end of the exposure, the arachnoid is then incised in the midline and opened toward the area of scarring. At that level, the arachnoid may become densely adherent to the cord

surface (Figs. 4.20i, 4.21d). With opening of the rostral and caudal subarachnoid space, CSF flushes into the surgical field and, often, the cord, which was distended by the syrinx, starts to pulsate and collapse at this point [94, 102]. The arachnoid scar is now resected further layer by layer leaving a last sheath of arachnoid on the cord surface to avoid injury to the cord or surface vessels (Figs. 4.20k, 4.21e, 4.22f). At that stage, the intradural dissection is completed and need not be extended further.

We emphasize the use of sharp dissection exclusively for this purpose. Blunt dissection carries the risk of rupturing small perforating vessels. No arachnoid dissection is performed laterally or anteriorly. The risk of injury or tearing spinal cord arteries is extremely high if the surgeon does not restrict his activities to the posterior aspect of the spinal canal [63]. This technique may not only achieve a free posterior CSF pathway but also decompression and untethering of the cord [47, 94, 119, 123] – provided the scar does not extend too far laterally or anteriorly (Fig. 4.20 e) [80, 149].

Any surgical intervention aiming at reducing scar tissue carries the risk of causing new scar formation which may even turn out to be worse than the preoperative one. Considerable experience is needed to be successful with this surgical technique. The more focussed the surgery, the less scarring may result. If unnecessary steps are taken, such as a too extensive dura opening, or the surgical field is contaminated with considerable amounts of blood, postoperative scarring may counterbalance completely the effect of surgery. However, if the dura opening is not wide enough to gain access to the normal subarachnoid space above and below the level of obstruction, the procedure is insufficient. As always, it is the right measure that counts.

In patients with a history of spinal meningitis, CSF flow may be obstructed throughout almost the entire spinal canal. In such instances, surgery aiming at improvement of CSF flow is no option. But axial MRI scans should be performed covering the affected spinal segments. Sometimes an area of cord compression due to an arachnoid cyst or pouch can be identified. Decompression by resection or at least wide fenestration of such a cyst may provide a significant benefit for the patient (Fig. 4.23).

To limit the risk of postoperative scar formation and tethering, an extensive duraplasty is inserted. For this purpose, a number of different materials have been used in the past: lyophilized dura, fascia lata, and Gore-Tex. Leaving the dura open as suggested by Williams [147, 188] has not given good results in our experience due to contamination of the subarachnoid space with wound exudate and blood. Similarly, autologous material carries a considerable risk of scarring as severe adhesions may form with the cord surface due to vascularization of the graft by pial vessels.

For these reasons, we prefer Gore-Tex [78, 118, 167, 193] for the duraplasty (Figs. 4.20k, 4.21f, 4.23). A few technical points should be followed to minimize the risk of CSF fistulas with the use of this material. Gore-Tex has a rather stiff texture. In order to avoid wrinkling of the duraplasty, the size of the graft should be fitted exactly to the dura opening. To avoid inadvertent injury of the cord during suturing, we leave the retention sutures in place. In this way, the size of the graft can be adjusted adequately and there is no risk to injure the cord during suturing. After a tight running suture has been applied, we perform "tenting sutures" to lift the dura graft off the cord surface. These sutures are anchored at intervertebral joint capsules or in epidural scar tissue (Figs. 4.22h, i). In this way, the suture line is elevated from the cord and pulled laterally to avoid scar formation. This maneuver also facilitates hemostasis, as epidural veins are compressed with this technique. Finally, the wound is closed layer by layer. Special attention is paid to a good, tight closure of the muscle layer to prevent any CSF from entering the epifascial space. In patients who have been operated on before, as in patients with PTS who underwent spinal instrumentation for instance, we place a lumbar drain prophylactically if the soft tissue is scarred and sparsely vascularized to avoid fistulas.

Similar surgical techniques have been proposed by several authors [41, 46, 51, 90, 95, 116, 119, 123, 136, 146, 147, 153, 188] using either fascia [46], lyophilized dura [153], or leaving the dura open [146, 147, 187, 188]. Shikata et al. [153] even performed spinal fusion to minimize spinal movements and the effect of cord tether-

ing. Other authors performed arachnoid dissections without a duraplasty [80, 98, 125] or inserted an additional syrinx shunt [51, 94, 125].

4.1.4.2
Surgical Strategy for Patients with Additional Degenerative Spinal Disease, Kyphotic Angulations, or Spinal Instabilities

Patients with PTS may present with additional spinal instability or kyphotic angulations (Figs. 4.2, 4.19). In such instances, neurological progression may occur independently of the syrinx due to myelopathy [122, 123, 145]. Furthermore, anterior compression of the spinal canal may interfere with CSF flow to such a degree that posterior decompression alone, as outlined above, is not sufficient.

Depending on the kyphotic angle, it may be advisable to treat the spinal stenosis first with an anterior decompression and stabilisation. Once the spinal canal has been reconstructed CSF flow may improve sufficiently for the syrinx to decrease as well. However, arachnoid adhesions may prevent this effect so that these patients may require anterior and posterior surgery to achieve clinical stabilisation. We would advise to perform instrumentations and intradural arachnoid dissections in separate operations to avoid contamination of the subarachnoid space with blood.

Seven patients presented with degenerative diseases of the cervical spine in addition to a syrinx related to spinal arachnoid scarring. In these patients, radicular symptoms rather than signs of a myelopathy or the syrinx predominated the clinical picture. In three patients, the cervical spine was operated on before treating the syrinx, in four patients the syrinx had already been operated on.

The relevance of degenerative changes of the spine for patients with syringomyelia should not be underestimated [147]. Rather moderate spinal stenosis may be sufficient to cause significant neurological problems in patients with syringomyelia. In some instances, we even observed a decrease of the syrinx postoperatively after discectomy and ventral fusion [109, 130, 141, 147].

4.1.4.3
Implantation of a Syrinx Shunt

A syrinx drainage is indicated exclusively if the underlying disorder of CSF flow cannot be corrected, such as in patients with extensive arachnoid scarring after meningitis or multiple intradural surgeries. Any drainage requires a myelotomy, which may be performed in the midline or dorsal root entry zone. This may cause additional sensory deficits [191]. The silicon catheter may cause additional arachnoid scarring, tethering, and CSF flow disturbances [16, 22, 146, 147,

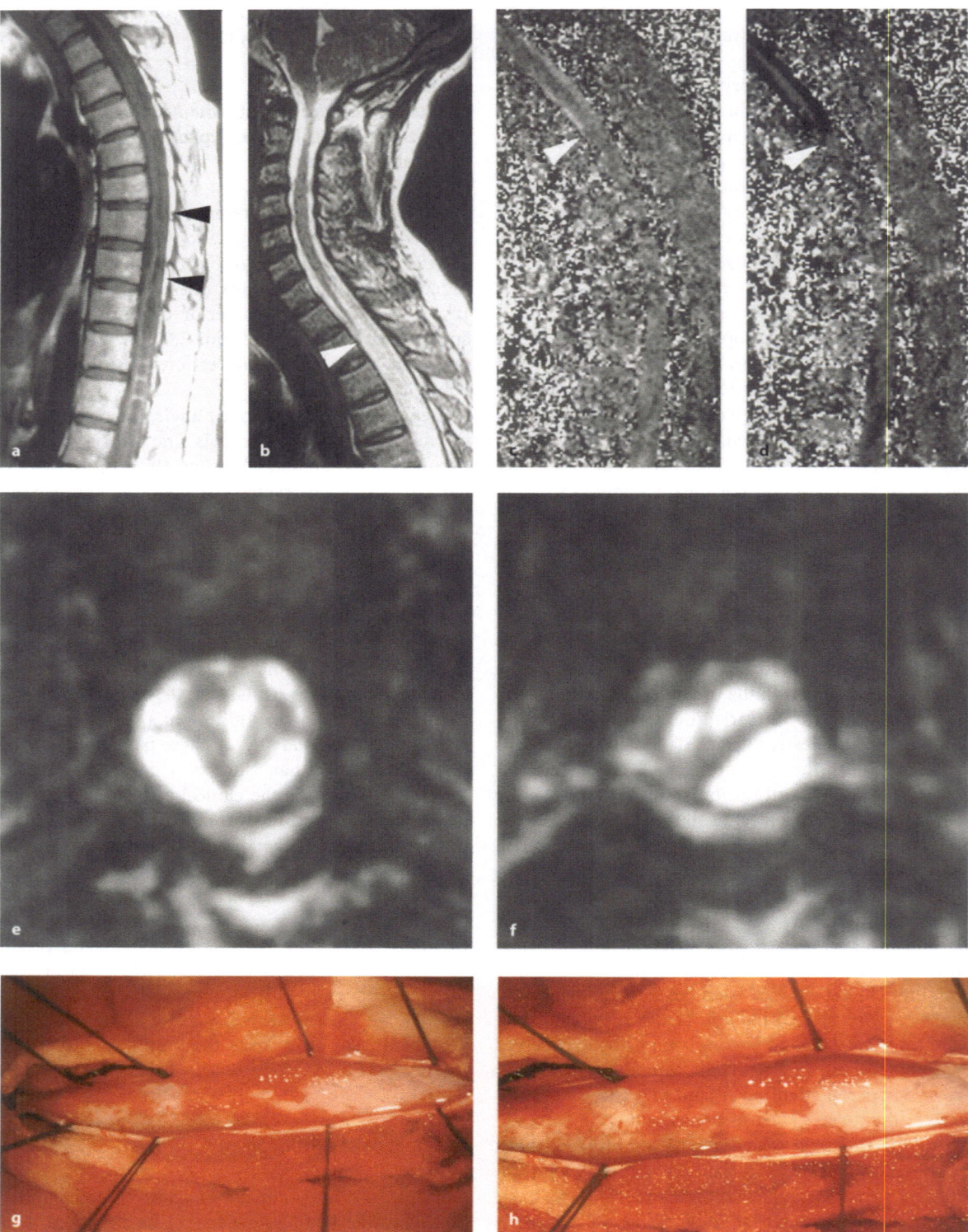

Fig. 4.23 a–n. This 39-year-old woman suffered from severe spinal meningitis related to intrathecal injection of a contaminated drug 6 years ago. After severe paraparesis initially she recovered fully. For three years she has experienced progressive gait ataxia and a spastic paraparesis with a sensory level at Th5

forcing her to use a wheelchair. **a** This T1-weighted sagittal MRI scan demonstrates a syrinx of the entire thoracic cord and a ventrally located arachnoid pouch at the level of Th8/9 (*arrows*). **b** The T2-weighted MRI scan of the cervical spine discloses the upper limit of the syrinx at C7. Note the ventral ad-

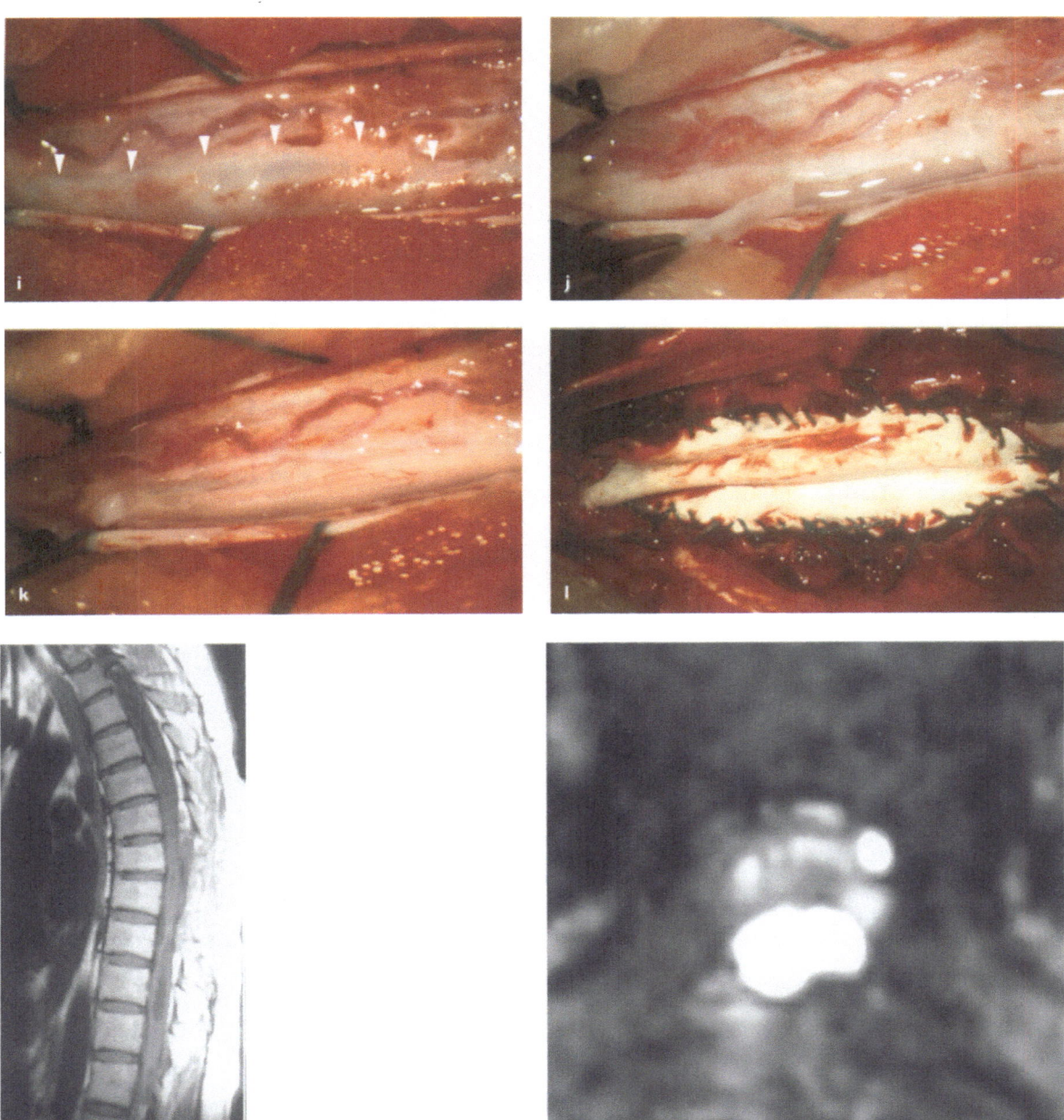

hesion of the cord at the level of Th2 (*arrow*). Caudally from this level the cord is irregularly defined indicating extensive arachnoid scarring. The cardiac gated cine-MRI studies in systole (**c**) and diastole (**d**) indicate no CSF flow signal distal to the level of Th2 (*arrow*). Axial T2-weighted scans of the thoracic cord show multiple septations within the subarachnoid space (**e**) but also an area of significant cord compression from an arachnoid cyst on the left side at the level of Th7 (**f**). **g** The intraoperative photograph displays the situation after laminectomy of Th7 and 8 and dura opening. The arachnoid is thickened throughout the exposure. **h** Higher magnification displays the area of cord compression. **i** With sharp dissection, part of the arachnoid scar is dissected off the cord. Now the arach-

noid cyst on the left side can be seen bulging out. *Arrows* mark the medial limit of this process. **j** With fenestration of the cyst wall CSF escaped under considerable pressure. Pulsations of the spinal cord related to respiration started to become evident and tibial-SEP improved instantly. **k** This view demonstrates the situation at the end of dissection. The cyst has been widely fenestrated. **l** A Gore-Tex duraplasty has been inserted. The postoperative sagittal T1-weighted scan shows the decompression at the level of Th6/7 (**m**). The axial T2-weighted scan demonstrates the posterior decompression at the level of operation (**n**). Within a few days, motor power improved considerably. At the time of discharge 3 weeks after surgery, the patient was again able to walk with a supporting person

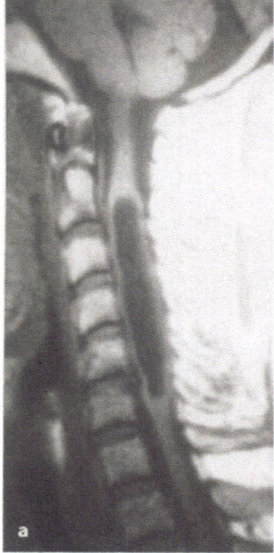
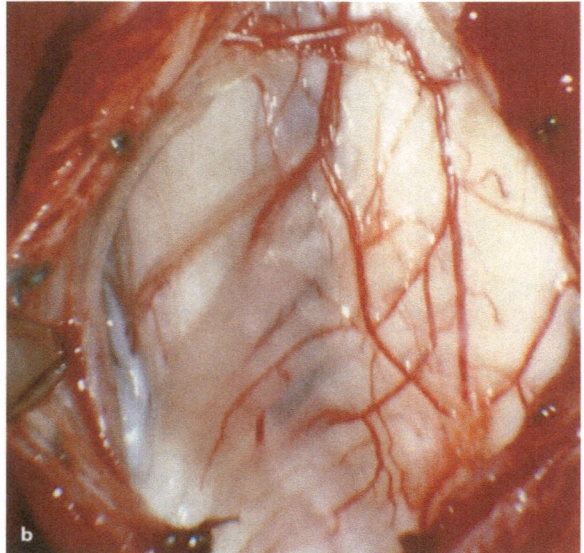
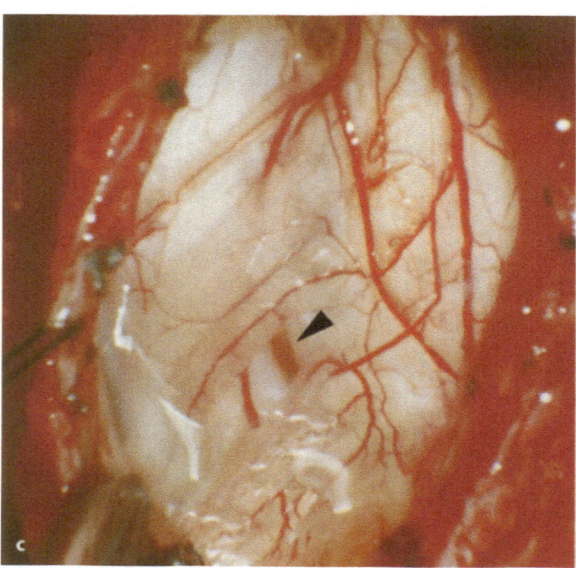
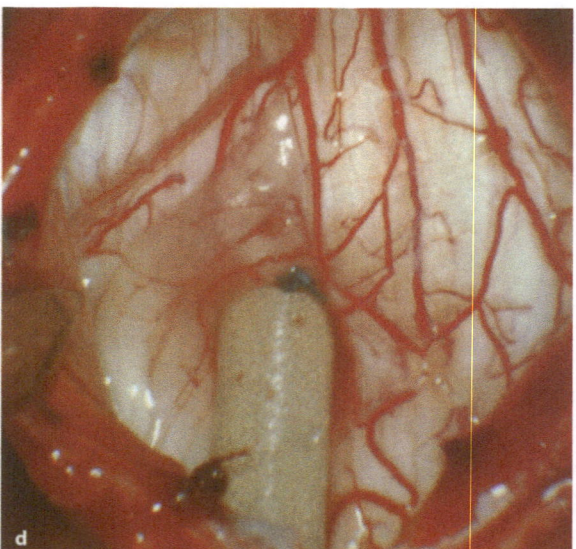

Fig. 4.24 a–f. This 45-year old man presented progressive dysesthesias, sensory deficits and motor weakness of his left hand. **a** The T1-weighted MRI discloses a syrinx between C2 and C6. At this time, syrinx shunts were still offered as first line of treatment in our institution. **b** The intraoperative view in the semi-sitting position at the level of C5/6 displays the distended spinal cord and the translucent pia revealing the underlying syrinx cavity along the left dorsal root entry zone. **c** A small incision (*arrowhead*) has been made in this area. The syrinx drained clear fluid. **d** A small syringosubarachnoid shunt catheter has been inserted and secured with a pia suture to prevent slipping. **e** The immediate postoperative MRI scan demonstrates complete disappearance of the cyst. **f** However, 6 months later a partial refilling is apparent

155, 157]. Therefore, the site of insertion has to be chosen very carefully. We avoid spinal areas of arachnoid scarring for shunt placement and adjust the myelotomy according to the sensory symptoms of the patient. Placement of syringosubarachnoid shunts into a subarachnoid space altered by arachnoiditis carries considerable risks of malfunction of the shunt [22, 70] as the distal end may become blocked.

If a shunt is indicated, we prefer syringosubarachnoid shunts to avoid the higher risk of postsurgical cord tethering associated with extrathecal shunts (Fig. 4.25). A laminectomy is performed at a level unaffected by arachnoiditis and the cord opened under the microscope at the thinnest area of the cord according to the preoperative sensory status of the patient (Fig. 4.24). Then a small silicon catheter as used for ventricular drains is inserted in cephalad direction. The distal part of the catheter is placed into a part of the subarachnoid space unaffected by arachnoid pathology.

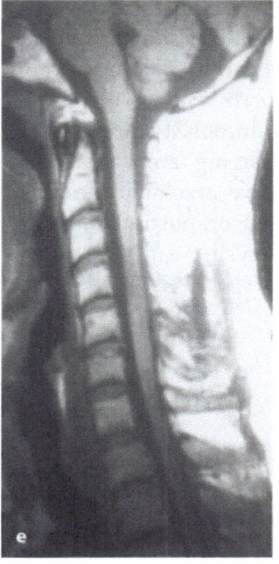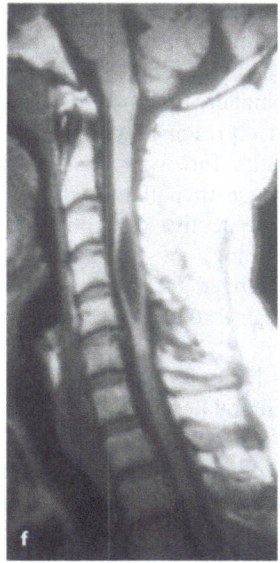

Fig. 4.24 e, f

Table 4.7. Complications for patients with posttraumatic and postinflammatory syringomyelia

Type of complication	Decompression	Shunt
Infection	–	–
Aseptic meningitis	4	–
CSF-leak, pseudomeningocele	3 (1)	2
Pleural collection, pneumothorax	–	2 (1)
Pneumonia	–	2
Urinary tract infection	1	1
Swallowing problems	1	2
Low pressure syndrome	–	1
Ileus	–	1
Deep vein thrombosis	1	–
Pulmonary edema	1	–
Brachial plexus palsy	1	–
Total	12 (17%)	11 (18%)

Numbers in brackets indicate operative revisions

4.1.5
Postoperative Outcome

Basically, two treatment groups can be distinguished in our series: syrinx drainage procedures and arachnolysis with duraplasty. Variations of the arachnolysis group, i.e., placing an additional shunt or leaving the dura open, were abandoned as soon as unfavorable postoperative results became apparent in these subgroups (Table 4.6).

4.1.5.1
Complications

In the great majority of publications on posttraumatic or postinflammatory syringomyelia, complications are hardly mentioned. Especially for syrinx draining operations, reports on complications and long-term malfunction rates have only appeared recently. Sgouros and Williams [147] gave a percentage of a 29.4% failure rate after shunting operations. For operations dealing with the arachnoid scar, the risk of cord damage is mentioned but no percentage rate is given [63].

Postoperative complications of our series are listed in Table 4.7. Postoperative aseptic meningitis was encountered exclusively in patients in whom the dura had been left open. Considering patients with arachnolysis and dura grafting separately reduces the complication rate to 14% (Table 4.7).

Among 16 patients Haberl et al. [64] observed seven new neurological deficits associated with shunting operations due to the myelotomy. Two catheters dislocated, one syringopleural shunt caused pneumothorax. Van Calenbergh and Van den Bergh [173] performed 23 syringosubarachnoid shunts and found seven postoperative sensory deficits due to myelotomy, two patients developed sphincter disturbances, four catheters dislocated, one catheter got blocked, and one patient reported persistent pain at the insertion site. One patient developed a postoperative hematoma and one patient died to postoperative apnea. Other complications such as intramedullary hematoma [174] or intramedullary abscess formation [22] have also been reported. Figure 4.24 provides an example of postoperative tethering after shunt implantation.

4.1.5.2
Radiological Results

Comparing radiological results of patients with arachnolysis and duraplasty with results from those who underwent syrinx drainage procedures revealed significantly better results for the arachnolysis group (Table 4.8) (Chi-square-test: $P=0.0087$). Interestingly, radiological results were better in the postinflammatory group after arachnolysis and duraplasty than in patients in the posttraumatic group undergoing the same procedure. For results after shunting, this relationship was reversed. However, for both groups, arachnolysis and duraplasty still brought superior results relative to shunting. In terms of different shunt

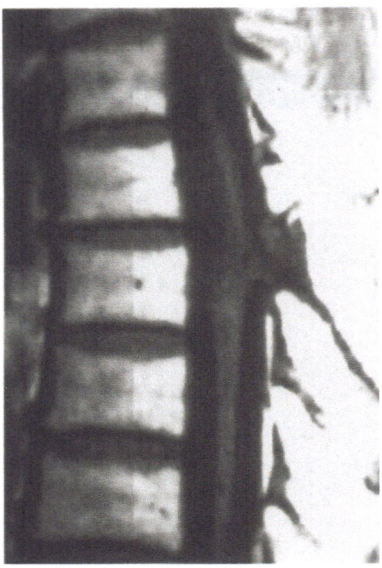

Fig. 4.25. This T1-weighted MRI scan shows tethering of the spinal cord at the site of a syringoperitoneal shunt. Since implantation of this device the patient complains about a sensory deficit in his left leg and irritating dysesthesias

Table 4.8. Radiological results for patients with syringomyelia associated with arachnoid scarring

Group	Arachnolysis + duraplasty	Syrinx shunt
Posttraumatic syringomyelia		
Syrinx smaller	41%	50%
Syrinx unchanged	23%	4%
Syrinx increased	36%	46%
Postinflammatory syringomyelia		
Syrinx smaller	60%	38%
Syrinx unchanged	33%	10%
Syrinx increased	7%	52%
Total		
Syrinx smaller	49%	45%
Syrinx unchanged	27%	6%
Syrinx increased	24%	49%

types, we observed no difference in radiological outcome for syringosubarachnoid, -peritoneal, or -pleural shunts.

Compared with results for patients with syringomyelia related to CMI, these results are less satisfactory. The major reason is the higher proportion of patients with a more extensive arachnoid pathology

in the group with spinal arachnoid scarring. For shunting procedures, the radiological outcome is not related to the grade of arachnoid scarring (syrinx smaller or unchanged for 43% and 56%, respectively). For arachnolysis and duraplasty, however, results for focal arachnoid scarring are superior to those in patients with extensive arachnoid scarring, irrespective of a posttraumatic or postinflammatory etiology of the scar [158] (syrinx smaller or unchanged for 83% and 64%, respectively; Chi-square-test: $P=0.021$).

4.1.5.3
Clinical Results

Patients with spinal arachnoid scarring were followed for an average time of 28±35 months. Quite often, the clinical outcome did not correlate with postoperative changes of syrinx size. This again emphasizes that treatment has to deal not just with the syrinx but also with the underlying arachnoid scar, associated tethering and compression of the cord and spinal stenosis or kyphotic angulations. Either of these mechanisms may continue to aggravate a myelopathy despite a free posterior passage of CSF and a collapsed syrinx.

4.1.5.3.1
Postoperative Clinical Results
Related to Preoperative Symptoms

Postoperative clinical results for patients with syringomyelia related to spinal arachnoid scarring are very much related to the preoperative neurological status in as much as no major changes or improvements should be expected. Stopping the progressive neurological deterioration is the realistic goal which can and should be achieved with successful therapy. After arachnolysis and dura grafting, slight postoperative improvements can be observed for sensory deficits, dysesthesias, pain, and bladder function. However, these improvements are marginal and usually not functionally significant. Therefore, the Karnofsky score remains unchanged during the first postoperative year (67±13 preoperatively and 68±14 after 1 year). After syrinx shunting, similar improvements may be seen for sensory deficits, dysesthesias, and pain, whereas the remainder of neurological symptoms is not altered. The Karnofsky score even tends to decrease in the first postoperative year (52±19 preoperatively and 49±20 after 1 year; Table 4.9).

After arachnolysis and duraplasty, 31% reported a better clinical situation postoperatively, 49% assumed their situation was unchanged, while 20% experienced a worse status than they had preoperatively. After shunting, the corresponding figures were 11%, 53%, and 35%, for improvement, unchanged status,

Table 4.9. Postoperative clinical results for patients with syringomyelia associated with spinal arachnoid scarring

Symptom and group	Preop.	Postop.	3 months	6 months	1 year	P
Sensory deficits						
Arachnolysis	3.0±0.9	3.0±1.0	3.1±1.0	3.1±1.0	3.1±1.0	n.s.
Shunt	2.4±1.1	2.5±1.2	2.5±1.3	2.5±1.3	2.5±1.3	n.s.
Dysesthesias						
Arachnolysis	3.6±1.0	3.9±0.7	3.9±0.8	3.9±0.8	3.8±0.9	n.s.
Shunt	3.4±1.2	3.6±1.1	3.7±1.0	3.7±1.1	3.6±1.1	n.s.
Pain						
Arachnolysis	3.7±0.9	3.9±0.6	3.9±0.7	3.9±0.7	3.9±0.9	n.s.
Shunt	3.4±1.0	3.7±0.9	3.9±0.7	3.9±0.7	3.8±0.7	0.009
Motor power						
Arachnolysis	3.7±1.2	3.5±1.3	3.6±1.2	3.7±1.2	3.7±1.2	n.s.
Shunt	2.9±1.3	2.9±1.4	2.9±1.4	2.9±1.4	2.9±1.5	n.s.
Gait ataxia						
Arachnolysis	3.5±1.1	3.4±1.1	3.4±1.2	3.5±1.2	3.5±1.2	n.s.
Shunt	2.1±1.6	2.0±1.5	2.1±1.6	2.1±1.6	2.0±1.6	n.s.
Bladder function						
Arachnolysis	3.7±1.2	3.8±1.2	3.9±1.2	3.9±1.2	3.9±1.2	n.s.
Shunt	2.4±1.7	2.5±1.7	2.5±1.7	2.4±1.7	2.4±1.6	n.s.
Bowel function						
Arachnolysis	4.0±1.3	4.0±1.3	4.0±1.2	4.0±1.2	4.0±1.2	n.s.
Shunt	2.6±1.7	2.6±1.7	2.6±1.7	2.6±1.7	2.6±1.7	n.s.
Karnofsky score						
Arachnolysis	67±13	66±13	68±14	68±14	68±14	n.s.
Shunt	52±19	50±20	51±20	51±20	49±20	n.s.

Preop. preoperatively, *Postop.* postoperatively, *P* P-value for comparison of pre- and postoperative scores after 1 year (paired *t*-test)

and worsening, respectively (Chi-square test: $P=0.0495$).

Special problems for this group of patients are burning type dysesthesias and pain syndromes which may behave completely different to the remainder of neurological symptoms. Some authors have recommended combination of a shunting procedure with coagulation of the dorsal root entry zone [110]. However, there appears to be accumulating evidence that pain described as a burning type and unrelated to physical activities may be centralized very early in the clinical course so that even successful treatment of the syrinx is no longer able to influence this type of pain [9]. As conventional analgesics are notoriously ineffective, this leaves each physician confronted with this problem in a dilemma. Tricyclic antidepressants, anticonvulsive drugs, and muscle relaxants may be useful in such instances. If these are not effective enough, opiates may be used. Whether additional neurosurgical options for treatment of pain, such as thalamic stimulators, etc., offer any benefit has not been established [9]. However, pain related to particular physical activities may be related to the arachnoid scarring and cord tethering. Its distribution corresponds to the nerve roots affected by the scarring. If untethering of the cord succeeds at surgery, this type of pain may improve considerably. Similarly, pain provoked by coughing or a Valsalva maneuver may be experienced in dermatomes corresponding to the spinal representation of the syrinx. This type of pain is the one most

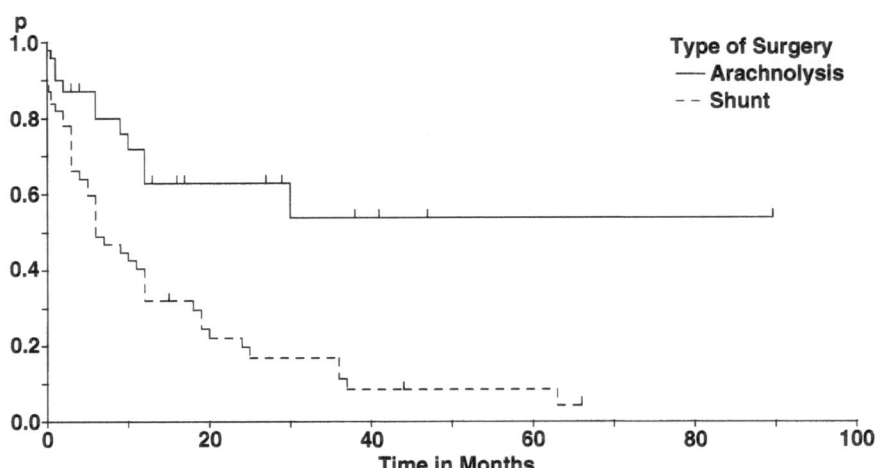

Fig. 4.26. Kaplan-Meier analysis of clinical recurrences for patients with posttraumatic and postinflammatory syringomyelia for comparison of syrinx shunts and arachnolysis with duraplasty (log-rank test: $P=0.0003$)

likely to improve postoperatively with successful treatment of the syrinx as it is caused by sudden pressure changes inside the spinal cord due to the CSF flow obstruction.

4.1.5.3.2
Postoperative Clinical Results Related to Type of Operation

The different surgical groups are listed in Table 4.6. Patients who underwent cervical fusions for signs of radicular compression did not demonstrate a postoperative change of the syrinx or of symptoms related to it. Radicular symptoms were influenced only. Since such maneuvers as implanting an additional shunt or leaving the dura open after arachnolysis have been employed in a small number of patients only, we will concentrate our analysis mainly on patients treated by arachnolysis and dura grafting and patients with syrinx shunts.

As one might expect from the analysis of radiological results, postoperative clinical results in terms of clinical recurrence rates were better for the group who underwent arachnolysis and a duraplasty (Fig. 4.26) (log-rank test: $P=0.0003$) [119, 123]. Results for shunting procedures were particularly disappointing. A considerable number of treatment failures were due to mechanical shunt problems, i.e., dislocations or obstructions. Just 8% of patients were in at least as good a clinical condition as they had been preoperatively 5 years after shunting, while 92% had experienced some progression in the meantime. Interestingly, results for shunting tended to be better if the shunt was inserted at a spinal level without arachnoid scarring than at a level with arachnoid scarring (26% and 0% free of recurrence after 5 years, respectively; not significant). In contrast, 46% of patients who underwent arachnolysis and dura grafting for treatment of the arachnoid scarring remained stabilized or improved

for at least 5 years. This again is a considerably worse result than in patients with syringomyelia and CMI, for instance. Leaving the dura open or implanting a shunt in addition to arachnolysis was associated with a worse outcome than arachnolysis and duraplasty.

Shunting is still considered the treatment of choice by many authors describing their treatment of posttraumatic [4, 7, 39, 57, 70, 76, 82, 99, 121, 129, 130, 135, 141, 160, 165] or postinflammatory syringomyelia [4, 16, 76, 83, 121, 160, 165, 166]. However, Sgouros and Williams [146] reported frustrating results with any form of syrinx shunting if long-term results were taken into account. Given the limitations of a comparison of results between different authors, the discrepancies between studies recommending shunts and our results may best be explained by differences of follow-up evaluation. Reading between the lines reveals a certain amount of dissatisfaction in publications favoring shunts. Several authors recommend shunting to either the pleural or peritoneal space instead of syringosubarachnoid shunting, as the former are thought to be associated with lower rates of malfunction [13, 16, 39, 55, 120, 127, 166, 176, 178, 182]. Shunts into the subarachnoid space are particularly vulnerable to obstruction due to arachnoid scarring which may be present at the site of shunt placement or induced by implantation of this foreign body [163]. Others noted that spinal arachnoiditis provided a worse prognosis for patients with PTS [166]. Extrathecal shunts may induce a low-pressure syndrome if excessive amounts of CSF are drained inadvertently [46] and are prone to cause cord tethering. Still another problem is presented with septations of a syrinx so that only a part of the cyst may be reached with a single catheter. This requires multiple shunts or perforation of the septations. The latter was suggested by Hüwel et al. [76] who used a small endoscope for this purpose. This technique, however, carries considerable risks. Some of these septations are vascularized so that intramedullary hemorrhages and spinal cord damage may be provoked if perforation is attempted. With collapse of the cyst during implantation of the shunt catheter, the cyst wall may adhere to the catheter and glial tissue may grow inside the tube blocking it completely. No matter what pathophysiological concept is considered to be responsible for the development of a syrinx, a shunt will never treat the cause and, thus, may not be able to prevent another cyst being formed, even if it drains successfully. These problems cannot be overcome with endoscopic methods either.

Most publications recommending syrinx shunts either lack sufficient follow up or they do not define what a successful operation is. With implantation of a catheter into a syrinx, the cyst is drained during surgery. Naturally, the patient will experience some relief immediately. After some time, the shunt may malfunction and need to be revised. Several authors mention this problem [70, 121, 178] but they do not consider shunt malfunctions as treatment failures or consider the possibility that shunts may not influence the prognosis in the long term. The immediate postoperative result does not mean anything for these patients. At least a year is required before the short term effect of a particular operation may be judged. In our opinion, at least a 5-year follow-up is necessary to establish which surgical strategy may be successful or superior to another.

Shunt malfunction rates in the literature vary between 10% [135], 13% [94], and 33% [83]. Edgar and Quail [46] estimated a percentage of as high as 50% depending on the experience of the surgeon. However, these figures mostly review short-term results and are not calculated according to survival statistics such as the Kaplan-Meier method. In reality, the malfunction rate will be even higher. Sgouros and Williams [146] and Batzdorf et al. [22] reviewed long-term results of shunting operations critically and concluded that the clinical recurrence rate after shunting operations is unacceptable.

Figures on morbidity associated with shunt implantations are rarely given. An old publication by Wetzel and Davis [183] mentioned two deaths among 28 patients. Edgar and Quail [46] estimated a morbidity of 3%. However, the number of patients experiencing additional sensory deficits due to the myelotomy is significant and almost never mentioned in the literature. Furthermore, any shunt may introduce another area of arachnoid scarring and cord tethering [146, 147, 155, 157, 184, 186, 191] and additional long-term morbidity (Fig. 4.25).

Vassilouthis et al. [175] and Suzuki et al. [161] proposed to insert thecoperitoneal shunts instead. Lowering subarachnoid pressure may actually cause a decrease of the syrinx. However, low-pressure syndromes may be induced with this technique and long-term studies will have to be done before this technique can be judged for its effectiveness.

Arachnoid dissection at the site of the arachnoid scar with the aim to provide a free CSF passage and to untether the cord offers the potential of a curative procedure. The underlying cause of the syrinx can be treated in this manner and clinical problems associated with the spinal cord tethering can be influenced as well. Both pathomechanisms can be attacked. This concept is not new. Victor Horsley [74] published the first series of 21 patients with focal arachnoid scarring in the spinal canal in 1909 which he treated by arachnoid dissection and suturing the dura into the muscles. Mauss and Krüger [102] used a similar approach for 14 patients with posttraumatic arachnopathies and progressive neurological symptoms in 1918. They sutured the dura after arachnoid dissection. They observed that pulsations of the cord often appeared only after the cord had been freed of the arachnoid tethering. No comment was made as to the possible presence of a syrinx in these patients or the postoperative outcome. The first attempt to treat a syrinx with arachnoid dissection at the site of scarring and leaving the dura open was published by Adelstein [2] in 1938. He achieved a short-term success for each of his three patients.

In general, however, the prognosis of spinal arachnoiditis is considered to be unfavorable irrespective of the type of surgical intervention by many authors [27, 63, 80, 119, 149]. There is a considerable risk of causing additional neurological deficits with attempts to dissect arachnoid scars [63]. In general, postoperative results of arachnolysis without duraplasty are worse than those with additional duraplasty. Elkington [47] reported on 41 patients in whom arachnolysis was performed. Only 12 showed a postoperative improvement, provided the preoperative history was short and no significant cord atrophy was present. Jenik et al. [80] operated on just 5 of 507 patients with spinal arachnoiditis reflecting a rather skeptical attitude towards surgery. Lombardi et al. [98] performed surgery on 31 of 41 patients without duraplasty. Seven patients improved postoperatively, 17 remained unchanged, and three deteriorated. Results of four patients are not known. The clinical course of unoperated patients was similar: one patient improved, six remained unchanged, and three deteriorated.

Some authors combined arachnolysis with puncture or drainage of the syrinx [4, 51, 93, 94, 105, 195]. Falci et al. [51] obtained a stabilization rate of 95.8% among 70 patients with PTS after arachnolysis and additional shunting. Lee et al. [94] described 34 patients with PTS. Their primary goal at surgery was untethering of the cord. If the syrinx collapsed after untethering, no further steps were taken apart form a duraplasty. Otherwise a syrinx shunt was placed. They found a success rate of 90% with this technique. Overall, clinical relapses were more common in the group with additional shunts. Alvisi and Cerisoli [4] reported postoperative improvement for 65% of their 26 patients treated by arachnolysis and cyst puncture. The other authors reported on single cases treated in this manner. For patients with PTS and complete spinal cord lesions, untethering of the cord may be achieved by transecting the cord [23, 148].

Williams and Page [188] reported on six postoperative improvements, ten stabilizations, and five deteriorations after arachnoid dissection, syrinx drainage, and leaving the dura open. In later publications, they advised against additional shunts, however [146, 147, 187]. Without additional shunting, 39 of 68 patients improved postoperatively, nine remained unchanged while ten deteriorated. Ten patients were not operated on due to a stable clinical situation. In one of their publications, they calculated the recurrence rate with the Kaplan-Meier method to be 17% after arachnolysis and 53% after shunting [147].

From our experience, we advise against leaving the dura open. Contamination of the subarachnoid space with blood, etc., may predispose to arachnoiditis and counteract the effect of surgery in the long term.

For treatment of arachnoid scarring and spinal cord tethering, arachnoid dissection alone is associated with a considerable risk of re-tethering [178]. Therefore, we would recommend combination of arachnoid dissection and untethering with a spacious duraplasty. As already outlined for patients with syringomyelia related to pathologies at the foramen magnum, we prefer artificial material for the duraplasty. Gore-Tex appears to be the best material according to our experience. Autologous material such as fascia lata may become vascularized by pial vessels and form dense adhesions with the spinal cord. Parker et al. [119] analyzed 29 patients with spinal arachnoid scarring and syringomyelia. After syrinx shunting, a clinical recurrence rate of 60% was observed compared with 33% after arachnolysis and duraplasty. Similar findings were reported by Schaller et al. [136] on 12 patients. They observed no clinical recurrences after arachnolysis and dura grafting but a recurrence rate of 30% after shunting. Shikata et al. [153] combined arachnoid dissection and duraplasty using lyophilized dura with fusion of the affected spinal levels to immobilize the spine and, thus, minimize the effects of tethering on the cord. They published a rate of 80% good results with this technique in 36 operations. Kramer and Levine [90] obtained good results for 21 patients. Dolan [42] found improvements for 15 patients, 19 remained unchanged, and seven got worse postoperatively. The largest series was published by Edgar and Quail [46] with 150 patients with posttraumatic arachnoid scarring and progressive neurological

symptoms. Unfortunately, they did not provide detailed statistics about their postoperative results.

4.1.5.3.3
Postoperative Clinical Results Related to Etiology

Even though the above-mentioned differences according to types of surgery apply for posttraumatic and postinflammatory arachnoid scarring alike, we would like to add a separate analysis for these two groups as the overwhelming majority of publications still consider them as two different entities.

4.1.5.3.3.1
Posttraumatic Syringomyelia

Comparing results of the two treatment strategies, Table 4.10 reveals almost no difference if short-term results are considered. Shunting as well as arachnolysis combined with a duraplasty are capable of providing at least a short-term benefit for this group of patients. The Karnofsky score remains virtually unchanged during the first postoperative year. In contrast with the rather marginal clinical changes, still 31% of patients considered their situation improved relative to preoperatively in the group treated by arachnolysis and duraplasty. Fifty-four percent thought they were stable, while 15% experienced some neurological progression. In the shunt group, the corresponding figures were 12%, 56%, and 32% for postoperative improvement, stabilization, and deterioration, respectively. There was no statistically significant difference.

Looking at long-term results and clinical recurrence rates, the figures were significantly better for arachnolysis and duraplasty (Fig. 4.27) (log-rank test: $P=0.0348$). Fifty-five percent were improved or stabilized for at least 5 years relative to 14% in the shunted group.

4.1.5.3.3.2
Postinflammatory Syringomyelia

Compared with patients with PTS, this patient group was in a better preoperative neurological status. This was mainly due to the fact that no initial spinal cord damage was present. This is mainly reflected in higher scores for motor power, gait, and Karnofsky rating (Tables 4.10 and 4.11).

Unlike posttraumatic patients, where differences between treatment groups were apparent for long-term results only, arachnolysis and duraplasty offered a better outcome already within the first postoperative year. Slight improvements were observed for sensory deficits, pain, gait ataxia, and bladder function. Thirty percent considered their situation improved post-

Table 4.10. Postoperative clinical results for patients with posttraumatic syringomyelia

Group	Preop.	Postop.	3 months	6 months	1 year	P
Sensory deficits						
Arachnolysis	2.8±1.0	2.8±1.1	2.8±1.0	2.9±1.1	2.8±1.0	n.s.
Shunt	2.3±1.2	2.5±1.3	2.6±1.4	2.6±1.4	2.6±1.4	n.s.
Dysesthesias						
Arachnolysis	3.4±1.2	3.8±0.8	3.8±0.9	3.9±1.0	3.8±0.9	n.s.
Shunt	3.1±1.1	3.4±1.0	3.5±0.9	3.5±0.9	3.4±1.0	n.s.
Pain						
Arachnolysis	3.5±0.9	3.8±0.6	3.8±0.8	3.8±0.8	3.7±0.9	n.s.
Shunt	3.5±0.9	3.5±0.9	3.8±0.8	3.8±0.8	3.7±0.7	n.s.
Motor power						
Arachnolysis	3.4±1.3	3.1±1.2	3.3±1.2	3.3±1.2	3.4±1.2	n.s.
Shunt	2.6±1.4	2.7±1.5	2.7±1.6	2.7±1.6	2.7±1.6	n.s.
Gait ataxia						
Arachnolysis	3.3±1.4	3.0±1.4	3.0±1.4	3.1±1.4	3.0±1.4	n.s.
Shunt	1.5±1.5	1.5±1.4	1.5±1.5	1.5±1.4	1.4±1.5	n.s.
Bladder function						
Arachnolysis	3.3±1.4	3.2±1.4	3.3±1.4	3.3±1.4	3.3±1.4	n.s.
Shunt	2.2±1.6	2.4±1.7	2.4±1.7	2.3±1.7	2.3±1.6	n.s.
Bowel function						
Arachnolysis	3.4±1.4	3.3±1.6	3.4±1.4	3.4±1.4	3.5±1.5	n.s.
Shunt	2.3±1.6	2.4±1.7	2.4±1.7	2.4±1.7	2.4±1.7	n.s.
Karnofsky score						
Arachnolysis	63±16	61±14	63±15	63±15	63±15	n.s.
Shunt	45±17	43±19	45±18	44±19	44±19	n.s.

Preop. preoperatively, *Postop.* postoperatively, *P* P-value for comparison preoperative and postoperative scores after 1 year (paired *t*-test)

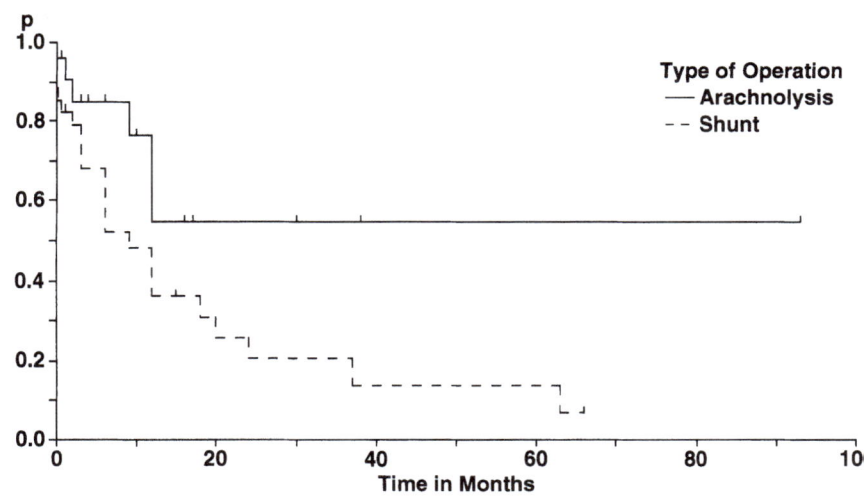

Fig. 4.27. Kaplan-Meier analysis of clinical recurrences for patients with posttraumatic syringomyelia for comparison of syrinx shunts and arachnolysis with duraplasty (log-rank test: *P*=0.0348)

Table 4.11. Postoperative results for patients with postinflammatory syringomyelia

Group	Preop.	Postop.	3 months	6 months	1 year	P
Sensory deficits						
Arachnolysis	3.1±0.8	3.2±0.9	3.4±0.9	3.3±0.9	3.3±0.9	n.s.
Shunt	2.4±0.9	2.4±1.0	2.4±1.1	2.4±1.1	2.4±1.1	n.s.
Dysesthesias						
Arachnolysis	3.8±0.8	4.0±0.7	4.0±0.7	3.9±0.7	3.8±0.8	n.s.
Shunt	3.8±1.2	3.9±1.2	4.0±1.1	3.9±1.2	3.8±1.3	n.s.
Pain						
Arachnolysis	3.8±0.8	4.0±0.7	4.1±0.6	4.1±0.6	4.0±0.9	n.s.
Shunt	3.3±1.0	3.8±0.9	4.1±0.7	4.1±0.7	3.9±0.8	0.04
Motor power						
Arachnolysis	3.9±1.1	3.8±1.3	3.9±1.2	3.9±1.1	3.9±1.2	n.s.
Shunt	3.2±1.1	3.2±1.1	3.3±0.9	3.3±1.0	3.1±1.3	n.s.
Gait ataxia						
Arachnolysis	3.6±0.7	3.6±0.7	3.8±0.9	3.9±0.9	3.8±0.9	n.s.
Shunt	2.9±1.4	2.9±1.4	2.9±1.4	3.0±1.4	2.8±1.6	n.s.
Bladder function						
Arachnolysis	4.1±1.0	4.3±0.7	4.4±0.7	4.4±0.7	4.4±0.7	n.s.
Shunt	2.7±1.8	2.6±1.7	2.6±1.7	2.6±1.7	2.6±1.7	n.s.
Bowel function						
Arachnolysis	4.5±0.9	4.5±0.7	4.5±0.7	4.5±0.7	4.5±0.8	n.s.
Shunt	3.1±1.8	3.0±1.7	3.0±1.7	2.9±1.7	2.9±1.7	n.s.
Karnofsky score						
Arachnolysis	71±9	72±10	73±12	74±10	73±11	n.s.
Shunt	62±17	61±18	61±19	61±19	58±21	n.s.

Preop. preoperatively, *Postop.* postoperatively, *P* P-value for comparison of preoperative and postoperative scores after 1 year (paired *t*-test)

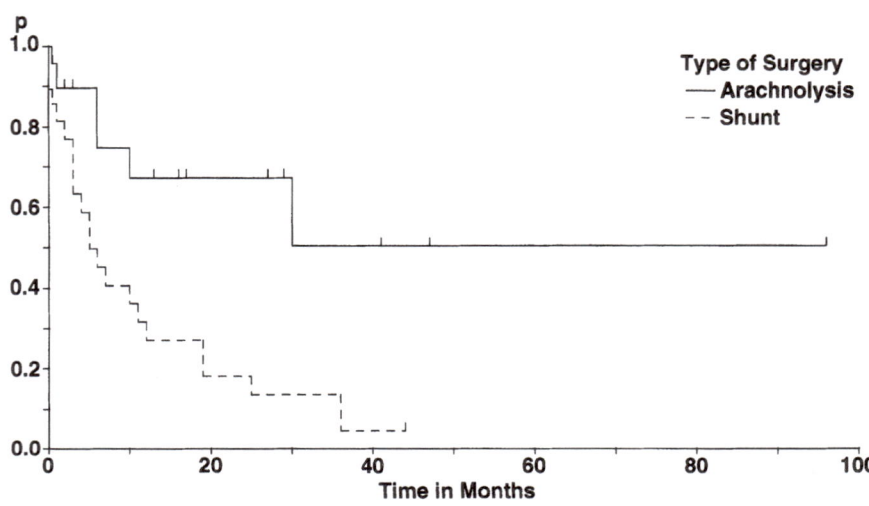

Fig. 4.28. Kaplan-Meier analysis of clinical recurrences for patients with postinflammatory syringomyelia for comparison of syrinx shunts and arachnolysis with duraplasty (log-rank test: *P*=0.0034)

operatively, 43% unchanged and 26% worse. The Karnofsky score tended to increase slightly. In contrast, shunting provided improvement for pain only. The Karnofsky score tended to decrease within the first postoperative year as did scores for motor power, gait, and sphincter functions. Just 11% thought shunting had improved their symptoms, 50% considered their status unaltered, while 39% reported postoperative worsening.

Looking at long-term results and clinical recurrence rates, this difference became even clearer. Fifty percent were improved or unchanged for at least 5 years after arachnolysis and duraplasty relative to just 5% in the shunted group (Fig. 4.28) (log-rank test: P=0.0034).

4.1.5.3.4
Postoperative Clinical Results Related to Grade of Scarring

Apart from the type of surgery and the preoperative neurological status, the grade of arachnoid scarring has a direct influence on postoperative outcome [31, 80, 88, 106, 119, 146, 149, 158, 187], irrespective of a traumatic or inflammatory origin. Except for dysesthesias, pain, and sphincter functions there was a correlation of preoperative symptoms to the grade of scarring (Table 4.12). Again, short-term results did not reveal a major difference between each treatment modality. However, the Karnofsky scores tended to increase slightly in the postoperative year for patients treated by arachnolysis and duraplasty, whereas they tended to decrease after shunting.

The analysis of long-term results revealed that patients with focal arachnoid scarring are the best candidates for arachnolysis and duraplasty (log-rank test: P=0.0018) [88, 119]. Eighty-one percent in this group were stabilized for at least 5 years compared with 26% in the group with extensive arachnoid scarring. The outcome after shunting, however, was not influenced by the degree of scarring. The rate of stabilized patients was low regardless (9% and 8%, respectively) (Fig. 4.29). The subjective postoperative reports of the patients reflect these long-term results quite accurately as depicted in Table 4.13 (Chi-square test: P=0.0382).

4.1.6
Management of Clinical Recurrences of Spinal Arachnoid Scarring

Seventy operations among 43 patients were secondary surgeries in our series. Compared with patients with syringomyelia related to foramen magnum diseases, this is a much higher proportion and emphasizes the therapeutic problems with this entity. Two major groups have to be distinguished in this subset of patients: patients who have undergone a syrinx shunting operation (Fig. 4.29) and have not been treated yet for the arachnoid scarring and patients in whom a first attempt to treat the arachnoid scarring has failed (Fig. 4.30). Nine patients underwent arachnolysis combined with a duraplasty more than once. Seventeen patients were operated on with this method after syrinx shunting. Twenty-five patients underwent syrinx shunts as a secondary operation after various types of primary operations. Six patients underwent cervical fusions (four patients), arachnolysis without duraplasty (one patient), or implantation of a thalamic stimulator for pain treatment (one patient) as a secondary procedure.

For patients who underwent a first attempt of arachnolysis, management guidelines are similar to those outlined for secondary foramen magnum operations. The major influence on surgical risks and clinical outcome is the extent and severity of the arachnoid scarring. For spinal arachnoid scarring, the severity and extent of the scarring can be estimated according to the clinical history and the operation notes of the first intervention. In general, severe forms of arachnoiditis will be encountered in this group. According to the above-mentioned results in relation to grade of arachnoid scarring, it can be expected that chances for a satisfactory long-term result are significantly reduced compared with a first operation.

If autologous material was inserted for grafting at the first operation, microsurgical dissection may be particularly dangerous as the dura graft may be densely adherent to the cord surface and may receive part of its blood supply from pial vessels making separation of dura patch and cord virtually impossible without damaging the cord surface (Fig. 4.30). Therefore, we would indicate a secondary operation in this group of patients only, if there is significant clinical deterioration and evidence on MRI that the obstruction of CSF flow is limited to a small area. If the preoperative MRI suggests extensive adherence of an autologous graft to the cord surface or the patient has severe neurological deficits related to the initial trauma or a severe arachnoiditis, we consider reoperation at that spinal level to be contraindicated. From our experience, the risks of reexploration – even opening the dura – are way too high to warrant this strategy. In such an instance, we would either implant a syrinx shunt at a different spinal level or even advise against surgery despite clinical progression. However, if artificial material was used for dura grafting, the risks of microsurgical dissection are much lower and chances for achieving a better result with secondary surgery may be more favorable.

Comparing the preoperative status of patients who underwent arachnolysis and duraplasty as a secondary

Table 4.12. Postoperative clinical results for patients with spinal arachnoid scarring related to grade of scarring

Group	Preop.	Postop.	3 months	6 months	1 year	P
Sensory deficits						
Arachnolysis I + II	3.1±1.0	3.1±1.1	3.1±1.0	3.3±1.0	3.3±1.0	n.s.
Arachnolysis III + IV	2.7±0.8	2.8±0.9	3.0±1.0	2.9±0.9	2.8±0.9	n.s.
Shunt I + II	2.6+0.9	2.8+1.0	2.8+1.2	2.8+1.2	2.8+1.2	n.s.
Shunt III + IV	2.2+1.1	2.3+1.2	2.3+1.3	2.3+1.3	2.3+1.3	n.s.
Dysesthesias						
Arachnolysis I + II	3.5±1.0	3.8±0.8	3.7±0.7	3.7±0.9	3.7±0.9	n.s.
Arachnolysis III + IV	3.8±1.0	4.1±0.7	4.2±0.8	4.2±0.8	3.9±0.8	n.s.
Shunt I + II	3.5±1.0	3.7+1.0	3.8+1.0	3.8+1.0	3.6+1.0	n.s.
Shunt III + IV	3.3+1.3	3.5+1.2	3.6+1.1	3.6+1.1	3.5+1.2	n.s.
Pain						
Arachnolysis I + II	3.4±0.8	3.8±0.6	3.7±0.6	3.7±0.6	3.6±0.8	n.s.
Arachnolysis III + IV	4.0±0.8	4.1±0.7	4.3±0.7	4.3±0.7	4.2±0.9	n.s.
Shunt I + II	3.6+0.9	3.8+0.8	4.0+0.5	4.0+0.5	3.8+0.5	n.s.
Shunt III + IV	3.3+1.0	3.6+1.0	3.9+0.9	3.8+0.9	3.7+0.9	0.015
Motor power						
Arachnolysis I + II	4.2±1.2	3.9±1.3	4.0±1.3	4.1±1.2	4.1±1.1	n.s.
Arachnolysis III + IV	3.0±1.0	2.8±1.0	3.0±1.0	3.1±0.9	3.0±0.9	n.s.
Shunt I + II	3.1+1.3	3.4+1.4	3.4+1.5	3.4+1.5	3.4+1.5	n.s.
Shunt III + IV	2.7+1.3	2.5+1.3	2.6+1.2	2.6+1.2	2.5+1.3	n.s.
Gait ataxia						
Arachnolysis I + II	3.7±1.2	3.5±1.3	3.5±1.3	3.6±1.3	3.6±1.3	n.s.
Arachnolysis III + IV	3.2±1.0	3.2±1.0	3.3±1.1	3.4±1.1	3.2±1.1	n.s.
Shunt I + II	2.4+1.7	2.4+1.7	2.3+1.7	2.3+1.7	2.3+1.8	n.s.
Shunt III + IV	1.9+1.5	1.8+1.4	1.9+1.5	2.0+1.5	1.8+1.6	n.s.
Bladder function						
Arachnolysis I + II	3.7±1.3	3.7±1.4	3.7±1.4	3.7±1.4	3.7±1.4	n.s.
Arachnolysis III + IV	3.7±1.1	3.9±0.9	4.1±0.8	4.1±0.8	4.1±0.8	n.s.
Shunt I + II	2.7+1.7	2.9+1.8	2.9+1.8	2.8+1.7	2.7+1.7	n.s.
Shunt III + IV	2.2+1.7	2.2+1.6	2.2+1.6	2.2+1.6	2.2+1.6	n.s.
Bowel function						
Arachnolysis I + II	3.9±1.5	3.8±1.6	3.9±1.5	3.9±1.5	3.9±1.5	n.s.
Arachnolysis III + IV	4.1±0.9	4.2±0.8	4.2±0.8	4.2±0.8	4.2±0.8	n.s.
Shunt I + II	3.1+1.8	3.1+1.8	3.1+1.8	3.1+1.8	3.1+1.8	n.s.
Shunt III + IV	2.3+1.6	2.3+1.6	2.3+1.6	2.3+1.6	2.3+1.6	n.s.
Karnofsky score						
Arachnolysis I + II	69±13	69±14	69±16	69±16	70±16	n.s.
Arachnolysis III + IV	64±13	64±13	66±12	67±12	66±12	n.s.
Shunt I + II	54+22	54+22	54+22	54+22	53+22	n.s.
Shunt III + IV	50+18	48+19	49+19	49+19	47+19	n.s.

Preop. preoperatively, *Postop.* postoperatively, *P* P-value for comparison of preoperative and postoperative scores after 1 year (paired *t*-test)

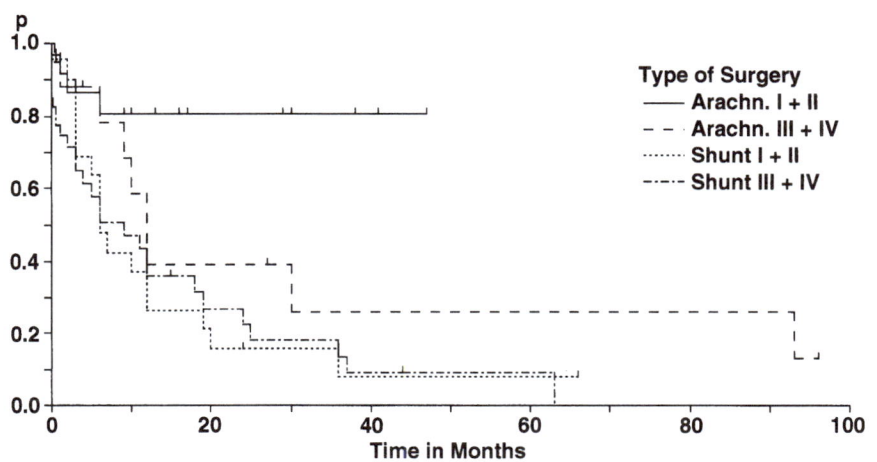

Fig. 4.29. Kaplan-Meier analysis of clinical recurrences for patients with posttraumatic and postinflammatory arachnoid scarring related to grade of arachnoid pathology (log-rank test: P=0018) (*Arachn.* arachnoid scarring)

Table 4.13. Postoperative results for patients with spinal arachnoid scarring

Result	Arachnolysis + duraplasty Grade I + II	Arachnolysis + duraplasty Grade III + IV	Shunt Grade I + II	Shunt Grade III + IV
Improved	33%	26%	9%	13%
Unchanged	57%	37%	64%	48%
Worse	10%	37%	27%	40%

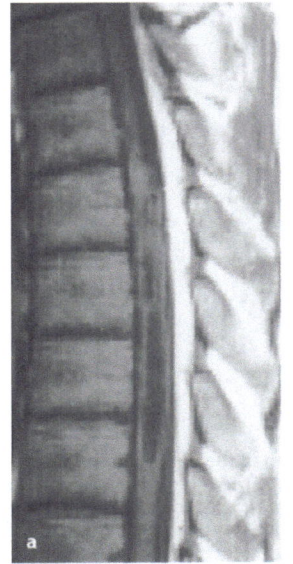
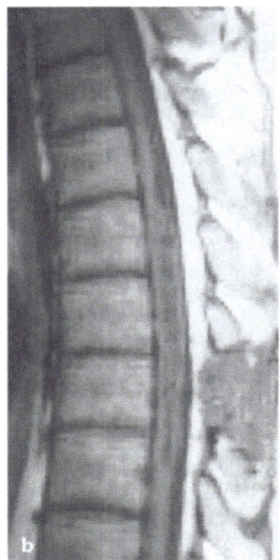
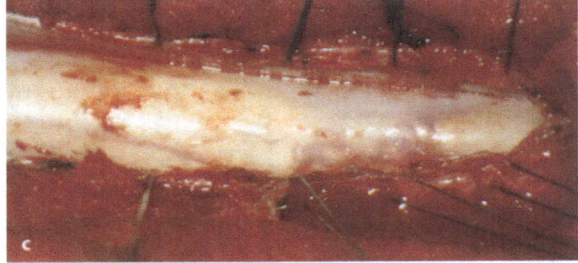
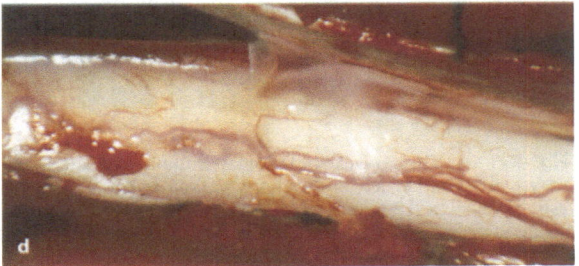

Fig. 4.30 a–g. a This T1-weighted MRI scan of a 35-year old man with progressive gait ataxia shows a syrinx between Th6 and Th9. The spinal cord image at the upper pole of the syrinx displays irregularities suggesting arachnoid scarring at this level. **b** After placement of a syringosubarachnoid shunt at Th8 in another hospital no clinical benefit was obtained. Gait pro-blems progressed to the point that he needed crutches to move around. **c** The surgical exploration extended from Th6 to Th8. After dura opening the arachnoid scarring becomes visible. **d** In usual technique layer by layer of scarring could be resected in the area of shunt implantation (continued on next page)

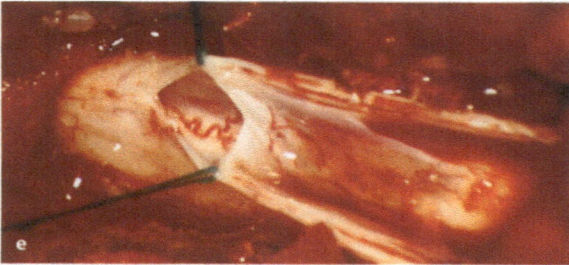

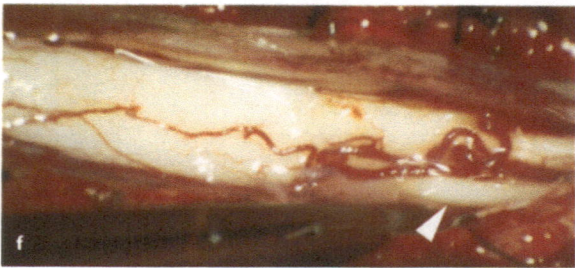

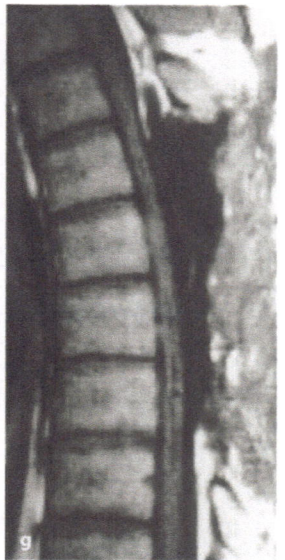

Fig. 4.30 e–g. e Finally, the area of Th5 was reached where an arachnoid web caused a complete block of CSF passage. After resection of this web, the cord collapsed and started to pulsate. **f** The final view shows the free CSF space throughout the exposure. The shunt catheter (*arrow*) was tightly adherent in arachnoid scar tissue laterally and was left in place. A large duraplasty was inserted. **g** The postoperative T1-weighted MRI scan demonstrates a marked decrease of the syrinx and a free posterior CSF pathway. The patient improved considerably and could walk without an aid 6 months later

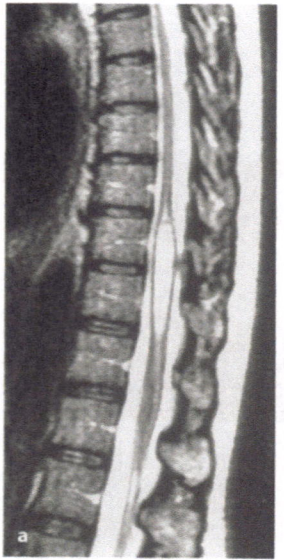

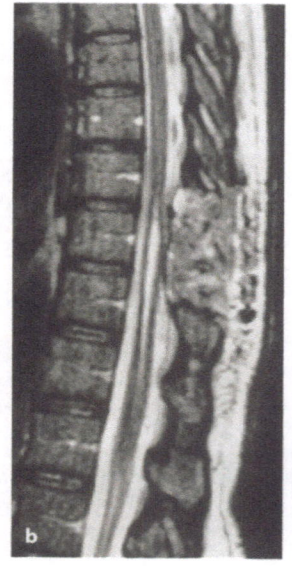

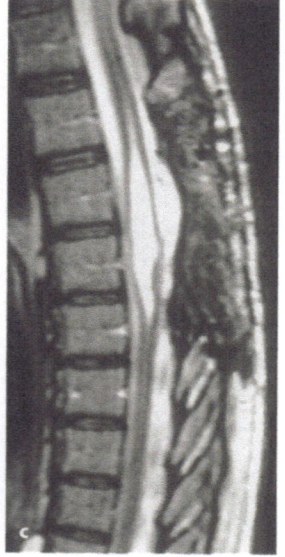

Fig. 4.31 a–j. This 42-year-old woman complained about sensory deficits in her left lower abdomen and burning type dysesthesias. **a** The T2-weighted MRI scan before surgery demonstrates a syrinx at Th8/9 and a small area of arachnoid scarring (*arrow*). **b** Postoperatively, the patient's symptoms improved and a MRI control revealed a decreased size of the syrinx. However, the fascia lata duraplasty appears in contact with the underlying spinal cord. **c** One year later, symptoms worsened again and this MRI showed an increase of the syrinx and a possible adhesion between graft and spinal cord in the lower half of the exposure. **d** This intraoperative view demonstrates the fascia dura graft before incision. With ultrasound an appropriate area was selected so that injury to the underlying cord could be avoided. **e** After insertion of the dura graft in the midline, thus avoiding the suture line, a pseudomembrane becomes apparent. **f** Incision at the cranial part of the exposure reveals the underlying spinal cord relatively unaffected by arachnoid scarring. **g** At the caudal part of the exposure, however, thick and densely adherent scar tissue bound the dura graft to the spinal cord surface. **h** This view demonstrates the final result with scar still covering the cord in the caudal part of the exposure obscuring blood vessels of the spinal cord surface. **i** A large Gore-Tex graft was inserted. **j** The postoperative MRI-scan 3 months later shows a free CSF passage but no significant change of the syrinx size. The patient still suffers from severe dysesthesias

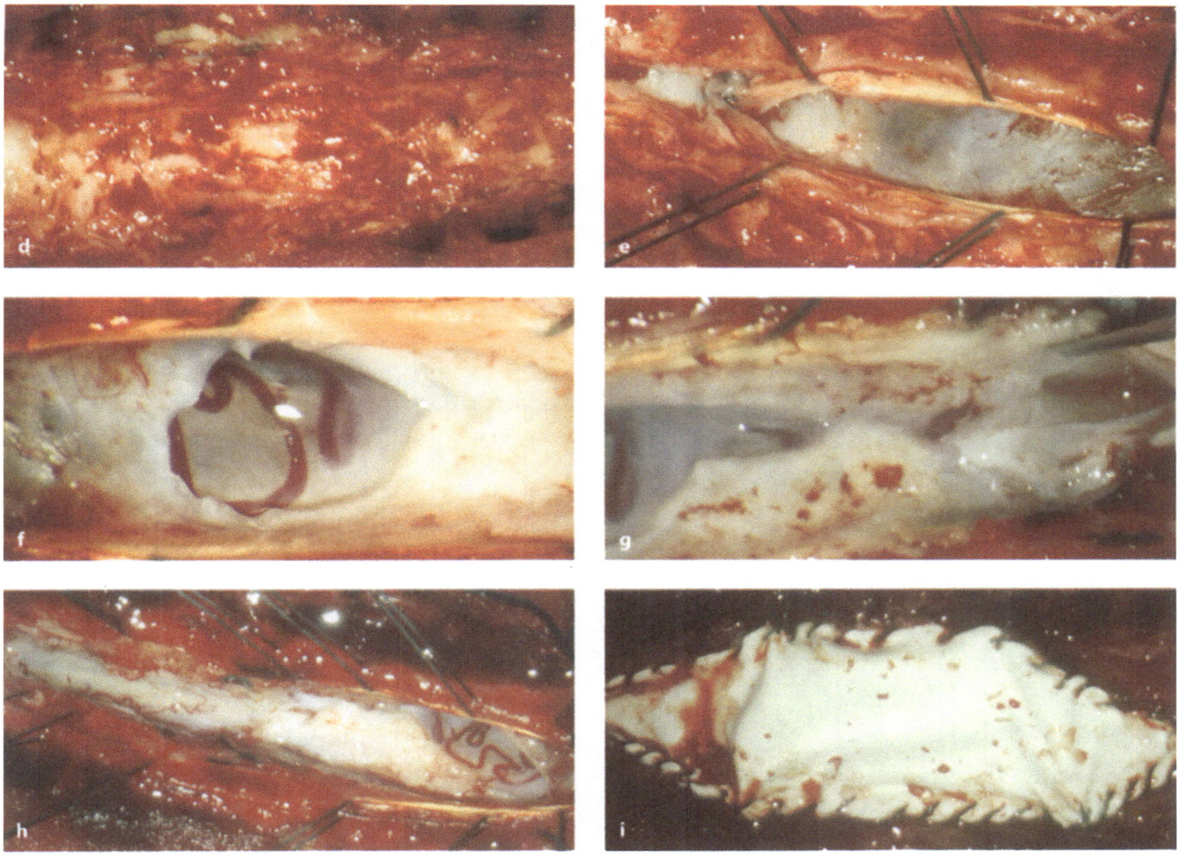

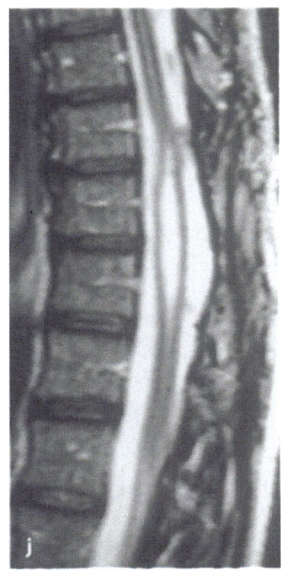

Fig. 4.31 d–j

operation after a first surgical attempt at the same spinal level to patients undergoing this surgery as the primary operation did not reveal significant differences for any symptom or the Karnofsky score (63±10 and 66±14, respectively). Patients in worse clinical condition underwent syrinx shunting procedures, if a second operation was required. Their preoperative scores were significantly lower than in those undergoing primary shunting operations (Karnofsky score 48±18 and 58±21, respectively; *t*-test: *P*=0.0013).

The patient is operated on while in the prone position. The old wound is reopened extending the exposure cranially and caudally for one spinal segment. The spinal laminae of these segments are exposed first and the remainder of the epidural dissection is performed after these two laminae have been identified. Extending the laminectomy for a few millimeters in either direction allows easy identification of the dura. In this manner, it is much easier and safer to dissect the epidural scar off the dura graft. Coming from an unoperated area, the dura can be followed around the dura patch laterally. This is much easier and safer than trying to dissect in the midline. Once the dura

Table 4.14. Postoperative clinical results for secondary operations in patients with spinal arachnoid scarring

Group	Preop.	Postop.	3 months	6 months	P
Sensory deficits					
Arach. Group A	3.3±0.5	3.5±0.6	3.5±1.0	3.5±1.0	n.s.
Arach. Group B	2.4±0.9	2.6±0.9	2.6±0.9	2.6±0.9	n.s.
Shunt	2.2±1.3	2.2±1.3	2.3±1.4	2.3±1.4	n.s.
Dysesthesias					
Arach. Group A	4.0±1.2	4.5±0.6	4.3±1.0	4.3±1.0	n.s.
Arach. Group B	3.1±1.3	3.6±1.0	3.6±1.0	3.7±1.0	n.s.
Shunt	3.4±1.2	3.6±1.1	3.8±1.1	3.8±1.1	n.s.
Pain					
Arach. Group A	4.8±0.5	4.0±0.8	4.5±0.6	4.8±0.5	n.s.
Arach. Group B	3.7±1.1	4.1±0.8	4.2±0.8	4.2±0.8	n.s.
Shunt	3.4±1.0	3.6±1.0	3.9±0.9	3.9±0.9	0.0007
Motor power					
Arach. Group A	3.3±1.0	3.5±0.6	3.5±0.6	3.5±0.6	n.s.
Arach. Group B	2.9±0.8	3.0±0.9	3.1±0.8	3.2±0.8	n.s.
Shunt	2.5±1.2	2.5±1.3	2.6±1.3	2.6±1.3	n.s.
Gait ataxia					
Arach. Group A	3.0±0.8	2.8±1.3	3.0±0.8	3.0±0.8	n.s.
Arach. Group B	2.6±1.2	2.6±1.4	2.7±1.4	2.8±1.4	n.s.
Shunt	1.8±1.5	1.8±1.4	1.9±1.5	1.8±1.5	n.s.
Bladder function					
Arach. Group A	2.8±1.7	3.0±1.8	3.0±1.8	3.0±1.8	n.s.
Arach. Group B	3.0±1.5	3.0±1.7	3.2±1.6	3.2±1.6	n.s.
Shunt	2.2±1.7	2.4±1.7	2.4±1.7	2.4±1.7	n.s.
Bowel function					
Arach. Group A	4.3±1.0	4.3±1.0	4.3±1.0	4.3±1.0	n.s.
Arach. Group B	3.6±1.2	3.4±1.3	3.5±1.3	3.5±1.3	n.s.
Shunt	2.4±1.7	2.4±1.7	2.5±1.7	2.5±1.7	n.s.
Karnofsky score					
Arach. Group A	63±10	63±10	65±13	63±17	n.s.
Arach. Group B	56±17	57±17	60±16	61±16	0.0143
Shunt	48±18	46±20	47±21	47±21	n.s.

Arach. Group A secondary arachnolysis and duraplasty after primary arachnolysis, *Arach. Group B* secondary arachnolysis and duraplasty after shunting, *shunt* shunt syrinx, *P* P-value for comparison of preoperative and postoperative scores after 6 months (paired *t*-test)

has been identified around the entire dura patch, the epidural scar on the graft can be resected layer by layer under the microscope. Ultrasound is then used to identify a safe spot for the initial dura opening avoiding an area where the cord is directly adherent to the dura or graft. As outlined above, the dura should be opened without simultaneously opening the arachnoid wherever possible. In the area of the graft, however, this may not be possible. Here, arachnoid and graft may no longer be separable and may form one layer of scar tissue. In such a case it is better to cut the dura around the graft leaving the graft adherent to the cord surface at first. In other instances, a pseudomembrane may have formed which can be used as a protective layer toward the underlying cord during dura opening (Fig. 4.31e). The dura is then held open with retention sutures. The arachnoid can now be opened on either end of the exposure gaining access to the subarachnoid space above and below the scarring. The scar and graft adherent to the cord surface can then be approached safely. Only if artificial material was used for duraplasty may it be possible to dissect it off without risking any cord damage. With dense adhesions to the cord surface, no attempts should be undertaken to resect such a scar off the cord surface. We prefer to leave such a piece of scar, i.e., part of the former dura patch, undisturbed (Fig. 4.31h). Dissection is strictly limited to the posterior part of the spinal canal. Untethering of the cord in secondary operations is not possible in the overwhelming majority of cases and should not be attempted unless the tethering is limited to the posterior aspect of the cord.

Finally, a spacious Gore-Tex patch is inserted. The graft may be fashioned to provide even enough space

for CSF flow in cases where parts of the former graft had to be left attached to the cord surface (Fig. 4.31i). The epidural soft tissue is closed tightly layer for layer, and a lumbar drain is inserted routinely in secondary cases to avoid CSF fistulas.

For patients who underwent a syrinx shunt as the first line of therapy, the same strategy applies if the shunt was inserted at the spinal level of arachnoid scarring. However, if the shunt had been placed at a different level, surgery of the arachnoid scarring can be undertaken as in a primary operation.

Short-term clinical results are presented in Table 4.13 and 4.14. As may be expected, the best results could be achieved in patients who underwent arachnolysis and duraplasty after shunting. The Karnofsky score increased from 56±17 to 61±17 6 months after surgery.

Looking at long-term results and clinical recurrence rates, the worst outcome was observed for patients who underwent a second attempt of arachnolysis and duraplasty. All patients experienced a clinical recurrence within 12 months. If arachnolysis and duraplasty was performed after shunting, 33% of patients were at least stabilized for 5 years. This outcome was still significantly worse, however, if compared with patients undergoing arachnolysis and duraplasty as the first line of treatment. In that group, 67% were stabilized for at least 5 years (log-rank test: $P=0.05$) (Fig. 4.32).

For patients undergoing syrinx shunts as secondary interventions, no significant differences were observed depending on the type of previous operation or whether secondary and primary operations were compared, even though there was a trend for a better outcome if the shunt had been placed after arachnolysis

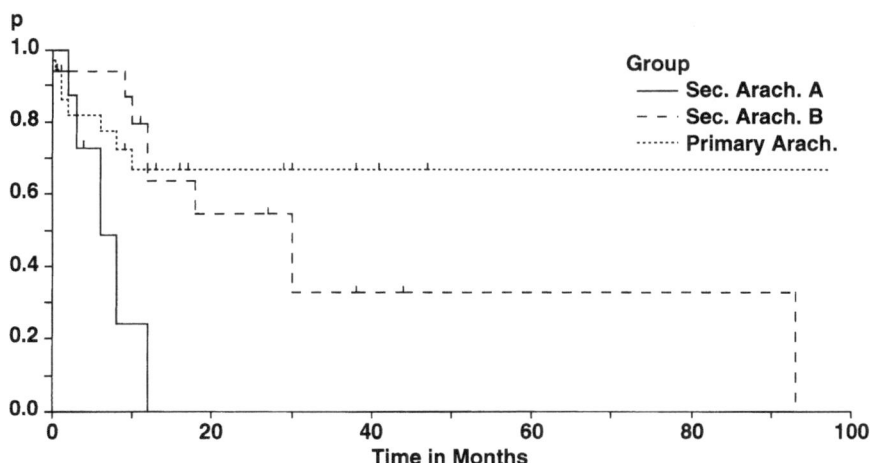

Fig. 4.32. Kaplan-Meier analysis of clinical recurrences for patients with posttraumatic and postinflammatory syringomyelia comparing patients with primary and secondary attempts of arachnolysis and duraplasty. Group A patients underwent a second attempt of arachnoid dissection after a failed first one. Group B patients underwent this procedure after a previous shunt (log-rank test: $P=0.05$) (*Sec. Arach.* secondary arachnolysis and duraplasty, *Primary Arach.* primary arachnolysis and duraplasty)

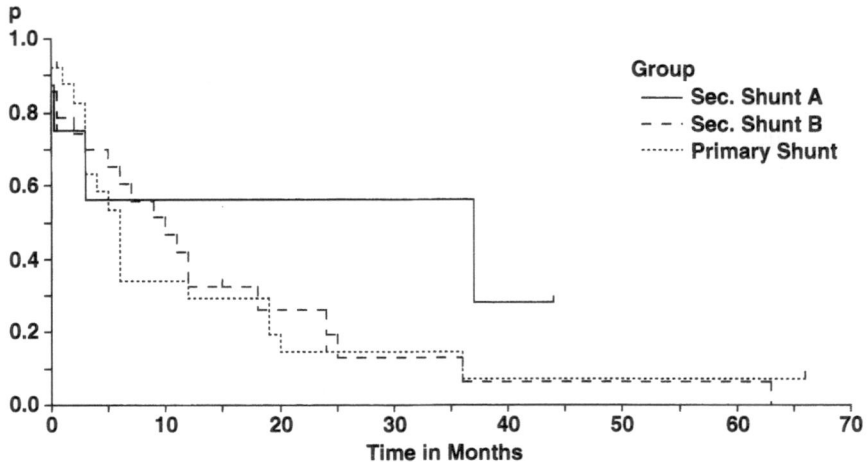

Fig. 4.33. Kaplan-Meier analysis of clinical recurrences for patients with posttraumatic and postinflammatory syringomyelia comparing patients with primary and secondary attempts of syrinx shunting. Group A patients underwent shunting after a failed attempt of arachnolysis and duraplasty. Group B patients underwent shunting revisions (log-rank test: not significant) (*Sec. Shunt* secondary shunt)

and duraplasty (5-year stabilization rate 28% compared with 7%) (Fig. 4.33).

This analysis reveals quite clearly that arachnolysis and duraplasty should be the treatment of choice for patients with syringomyelia associated with arachnoid scarring unless a previous intradural surgery was undertaken at the spinal level of scarring. In that particular subgroup of patients, long-term results are better if shunting is performed as the secondary procedure rather than re-exploring the site of arachnoid scarring.

4.1.7
Conclusions for Patients with Spinal Arachnoid Scarring

Posttraumatic and postinflammatory syringomyelia are caused by arachnoid scarring. CSF flow obstruction, spinal cord compression and tethering may lead to a combination of a local myelopathy and syringomyelia extending from the area of scarring in a cranial or caudal direction. A primary cord injury is not required for the development of PTS. Thus, a minor trauma may be sufficient to cause this complication provided an arachnoid scar is formed at the level of the impact. The percentage of patients developing syringomyelia after arachnoid scarring is still not precisely known.

Neuroradiological diagnosis of the localization, severity and extent of the arachnoid scar remains to be a challenge but is essential for precise surgical planning. The realistic goal of surgical treatment in this group of patients is stabilization of the neurological status with arachnolysis and duraplasty. Therefore, patients with PTS or PIS are candidates for surgery once neurological symptoms start to progress.

For focal arachnoid scarring, we recommend that the dissection be performed using microsurgical techniques aimed at obtaining free CSF flow and untethering of the cord. With more extensive forms of arachnoid scarring, a free passage of CSF can still be obtained posteriorly, but untethering of the cord is almost impossible to achieve. In selected cases, spinal cord decompression by resection of arachnoid cysts or pouches may be an alternative option. If primary attempts to improve CSF flow and to decompress the spinal canal have failed, shunting of a syrinx may be indicated as a secondary intervention. If a shunt is implanted, it should be inserted at a spinal level unaffected by arachnoid changes.

References

1. Abbe R, Coley WB (1892) Syringomyelia; operation, exploration of the cord; withdrawal of fluid. J Nerv Ment Dis 19:512–520
2. Adelstein LJ (1938) Surgical treatment of syringomyelia. Am J Surg 40:384–395
3. Alajouanine T, Hornet T, Thurel R, Andre R (1935) Le feutrage arachnoidien postérieur dans la syringomyélie (sa place dans la pathologie des leptoméninges). Rev Neurol (Paris) 64:91–98
4. Alvisi C, Cerisoli M (1984) Longterm results of the surgical treatment of syringohydromyelia. Acta Neurochir (Wien) 71:133–140
5. Aminoff MJ, Wilcox CS (1972) Autonomic dysfunction in syringomyelia. Postgrad Med J 48:113–115
6. Anderson NE, Willoughby EW, Wrightson P (1986) The natural history of syringomyelia. Clin Exp Neurol 22:71–80
7. Anton HA, Schweigel JF (1986) Posttraumatic syringomyelia: the British Columbia experience. Spine 11:865–868
8. Assenmacher DR, Ducker TB (1971) Experimental traumatic paraplegia. The vascular and pathological changes seen in reversible and irreversible spinal cord lesions. J Bone Joint Surg Am 53:671–680
9. Attal N, Brasseur L, Parker F, Tadie M, Bouhassira D (1999) [Characterization of sensation disorders and neuropathic pain related to syringomyelia. A prospective study]. Neurochirurgie 45 [Suppl 1]:84–94
10. Aubin ML, Vignaud J, Jardin C, Bar D (1981) Computed tomography in 75 clinical cases of syringomyelia. AJNR Am J Neuroradiol 2:199–204
11. Aubin ML, Baleriaux D, Cosnard G, Crouzet G, Doyon D, Halimi P, Manelfe C (1987) MRI in syringomyelia of

congenital, infectious, traumatic or idiopathic origin. A study of 142 cases. J Neuroradiol 14:313–336

12. Backe HA, Betz RR, Mesgarzadeh M, Beck T, Clancy M (1991) Post-traumatic spinal cord cysts evaluated by magnetic resonance imaging. Paraplegia 29:607–612

13. Barbaro NM, Wilson CB, Gutin PH, Edwards MSB (1984) Surgical treatment of syringomyelia. J Neurosurg 61:531–538

14. Barnett HJ, Botterell EH, Jousse AT, Wynne-Jones M (1966) Progressive myelopathy as a sequel to traumatic paraplegia. Brain 89:159–174

15. Barnett HJM (1973) Syringomyelia associated with spinal arachnoiditis. In: Barnett HJM, Foster JB, Hudgson P (eds) Syringomyelia. Major problems in neurology, vol 1. Saunders, London, pp 220–244

16. Barnett HJM (1973) The pathogenesis of syringomyelic cavitation associated with arachnoiditis localised to the spinal cord. In: Barnett HJM, Foster JB, Hudgson P (eds) Syringomyelia. Major problems in neurology, vol 1. Saunders, London, pp 245–260

17. Barnett HJM, Jousse AT (1973) Syringomyelia as a late sequel to traumatic paraplegia and quadriplegia – clinical features. In: Barnett HJM, Foster JB, Hudgson P (eds) Syringomyelia. Major problems in neurology, vol 1. Saunders, London, pp 129–153

18. Barnett HJM, Jousse AT (1976) Posttraumatic syringomyelia cystic myelopathy. In: Vinken PJV, Bruyn GW (eds) Handbook of clinical neurology, vol 26. II. Injuries of the spine and spinal cord. North Holland Publishing Company, Amsterdam, pp 113–157

19. Barnett HJM, Jousse AT, Ball MJ (1973) Pathology and pathogenesis of progressive cystic myelopathy as a late sequel to spinal cord injury. In: Barnett HJM, Foster JB, Hudgson P (eds) Syringomyelia. Major problems in neurology, vol 1. Saunders, London, pp 179–219

20. Bastian HC (1867) On a case of concussion-lesion with extensive secondary degeneration of the spinal cord. Proc R Med Chir Soc London 50:499

21. Batten FE (1916) Paraplegia following cerebrospinal meningitis: laminectomy. Proc R Soc Med (Neurol Sect) 9:63

22. Batzdorf U, Klekamp J, Johnson JP (1998) A critical appraisal of syrinx cavity shunting procedures. J Neurosurg 89:382–388

23. Berrington NR (1993) Posttraumatic spinal cord tethering. Case report. J Neurosurg 78:120–121

24. Betz RR, Gelman AJ, DeFilipp GJ, Mesgarzadeh M, Clancy M, Steel HH (1987) Magnetic resonance imaging in the evaluation of spinal cord injured children and adolescents. Paraplegia 25:92–99

25. Biyani A, El Masry WS (1994) Post-traumatic syringomyelia: a review of the literature. Paraplegia 32:723–731

26. Bleasel A, Clouston P, Dorsch N (1991) Post-traumatic syringomyelia following uncomplicated spinal fracture. J Neurol Neurosurg Psychiatry 54:551–553

27. Bourne IHJ (1990) Lumbo-sacral adhesive arachnoiditis: a review. J R Soc Med 83:262–265

28. Brammah TB, Jayson MIV (1994) Syringomyelia as a complication of spinal arachnoiditis. Spine 19:2603–2605

29. Brouwer B (1931) Über Arachnoiditis adhesiva circumscripta. Dtsch Z Nervenheilkd 117–119:38–66

30. Brugieres P, Iffenecker C, Hurth M, Parker F, Fuerxer F, Idy-Peretti I, Bittoun J (1999) [Dynamic MRI in the evaluation of syringomyelic cysts]. Neurochirurgie 45 [Suppl 1]:115–129

31. Caplan LR, Norohna AB, Amico LL (1990) Syringomyelia and arachnoiditis. J Neurol Neurosurg Psychiatry 53:106–113

32. Chapman PH, Frim DM (1995) Symptomatic syringomyelia following surgery to treat retethering of lipomyelomeningoceles. J Neurosurg 82:752–755

33. Charcot JM, Joffroy A (1869) Deux cas d'atrophie musculaire progressive avec lésions de la substance grise et des faisceaux anterolatéraux de la moelle épinière. Arch Physiol Ser 1 2:354–367

34. Chiapparini L, Sghirlanzoni A, Pareyson D, Savoiardo M (2000) Imaging and outcome in severe complications of lumbar epidural anaesthesia: report of 16 cases. Neuroradiology 42:564–571

35. Collier J (1916) Gunshot wounds and injuries of the spinal cord. Lancet 1:711–716

36. Cushing HW (1898) Hematomyelia from gunshot wounds of the spine. A report of two cases, with recovery following symptoms of hemilesion of the cord. Am J Med Sci 115:654–683

37. Cusick JF, Bernardi R (1995) Syringomyelia after removal of benign spinal extramedullary neoplasms. Spine 20:1289–1293

38. Daif AK, al Rajeh S, Ogunniyi A, al Boukai A, al Tahan A (1997) Syringomyelia developing as an acute complication of tuberculous meningitis. Can J Neurol Sci 24:73–76

39. Davis CH, Symon L (1989) Mechanisms and treatment in post-traumatic syringomyelia. Br J Neurosurg 3:669–674

40. Di Benedetto M, Rossier AB (1977) Electrodiagnosis in posttraumatic syringomyelia. Paraplegia 14:286–295

41. Dolan EJ, Transfeld EE, Tator CH, Simmons EH, Hughes KF (1980) The effect of spinal distraction on regional spinal cord blood flow in cats. J Neurosurg 53:756–764

42. Dolan RA (1993) Spinal adhesive arachnoiditis. Surg Neurol 39:479–484

43. Donaldson I, Gibson R (1982) Spinal cord atrophy associated with arachnoiditis as demonstrated by computed tomography. Neuroradiology 24:101–105

44. Durward QJ, Rice GP, Ball MJ, Gilbert JJ, Kaufmann JCE (1982) Selective spinal cordectomy: clinicopathological correlation. J Neurosurg 56:359–367

45. Edelman RR, Wedeen VJ, Davis KR, Widder D, Hahn P, Shoukimas G, Brady TJ (1986) Multiphase MR imaging: a new method for direct imaging of pulsatile CSF flow. Radiology 161:779–783

46. Edgar R, Quail P (1994) Progressive post-traumatic cystic and non-cystic myelopathy. Br J Neurosurg 8:7–22

47. Elkington JSC (1936) Meningitis serosa circumscripta spinalis (spinal arachnoiditis). Brain 59:181–203

48. Enzmann DR, Pelc NJ (1991) Normal flow patterns with phase-contrast cine MRI imaging. Radiology 178:467–474

49. Enzmann DR, O'Donohue J, Rubin JB, Shuer L, Cogen P, Silverberg G (1987) CSF pulsations within nonneoplastic spinal cord cysts. AJR Am J Roentgenol 149:149–157

50. Errea JM, Ara JR, Alberdi J, Pascual C, Fayed N (1993)

[Syringomyelia due to arachnoiditis. Clinical-radiological description in 5 patients] Neurologia 8:226–230

51. Falci SP, Lammertse DP, Best L, Starnes CA, Prenger EC, Stavros AT, Mellick D (1999) Surgical treatment of posttraumatic cystic and tethered spinal cords. J Spinal Cord Med 22:173–181

52. Fehlings MG, Bernstein M (1992) Syringomyelia as a complication of tuberculous meningitis. Can J Neurol Sci 19:84–87

53. Feve A, Wallays C, Nicolle MH, Guillard A (1992) Syringomyelia as a late complication of paralytic poliomyelitis. Neurology 42:1421–1422

54. Fitt GJ, Stevens JM (1995) Postoperative arachnoiditis diagnosed by high resolution fast spin-echo MRI of the lumbar spine. Neuroradiology 37:139–145

55. Freckmann N, Westphal M, Winkler D, Valdueza JM, Herrmann HD (1993) Neurosurgical management of the syringohydromyelia-complex. Acta Neurochir (Wien) 123:201–203

56. Freund M, Aschoff A, Spahn B, Sartor K (1999) [Posttraumatic syringomyelia]. ROFO Fortschr Geb Rontgenstr Neuen Bildgeb Verfahr 171:417–423

57. Gebarski SS, Maynard FW, Gabrielsen TO, Knake JE, Latack JT, Hoff JT (1985) Posttraumatic progressive myelopathy. Radiology 157:379–385

58. Gerstmann J (1915) Beiträge zur Pathologie des Rückenmarks. Zur Frage der Meningitis serosa und serofibrosa circumscripta spinalis. Z Ges Neurol Psychiatry 29:97–167

59. Giminez-Roldan S, Esteban A, Benito C (1974) Communicating syringomyelia following cured tuberculous meningitis. J Neurol Sci 23:185–197

60. Greitz D (1993) Cerebrospinal fluid circulation and associated intracranial dynamics. A radiologic investigation using MR imaging and radionuclide cisternography. Acta Radiol Suppl 386:1–23

61. Greitz D, Franck A, Nordell B (1993) On the pulsatile nature of intracranial and spinal CSF-circulation demonstrated by MR imaging. Acta Radiol 34:321–328

62. Griffiths ER, McCormick CC (1981) Posttraumatic syringomyelia (cystic myelopathy). Paraplegia 19:81–88

63. Guyer DW, Wiltse LL, Eskay ML, Guyer BH (1989) The long-range prognosis of arachnoiditis. Spine 14:1332–1341

64. Haberl H, Zimmermann W, Schmiedek P, Stelzer S, Marguth F (1990) Comparison of syringoperitoneal and syringopleural shunting in patients with syringomyelia. Adv Neurosurg 18:131–136

65. Hackney DB, Asato R, Joseph PM, Carolin MJ, McGrath JT, Grossman RI, Kassab EA, DeSimone D (1986) Hemorrhage and edema in acute spinal cord compression: demonstration by MR imaging. Radiology 161:387–390

66. Harbitz F, Lossius E (1929) Extramedullary tumor. Arachnoiditis fibrosa cystica et ossificans. Gliosis of the medulla. Acta Psychiatr Neurol 4:51–64

67. Haughton VM, Nguyen CM, Ho KC (1993) The etiology of focal spinal arachnoiditis. An experimental study. Spine 18:1193–1198

68. Hertel G, Kramer S, Placzek E (1973) Die Syringomyelie. Klinische Verlaufsbeobachtungen bei 323 Patienten. Nervenarzt 44:1–13

69. Hetherington NJ, Dooley MJ (2000) Potential for patient harm from intrathecal administration of preserved solutions. Med J Aust 173:141–143

70. Hida K, Iwasaki Y, Imamura H, Abe H (1994) Posttraumatic syringomyelia: its characteristic magnetic resonance imaging findings and surgical management. Neurosurgery 35:886–891

71. Hoffman GS, Ellsworth CA, Wells EE, Frank WA, Mackie RW (1983) Spinal arachnoiditis: what is the clinical spectrum? II. Arachnoiditis induced by Pantopaque/autologous blood in dogs, a possible model for human disease. Spine 8:541–551

72. Holmes G (1915) The Goulstonian Lectures on spinal injuries of warfare. I. The pathology of acute spinal injury. BMJ 2:769–774

73. Holmes G, Kennedy RF (1909) Two anomalous cases of syringomyelia. Proc R Soc Med 2:1–7

74. Horsley V (1909) Chronic spinal meningitis: its differential diagnosis and surgical treatment. BMJ 1:513–517

75. Hort-Legrand C, Emery E (1999) [Evoked motor and sensory potentials in syringomyelia]. Neurochirurgie 45 [Suppl 1]:95–104

76. Hüwel N, Perneczky A, Urban V, Fries G (1992) Neuroendoscopic technique for the operative treatment of septated syringomyelia. Acta Neurochir Suppl (Wien) 54:59–62

77. Ikai T (1993) [Effects of caudal traction of the spinal cord on evoked spinal cord potentials in the cat.] Nippon Seikeigeka Gakkai Zasshi 67:275–288

78. Inoue HK, Kobayashi S, Ohbayashi K, Kohga H, Nakamura M (1994) Treatment and prevention of tethered and retethered spinal cord using a Gore-Tex surgical membrane. J Neurosurg 80:689–693

79. Itabashi T (1990) Quantitative analysis of cervical CSF and syrinx fluid pulsations. Nippon Seikeigeka Gakkai Zasshi 64:523–533

80. Jenik F, Tekle-Haimanot R, Hamory BH (1981) Nontraumatic adhesive arachnoiditis as a cause of spinal cord syndromes. Investigations of 507 patients. Paraplegia 19:140–154

81. Jourdan P, Pharaboz C, Ducolombier A, Pernod P, Desgeorges M (1987) Syringomyélie précoce après traumatisme cervical benin apport de l'I.R.M. post-opératoire. Neurochirurgie 33:57–61

82. Juzelevskij A (1935) Die operative Behandlung der Syringomyelie; ihre kritische Bewertung nach den unmittelbaren und den Fernresultaten. Dtsch Z Chir 244:503–520

83. Kamada K, Iwasaki Y, Hida K, Abe H, Isu T (1993) [Syringomyelia secondary to adhesive arachnoiditis: clinical profile and efficiency of shunt operations.] No Shinkei Geka 21:135–140

84. Kamm C, Exner G (1993) Review of 17 cases of posttraumatic syringomyelia concerning symptoms, incidence, diagnostic problems, and (operative) procedures. Acta Neurochir (Wien) 123:217–218

85. Kaynar MY, Kocer N, Gencosmanoglu BE, Hanci M (2000) Syringomyelia - as a late complication of tuberculous meningitis. Acta Neurochir (Wien) 142:935–938; discussion 938–939

86. Kikuchi I (1935) Nachtrag von drei Fällen der mit Laminektomie ganz erfolgreich behandelten Meningitis spinalis circumscripta chronica. Ztsch Jap Chir Ges 36:129–130

87. Klawans HL Jr (1968) Delayed posttraumatic syringomyelia. Dis Nerv Syst 29:525–528

88. Klekamp J, Batzdorf U, Samii M, Bothe HW (1997) Treatment of syringomyelia associated with arachnoid

scarring caused by arachnoiditis or trauma. J Neurosurg 86:233–240

89. Kok AJ, Verhagen WI, Bartels RH, van Dijk R, Prick MJ (2000) Spinal arachnoiditis following subarachnoid haemorrhage: report of two cases and review of the literature. Acta Neurochir (Wien) 142:795–798; discussion 798–799

90. Kramer KM, Levine AM (1997) Posttraumatic syringomyelia: a review of 21 cases. Clin Orthop 334:190–199

91. Laha RK, Malik HG, Langille RA (1975) Post-traumatic syringomyelia. Surg Neurol 4:519–522

92. La Haye PA, Batzdorf U (1988) Posttraumatic syringomyelia. West J Med 148:657–663

93. Lassman LP, Michael James CC, Foster JB (1968) Hydromyelia. J Neurol Sci 7:149–155

94. Lee TT, Alameda GJ, Gromelski EB, Green BA (2000) Outcome after surgical treatment of progressive posttraumatic cystic myelopathy. J Neurosurg 92:149–154

95. Levi AD, Sonntag VK (1998) Management of posttraumatic syringomyelia using an expansile duraplasty. A case report. Spine 23:128–132

96. Levy MR, Di Chiro G (1990) MR phase imaging and cerebrospinal fluid flow in the head and spine. Neuroradiology 32:399–406

97. Lloyd JH (1894) Traumatic affections of the cervical region of the spinal cord, simulating syringomyelia. J Nerv Ment Dis 21:345–358

98. Lombardi G, Passerini A, Migliavacca F (1962) Spinal arachnoiditis. Br J Radiol 35:314–320

99. Lyons BM, Brown DJ, Calvert JM, Woodward JM, Wriedt CHR (1987) The diagnosis and management of post traumatic syringomyelia. Paraplegia 25:340–350

100. Mackay R (1939) Chronic adhesive spinal arachnoiditis. A clinical and pathologic study. JAMA 112:802–808

101. Matsuzawa H, Hida K, Houkin K, Yoshinobu I, Abe H, Akino M, Saito H (1992) [Quantitative analysis of cerebrospinal fluid dynamics in syringomyelia using cine MRI with pre-saturation.] No To Shinkei 44:24–29

102. Mauss T, Krüger H (1918) Über die unter dem Bilde der Meningitis serosa circumscripta verlaufenden Kriegsschädigungen des Rückenmarks und ihre operative Behandlung. Dtsch Z Nervenheilkd 62:1–116

103. McComas CF, Frost JL, Schochet SS (1983) Posttraumatic syringomyelia with paroxysmal episodes of unconsciousness. Arch Neurol 40:322–324

104. McLean DR, Miller JDR, Allen PBR, Ezzedin SA (1973) Posttraumatic syringomyelia. J Neurosurg 39:485–492

105. Morota N, Sakamoto K, Kobayashi N (1992) Traumatic cervical syringomyelia related to birth injury. Child's Nerv Syst 8:234–236

106. Munro JC (1910) Circumscribed serous meningitis of the cord. Surg Gynecol Obstet 10:235–244

107. Nagahiro S, Matsukado Y, Hirata Y, Saito Y, Hamada J, Fukumura A, Itoyama Y (1987) [Pathogenesis and treatment of secondary syringomyelia.] No To Shinkei 39:143–149

108. Nagai M, Sakuma R, Aoki M, Abe K, Itoyama Y (2000) Familial spinal arachnoiditis with secondary syringomyelia: clinical studies and MRI findings. J Neurol Sci 177:60–64

109. Narumi S, Saiki I, Kidoguchi J, Kanaya H, Tomita Y,

110. Abe H (1990) [A case of traumatic syringomyelia that disappeared after anterior decompression: a suggestion for surgical treatment of syringomyelia.] No Shinkei Geka 9:851–854

110. Nashold BS Jr, Nashold JRB (1991) Dorsal root entry zone and the treatment of traumatic syringomyelia. Neurosurgery 28:769–770

111. Nicholas DS, Weller RO (1988) The fine anatomy of the human spinal meninges: a light and scanning electron microscopy study. J Neurosurg 69:276–282

112. Nogues M, Camarota A, Blanco M, Garcia H (1987) Evoked potentials in syringomyelia. Electroencephalogr Clin Neurophysiol 66:S74

113. Nogues MA, Pardal AM, Merello M, Miguel MA (1992) SEPs and CNS magnetic stimulation in syringomyelia. Muscle Nerve 15:993–1001

114. Nunomura M, Iwasaki Y, Isu T, Akino M, Abe H, Miyasaka K, Nomura M, Saiton H, Nakamura N (1991) Post-traumatic syringomyelia. Report of three cases. Neurol Med Chir 31:931–935

115. Oakley JC, Ojemann GA, Alvard EC Jr (1981) Posttraumatic syringo-myelia. Case report. J Neurosurg 55:276–281

116. Ohata K, Gotoh T, Matsusaka Y, Morino M, Tsuyuguchi N, Sheikh B, Inoue Y, Hakuba A (2001) Surgical management of syringomyelia associated with spinal adhesive arachnoiditis. J Clin Neurosci 8:40–42

117. Padilla CR (1982) Syringomyelia after spinal cord injury. Am Fam Physician 26:145–151

118. Park YK, Tator CH (1998) Prevention of arachnoiditis and postoperative tethering of the spinal cord with Gore-Tex surgical membrane: an experimental study with rats. Neurosurgery 42:813–823; discussion 823–824

119. Parker F, Aghakhani N, Tadie M (1999) [Non-traumatic arachnoiditis and syringomyelia. A series of 32 cases]. Neurochirurgie 45 [Suppl 1]:67–83

120. Pecker J, Gavalet A, Boutlelis A (1983) La dérivation syringopéritoneale. Neurochirurgie 29:171–173

121. Peerless SJ, Durward QJ (1982) Management of syringomyelia: a pathophysiological approach. Clin Neurosurg 30:531–576

122. Perrouin-Verbe B, Lenne-Aurier K, Robert R, Auffray-Calvier E, Richard I, Mauduyt de la Greve I, Mathe JF (1998) Post-traumatic syringomyelia and post-traumatic spinal canal stenosis: a direct relationship: review of 75 patients with a spinal cord injury. Spinal Cord 36:137–143

123. Perrouin-Verbe B, Robert R, Lefort M, Agakhani N, Tadie M, Mathe JF (1999) [Post-traumatic syringomyelia]. Neurochirurgie 45 [Suppl 1]:58–66

124. Pette H (1925) Über lokalisierte, unter dem Bilde eines raumbeschränkenden Prozesses verlaufende Spinalmeningitis. Arch Psychiatr Nervenkr 74:631–640

125. Phanthumchinda K, Kaoropthum S (1991) Syringomyelia associated with post-traumatic spinal arachnoiditis due to Candida tropicalis. Postgrad Med J 67:767–769

126. Philippe C, Oberthur J (1900) Contribution à l'étude de la syringomyélie. II. La forme pachyméningitique. Arch de Med Exp et d'Anat Path 12:607–651

127. Pillay PK, Awad IA, Little JR, Hahn JF (1991) Surgical management of syringomyelia: a five year experience in the era of magnetic resonance imaging. Neurol Res 13:3–9

128. Post MJD, Quencer R, Green BA, Montalvo BM, Eismont FJ (1986) Radiologic evaluation of spinal cord fissures. AJNR Am J Neuroradiol 7:329–335

129. Quencer RM, Green BA, Eismont FJ (1983) Posttraumatic spinal cord cysts: clinical features and characterization with metrizamide computed tomography. Radiology 146:415–423

130. Quencer RM, Morse BMM, Green BA, Eismont FS, Brost P (1984) Intraoperative spinal sonography: adjunct to metrizamide CT in the assessment and surgical decompression of posttraumatic spinal cord cysts. AJNR Am J Neuroradiol 5:71–79

131. Quencer RM, Post MJD, Hinks RS (1990) Cine MRI in the evaluation of normal and abnormal CSF flow: intracranial and intraspinal studies. Neuroradiology 32:371–391

132. Ragnarsson TS, Durward QJ, Nordgren RE (1986) Spinal cord tethering after traumatic paraplegia with late neurological deteoration. J Neurosurg 64:397–401

133. Rosenblath W (1893) Zur Casuistik der Syringomyelie und Pachymeningitis cervicalis hypertrophica. Dtsch Arch Klin Med 51:210–223

134. Rossier AB, Werner A, Wildi E, Berney J (1968) Contribution to the study of late cervical syringomyelic syndromes after dorsal or lumbar traumatic paraplegia. J Neurol Neurosurg Psychiatry 31:99–105

135. Rossier AB, Foo D, Shillito I, Dyro FM (1985) Posttraumatic cervical syringomyelia. Brain 108:439–461

136. Schaller B, Mindermann T, Gratzl O (1999) Treatment of syringomyelia after posttraumatic paraparesis or tetraparesis. J Spinal Disord 12:485–488

137. Schellinger D, Le Bihan D, Rajan SS, Cammarata CA, Patronas NJ, Deveikis JP, Levy LM (1992) MR of slow CSF flow in the spine. AJNR Am J Neuroradiol 13:1393–1403

138. Schliep G, Ritter U (1971) Klinik der Syringomyelie. Fortschr Neurol Psychiatr 39:53–82

139. Schon F, Bowler JV (1990) Syringomyelia and syringobulbia following tuberculous meningitis. J Neurol 237:122–123

140. Schroth G (1991) Physiologie und Pathologie der intrakraniellen Liquordynamik. Jahrbuch der Radiologie, pp 287–290

141. Schurch B, Wichmann W, Rossier AB (1996) Post-traumatic syringomyelia (cystic myelopathy): a prospective study of 449 patients with spinal cord injury. J Neurol Neurosurg Psychiatry 60:61–67

142. Schuster P (1915) Beitrag zur Kenntnis der Anatomie und Klinik der Meningitis serosa spinalis circumscripta. Monatschr Psychiatr Neurol 37:341–373

143. Schwarz E (1897) Präparate von einem Falle syphilitischer Myelomeningitis mit Höhlenbildung im Rückenmarke und besonderer degenerativen Veränderungen der Neuroglia. Wien Klin Wochschr 7:177–178

144. Seibert CE, Dreisbach JN, Swanson WB, Edgar RE, Williams P, Hahn H (1981) Progressive posttraumatic cystic myelopathy: neuroradiologic evaluation. AJR Am J Roentgenol 136:1161–1166

145. Sett P, Crockard HA (1991) The value of magnetic resonance imaging in the follow-up management of spinal injury. Paraplegia 29:396–410

146. Sgouros S, Williams B (1995) A critical appraisal of drainage in syringomyelia. J Neurosurg 82:1–10

147. Sgouros S, Williams B (1996) Management and outcome of posttraumatic syringomyelia. J Neurosurg 85:197–205

148. Shannon N, Symon L, Logue V, Cull D, Kang J, Kendall B (1981) Clinical features, investigation and treatment of post-traumatic syringomyelia. J Neurol Neurosurg Psychiatry 44:35–42

149. Shaw MDM, Russell JA, Grossart KW (1978) The changing pattern of spinal arachnoiditis. J Neurol Neurosurg Psychiatry 41:97–107

150. Sherman JL, Barkovich AJ, Citrin CM (1986) The MR appearance of syringomyelia: new observations. AJNR Am J Neuroradiol 7:985–995

151. Sherman JL, Citrin CM, Bowen BJ, Gangarosa RE (1986) MR demonstration of cerebrospinal fluid flow by obstructive lesions. AJNR Am J Neuroradiol 7:571–579

152. Sherman JL, Barkovich AJ, Citrin CM (1987) The MR appearance of syringomyelia: new observations. AJR Am J Roentgenol 148:381–391

153. Shikata J, Yamamuro T, Iida H, Sugimoto M (1989) Surgical treatment for symptomatic spinal adhesive arachnoiditis. Spine 14:870–875

154. Silberstein M, Hennessy O (1992) Cystic cord lesions and neurological deterioration in spinal cord injury: operative considerations based on negative magnetic resonance imaging. Paraplegia 30:661–668

155. Smith KA, Rekate HL (1994) Delayed postoperative tethering of the cervical spinal cord. J Neurosurg 81:196–201

156. Spiller WG (1908) The association of syringomyelia with tabes dorsalis. J Med Res 18:149–158

157. Steinmetz A, Aschoff A, Kunze S (1993) The iatrogenic tethering of the cord. Acta Neurochir (Wien) 123:219–220

158. Stookey B (1927) Adhesive spinal arachnoiditis simulating spinal cord tumor. Arch Neurol Psychiatr 17:151–178

159. Strowitzki M, Schwerdtfeger K, Donauer E (1993) The value of somato-sensory evoked potentials in the diagnosis of syringomyelia. Acta Neurochir (Wien) 123:184–187

160. Suzuki M, Davis C, Symon L, Gentili F (1985) Syringoperitoneal shunt for treatment of cord cavitation. J Neurol Neurosurg Psychiatry 48:620–627

161. Suzuki S, Chiba Y, Hidaka K, Nishimura S, Noji M (1998) [A new operative technique of posttraumatic syringomyelia: thecoperitoneal shunt]. No Shinkei Geka 26:541–546

162. Tabor EN, Batzdorf U (1996) Thoracic pantopaque cyst and associated syrinx resulting in progressive spastic paraparesis: case report. Neurosurgery 39:1040–1042

163. Takayasu M, Shibuya M, Konketsu N, Suzuki Y (1996) Rapid enlargement of a syringomyelia cavity following syringo-subarachnoid shunt: case report. Surg Neurol 45:366–369

164. Tamaki K, Lubin AJ (1938) Pathogenesis of syringomyelia: case illustrating the process of cavity formation from embryonic cell rests. Arch Neurol Psychiatr 40:748–761

165. Tator CH, Meguro K, Rowed DW (1982) Favorable results with syringosubarachnoid shunts for treatment of syringomyelia. J Neurosurg 56:517–523

166. Tator CH, Briceno C (1988) Treatment of syringomyelia with a syringosubarachnoid shunt. Can J Neurol Sci 15:48–57

167. Thompson DN, Taylor WF, Hayward RD (1994) Silastic dural substitute: experience of its use in spinal and foramen magnum surgery. Br J Neurosurg 8:157–167
168. Tobimatsu Y, Nihei R, Kimura T, Suyama T, Tobimatsu H (1991) [A quantitative analysis of cerebrospinal fluid flow in posttraumatic syringomyelia.] Nippon Seikei-geka Gakkai Zasshi 65:505–516
169. Tobimatsu Y, Nihei R, Kimura T, Suyama T, Kimura H, Tobimatsu H, Shirakawa T (1995) A quantitative analysis of cerebrospinal fluid flow in post-traumatic syringomyelia. Paraplegia 33:203–207
170. Treede RD, Lankers J, Frieling A, Zangemeister WH, Kunze K, Bromm B (1991) Cerebral potentials evoked by painful laser stimuli in patients with syringomyelia. Brain 114:1595–1607
171. Tsuchiya K (1988) [Syringomyelia following tuberculous meningitis – report of three cases diagnosed by MR imaging.] Rinsho Hoshasen 33:1589–1592
172. Umbach I, Heilporn A (1991) Review article: post-spinal cord injury syringomyelia. Paraplegia 29:219–221
173. Van Calenbergh F, Van den Bergh R (1993) Syringo-peritoneal shunting: results and problems in a consecutive series. Acta Neurochir (Wien) 123:203–205
174. Van Velthoven V, Jost M, Siekmann R, Eggert HR (1993) Surgical strategies and results in syringomyelia. Acta Neurochir (Wien) 123:199–201
175. Vassilouthis J, Papandreou A, Anagoustaras S (1994) The coperitoneal shunt for posttraumatic syringomyelia. J Neurol Neurosurg Psychiatry 57:755–756
176. Vernet O, Farmer JP, Montes JL (1996) Comparison of syringopleural and syringosubarachnoid shunting in the treatment of syringomyelia in children. J Neurosurg 84:624–628
177. Vernon JD, Silver JR, Ohry A (1982) Post-traumatic syringomyelia. Paraplegia 20:339–364
178. Vernon JD, Silver JR, Symon L (1983) Post-traumatic syringomyelia: the results of surgery. Paraplegia 21:37–46
179. Wagner FC Jr, Van Gilder JC, Dohrmann GJ (1977) The development of intramedullary cavitation following spinal cord injury. An experimental pathological study. Paraplegia 14:245–250
180. Wagner W, Peghini-Halbig L, Maeurer JC, Hüwel NM, Perneczky A (1995) Median nerve somatosensory evoked potentials in cervical syringomyelia: correlation of preoperative versus postoperative findings with upper limb somatosensory function. Neurosurgery 36:336–345
181. Watson N (1981) Ascending cystic degeneration of the cord after spinal cord injury. Paraplegia 19:89–95
182. Westphal M, Winkler D, Cristante L, Herrmann HD (1990) Syringomyelia: aspects of therapeutic decisions. Adv Neurosurg 16:113–118
183. Wetzel N, Davis L (1954) Surgical treatment of syringomyelia. Arch Surg 68:570–573
184. Wiart L, Dautheribes M, Pointillart V, Gaujard E, Petit H, Barat M (1995) Mean term follow-up of a series of post-traumatic syringomyelia patients after syringo-peritoneal shunting. Paraplegia 33:241–245
185. Williams B (1980) On the pathogenesis of syringomyelia: a review. J R Soc Med 73:798–806
186. Williams B (1992) Pathogenesis of post-traumatic syringomyelia. Br J Neurosurg 6:517–520
187. Williams B (1995) Surgical management of non-hindbrain-related and posttraumatic syringomyelia. In:
Schmidek HH, Sweet WH (eds) Operative techniques in neurosurgery, 3rd edn. Saunders, Philadelphia, pp 2119–2138
188. Williams B, Page N (1987) Surgical treatment of syringomyelia with syringopleural shunting. Br J Neurosurg 1:63–80
189. Williams B, Terry AF, Jonas HWF, McSweeney T (1981) Syringomyelia as a sequel to traumatic paraplegia. Paraplegia 19:67–80
190. Wilske J (1989) Rückenmarkstrauma. In: Cervos-Navarro J, Ferszt R (eds) Klinische Neuropathologie. Thieme, Stuttgart, pp 319–335
191. Wisoff JH, Epstein F (1989) Management of hydromyelia. Neurosurgery 25:562–571
192. Wozniewicz B, Filipowicz K, Swideska SK, Deraka K (1983) Pathophysiological mechanism of traumatic cavitation of the spinal cord. Paraplegia 21:312–317
193. Yamagata S, Goto K, Oda Y, Kikuchi H (1993) Clinical experience with expanded polytetrafluoroethylene sheet used as an artificial dura mater. Neurol Med Chir 33:582–585
194. Yasuda T (1937) Zur Frage der Arachnopathia fibrosa cystica proliferans. Dtsch Z Nervenheilkd 143:61–76
195. Zdrojewski B, Werner A, Rossio A (1969) Syndrome syringomyélique cervical tardif après paraplégie traumatique dorsale. Neurochirurgie 15:153–163

4.2
Syringomyelia Related to Tumors of the Spinal Canal

Between 1977 and 2000, a total of 886 spinal tumors were operated on. Among 160 intramedullary tumors, 339 extramedullary tumors, 65 dumbbell tumors, and 322 epidural tumors, the rates of accompanying syringomyelia were determined. Whereas syringomyelia was quite commonly associated with intramedullary tumors (47%) [3, 12, 13, 19, 23, 26, 46, 47], it was found to be a rarity with the remaining pathologies (1.8% among extramedullary tumors, none among dumbbell or epidural tumors). Among spinal hamartomas associated with spina bifida, 23% demonstrated a syrinx. Sizable or symptomatic syringomyelic cavities were only observed for intramedullary tumors. Extramedullary and epidural tumors were mostly associated with what looked like small dilatations of the central canal.

4.2.1
Intramedullary Tumors

Intramedullary cysts are so often associated with intramedullary tumors that each clinical and radiological examination of a patient with syringomyelia requires looking for this pathology. Any cystic process in the spinal cord should be considered as an intramedullary tumor until proven otherwise. Forty-seven percent of patients with intramedullary tumors demonstrated an additional syrinx on MRI. Similar percentages were given in the literature [3, 19, 26, 46, 47].

4.2.1.1
Clinical Presentation

Comparing the clinical histories of patients with intramedullary tumors with or without an associated syrinx does not disclose any differences. For the overwhelming majority, the syrinx is clinically of minor importance and neurological symptoms can be attributed exclusively to the tumor. We observed two patients with thoracic ependymomas and large cysts extending into the cervical cord who presented with dysesthesias and sensory deficits in their upper extremities before there were any clinical signs of the tumor. In most instances, the first symptom is local or radicular pain related to the spinal level of the tumor (34%). Motor weakness (17%), gait problems (21%), dysesthesias (14%), or sensory disturbances (14%) are less often reported at the beginning. On average, 28±36 months elapse without syringomyelia and 26±31 months with syringomyelia, before the patient undergoes neuroradiological examinations and presents to a neurosurgeon. The average age at presentation was 38±17 years [39, 56]. At the time of surgery, there were again no significant differences in neurological presentation or status. The major clinical problem was related to gait for 40% of patients. Motor weakness (22%), pain (16%), sensory deficits (11%), dysesthesias (9%), and sphincter disturbances (1%) were less often mentioned as the major complaint.

Table 4.15 gives an overview on the percentage of patients who demonstrated a particular symptom or sign before surgery. The figures for each of these symptoms are virtually identical. Looking at preoperative Karnofsky scores, there was no significant difference between the two groups (66±17 with and 65±19 without syringomyelia, respectively).

4.2.1.2
Neuroradiology

With the introduction of MRI, an increasing number of patients with intramedullary tumors is diagnosed at an early stage of the disease. Other diagnostic modalities like myelography or angiography, which were used in the past, have almost completely lost their role in preoperative imaging of intramedullary tumors. Without any doubt MRI has revolutionized our preoperative possibilities to establish the diagnosis, determine the exact extent of the tumor, and visualize associated cysts or tumor hemorrhages. Nobody will operate on an intramedullary tumor anymore without an adequate preoperative MRI scan. However, as informative a MRI scan is, it does not give an answer to the question almost every patient will ask when confronted with the diagnosis: is the

Table 4.15. Clinical presentation of patients with intramedullary tumors

Symptom	With syringomyelia	Without syringomyelia
Gait ataxia	85%	80%
Motor weakness	75%	83%
Pain	53%	47%
Sensory deficits	89%	86%
Dysesthesias	56%	61%
Sphincter disturbances	39%	36%

tumor completely resectable? Although there are signs that may suggest that the tumor may be well demarcated, such as a bright enhancement with gadolinium, we have been unable to define radiological criteria that allow prediction of what the surgeon will find at operation.

The MRI scan has to demonstrate the exact extent of the solid tumor part and the presence of tumor cysts or hemorrhages. An examination with and without gadolinium in at least two planes is mandatory to obtain some information on the vascularization of the tumor and the presence of a cystic tumor part. The wall of a tumor cyst will take up some contrast in most instances, whereas the glial tissue lining a syrinx cavity will not. This information is essential for adequate exposure of the tumor. With accompanying syringomyelia, only the solid tumor part has to be accessed. With a cystic tumor part, the exposure has to include the spinal levels of the cyst to be able to achieve a radical resection.

The differential diagnosis of some intramedullary tumors may not only be difficult to distinguish from syringomyelia. Another diagnostic problem is intramedullary signal changes mimicking tumors, such as demyelinating diseases or inflammatory processes [5, 37]. Two crucial points should be sought in such instances: is there a space-occupying effect of the lesion in question [37]? Did clinical symptoms evolve acutely or slowly? Non-tumorous lesions characteristically lack a space-occupying effect, even though a large spinal multiple sclerosis lesion with accompanying syringomyelia has been described in the literature [5]. Intramedullary tumors do not cause acute symptoms unless there is a tumor-associated intramedullary hemorrhage. Demyelinating and inflammatory lesions generally cause an acute onset of symptoms which then may fluctuate in intensity and radicular distribution. If in doubt, the best policy is to wait for a few weeks or months and repeat the MRI scan. A tumor will not have changed its signal pattern, whereas non-tumorous lesions often change their radiological appearance.

Table 4.16. Syringomyelia and intramedullary tumors

Histology	Cervical	Thoracic	Conus	Total
Ependymomas				
With syrinx	72%	63%	–	63%
No syrinx	28%	37%	100%	37%
Astrocytomas				
With syrinx	25%	24%	46%	29%
No syrinx	75%	76%	54%	71%
Angioblastomas				
With syrinx	89%	80%	–	86%
No syrinx	11%	20%	–	14%
Cavernomas				
With syrinx	–	50%	–	50%
No syrinx	–	50%	–	50%
Other tumors				
With syrinx	–	30%	–	16%
No syrinx	100%	70%	100%	84%
All tumors				
With syrinx	56%	46%	33%	47%
No syrinx	44%	54%	67%	53%

In terms of the underlying histology and the spinal distribution [36] of the tumors, we found remarkable features (Table 4.16). Interestingly, there was a tendency for a higher proportion of associated syrinx cavities with higher spinal levels of the intramedullary tumor irrespective of the histology [3, 23]. However, this trend was not statistically significant. In terms of tumor histology, we observed a higher rate of syringomyelia in association with ependymomas, angioblastomas, and cavernomas, i.e., tumors that compress spinal cord tissue rather than invade it. In other words, an associated syrinx is an indirect indicator that the tumor should be surgically resectable [8, 52]. A tumor-associated syrinx was found more often in adults than children (50.1% and 21.1%, respectively) reflecting the higher proportion of astrocytomas in the pediatric age group.

As to the relationship between spinal level of the tumor and orientation of the syrinx, similar figures to those associated with spinal arachnoid scarring were observed: 56% were found above and below the tumor, 34% above and 10% below the level of the tumor.

4.2.1.3
Surgical Management

The exposure of an intramedullary tumor is done almost exclusively from the posterior. Neurophysiological monitoring of sensory evoked potentials is used throughout surgery and started before positioning of the patient [43]. Except for cervical tumors, we operate with the patient in the prone position. The correct spinal level is determined by fluoroscopic control. The exposure is performed as described in Chap. 4.1 for spinal arachnoid scarring. A medial laminectomy about 15 mm wide is sufficient for tumor removal. For cervical tumors, we use a laminotomy. For this purpose, we cut the vertebral arches with a small oscillating saw or a small craniotome and remove all laminae including interspinous ligaments together. To avoid shrinkage of the interspinous ligaments, we keep them moist and under tension during the remainder of the procedure.

To ensure an adequate dural exposure, ultrasound may be used to determine the extent of the tumor. The dural opening and the remainder of the operation is done under the microscope. Particularly with recurrent tumors, ultrasound may be useful to determine areas of intradural scarring which may attach the cord to the dura posteriorly. The dura is opened in the midline and dural retention sutures applied. Figures 4.34 and 4.35 give examples for the removal of intramedullary tumors associated with syringomyelia. Once the arachnoid is opened, the cord is inspected for a suitable area for entry. Ultrasound may indicate the exact extension of the tumor even if no signs of an intramedullary tumor are visible on the surface of the cord. Usually, the cord is opened in the midline. If the tumor is located laterally, the dorsal root entry zone may be used. With exophytic tumors, the exit area of the tumor may be used for entry into the cord.

We recommend opening the cord over the entire tumor before attempting to identify dissection planes. We use a diamond knife to transect the pia mater for this purpose. Depending on the required depth, it may be possible to spread overlying cord fibers apart with two microdissectors avoiding any sharp dissection to reach the tumor. We use 6–0 sutures which we anchor in the pia mater and connect to the dura to keep the cord open. This may facilitate the determination of tissue planes considerably.

Whether a dissection plane between tumor and cord can be determined is of paramount importance. Several techniques may be used to achieve this goal. With fine forceps and microdissectors, it may be possible to almost wipe the thin covering layer of spinal cord tissue off the tumor in some instances. Once small tumor feeding vessels are identified, they are coagulated and cut with microscissors. Obviously, this

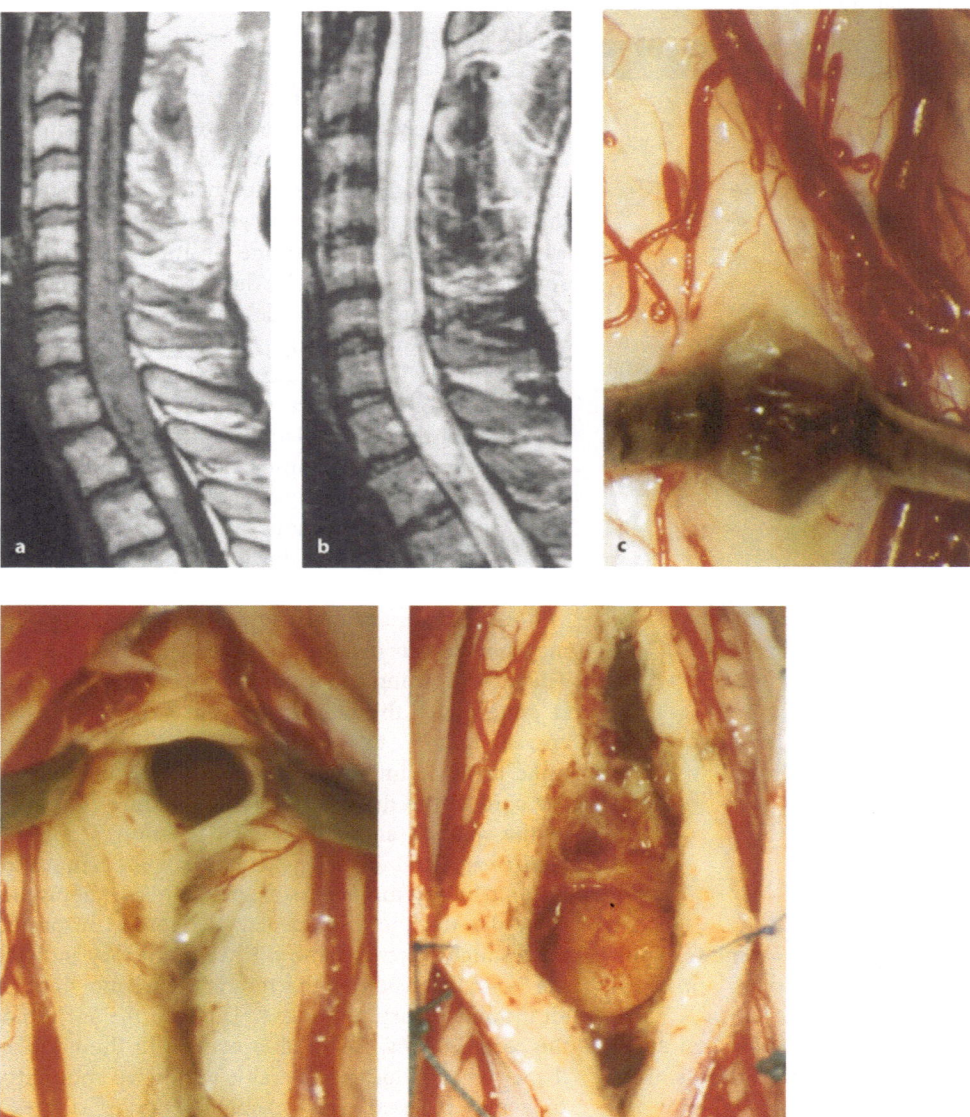

Fig. 4.34 a–l. This 32-year old man presented with a 18-month history of radicular pain and sensory problems of his right arm. No other symptoms were discovered. The sagittal T1- (**a**) and T2-weighted (**b**) MRI scans show a solid tumor between C4 and Th1 with a syrinx at either end. At the lower end of the solid tumor a small intramedullary hemorrhage can be seen. The patient was operated in the semi-sitting position. **c** After dura opening the pia mater has been incised in the midline and the posterior surface of the tumor can be reached by gently spreading the medullary tissue sideways with two microdissectors. This is done over the entire extent of the tumor. **d** The syringomyelia at the upper pole of the tumor is opened. **e** Pia retention sutures have been applied and the upper part of the partly cystic ependymoma is visible with a clear demarcation towards the cord tissue

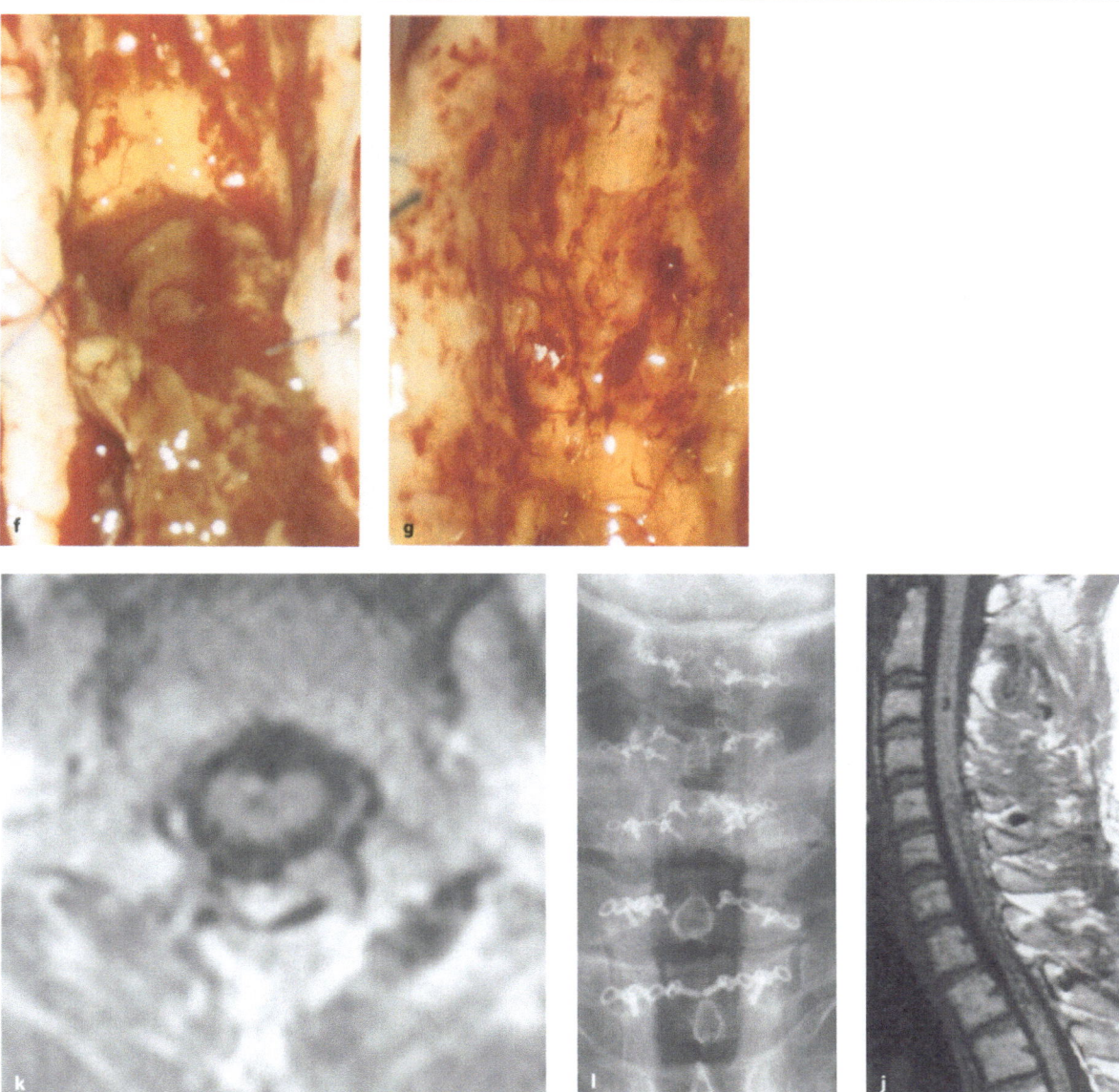

Fig. 4.34 f–j. f The tumor is removed with blunt dissection and intermittent debulking. Tumor feeding vessels are isolated, coagulated and transected. **g** The upper part of the tumor bed is shown after complete resection of the tumor. **h** With suture of the pia mater adhesion of the tumor bed to the dura can be prevented. i The laminae have been reinserted with miniplates. j The postoperative T1-weighted MRI scan shows the complete tumor resection and collapse of both syrinx cavities (continued on next page)

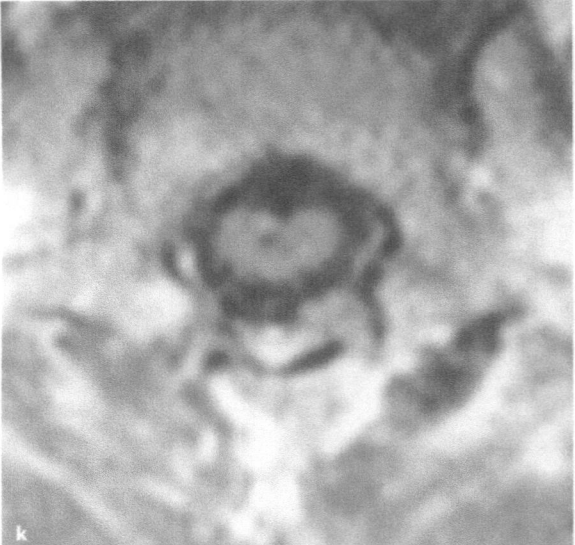
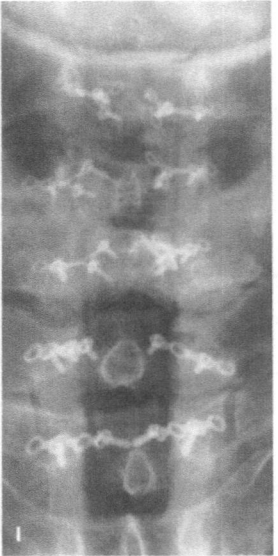

Fig. 4.34 k, l. k In the axial plane, the cord has regained its normal shape with no adhesion to the dura mater. **l** The postoperative X-ray control shows the realignment of the laminae. Postoperatively, the patient complained about aggravated sensory changes but acquired no other neurological deficits. Three years later the patient is still working as a truck driver and free of a clinical or radiological recurrence

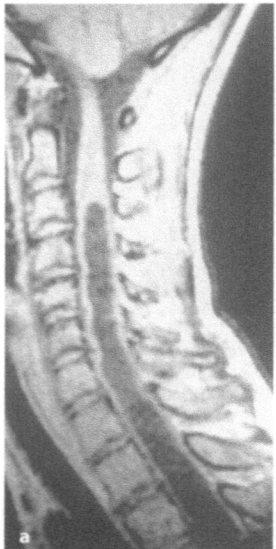
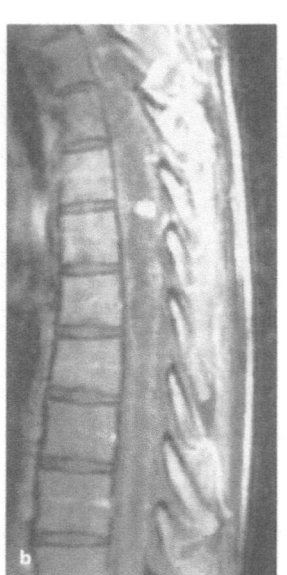
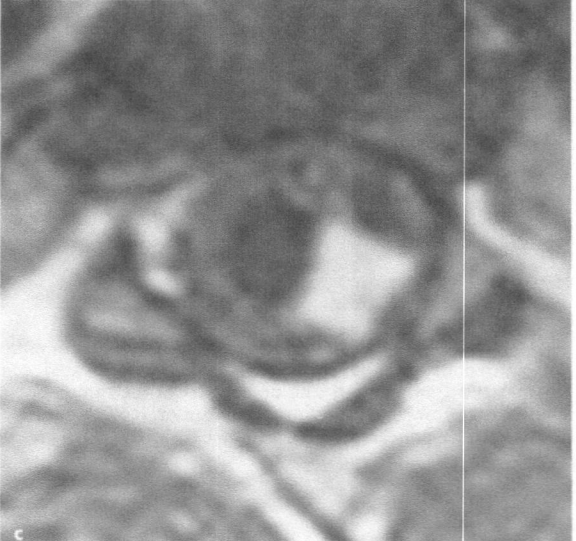

Fig. 4.35 a–j. This 23-year old woman with von Hippel-Lindau disease presented a 13-month history of sensory deficits and gait ataxia without any motor weakness or pain. The T1-weighted MRI scan with gadolinium demonstrates a syrinx of the entire cord (**a, b**) and a small enhancing lesion at the level of Th5/6 (**b**). **c** The axial plane reveals the lesion approaching the cord surface on the left side

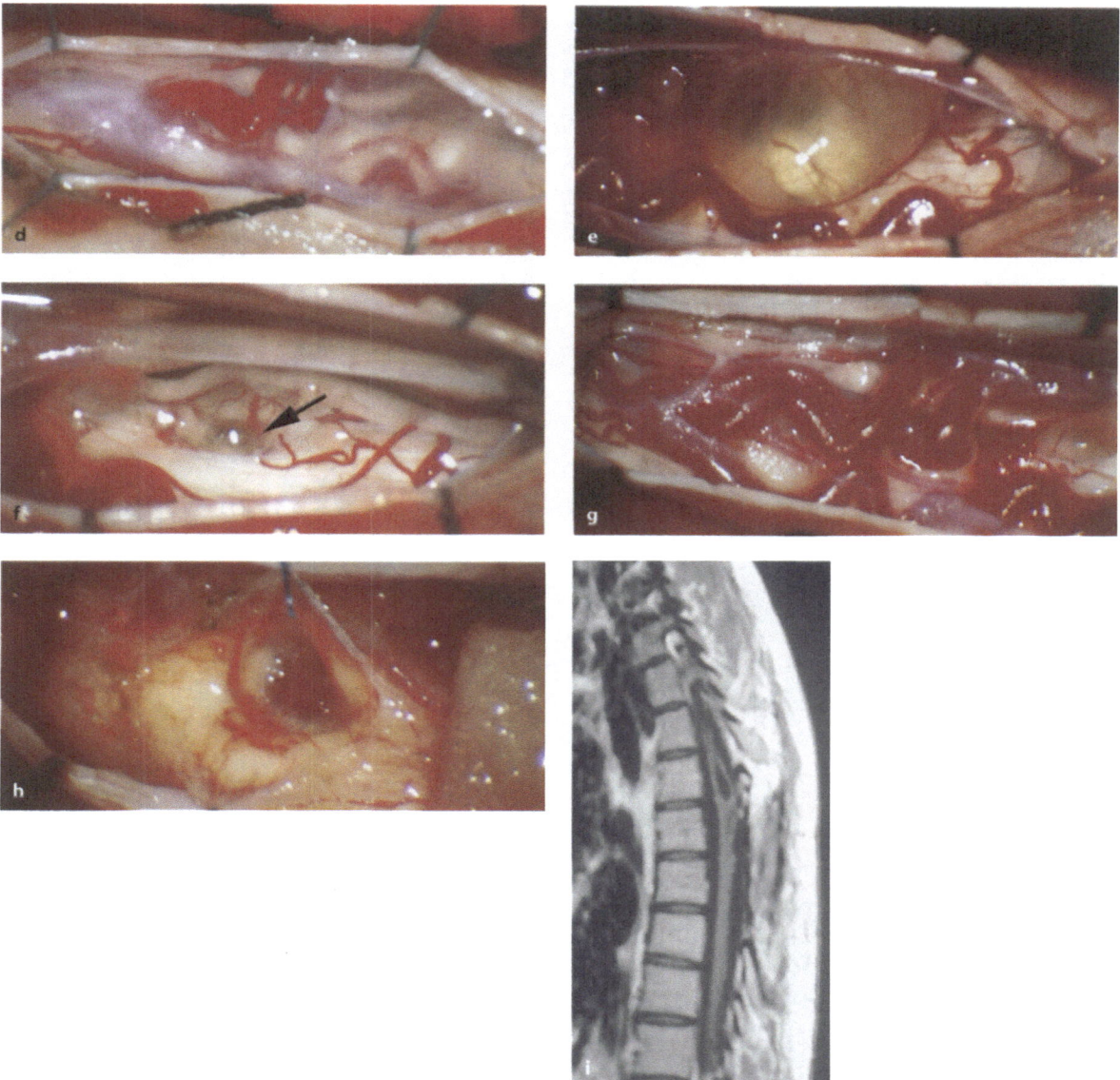

Fig. 4.35 d–i. d This intraoperative photograph demonstrates the situation after dura opening with the arachnoid intact. The tumor is covered by thickened arachnoid in the left half of the exposure. **e** After arachnoid opening, this cystic process protruding out of the spinal cord below the angioblastoma, which can be seen in its characteristic orange color to the left, was discovered. This extramedullary cyst is part of the syrinx which has penetrated the pia mater in the area of the dorsal root entry zone on the right side. Presumably, a spontaneous rupture of this part of the syrinx which is lined by gliotic tissue would have drained the syrinx at a later stage of the disease. **f** After resection of this extramedullary part of the syrinx the communication with its intramedullary part is apparent (*arrow*). **g** The arterialized veins around the angioblastoma are visible and some have to be coagulated to remove the tumor which reaches the cord surface in the right half of the picture. **h** The tumor has been removed in toto. **i** The postoperative T1-weighted MRI scan after 1 year shows collapse of the syrinx and no evidence of residual or recurrent tumor. Postoperatively, her sensory disturbances were aggravated but no other deficit appeared. She made a full recovery. However, 3 years after surgery extramedullary angioblastomas have appeared at different spinal levels due to her genetically based disease

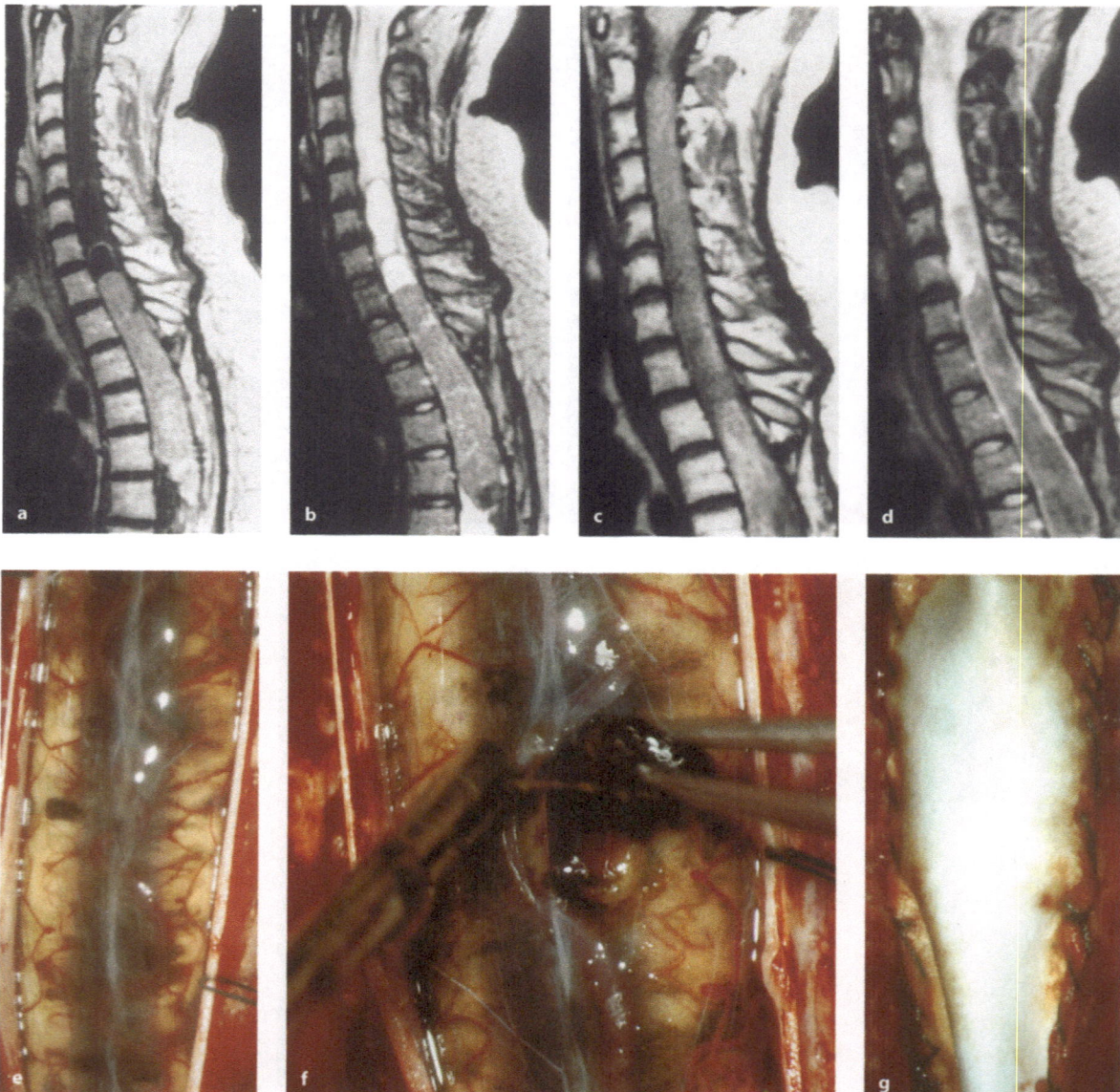

Fig. 4.36 a–h. This 26-year old paraplegic woman had undergone two attempts to remove an intramedullary melanocytoma
extending from Th1 to Th7 with asymptomatic syringomyelia
above the tumor extending into the cervical cord. Due to high
vascularity and invasive growth tumor removal was partial. She
developed subarachnoid dissemination with multiple intracranial and intraspinal tumors. These T1- (**a**) and T2-weighted (**b**)
MRI scans show the situation 1 year after the second operation. Despite radiation the tumor seeded in the subarachnoid
space of the spine as well as intracranially. Due to this widespread disease, she refused any further attempts of tumor
resections. These T1- (**c**) and T2-weighted (**d**) MRI scans without contrast were performed under emergency conditions

due to acute ascending tetraparesis and impeding respiratory
failure due to an enormous hematomyelia. **e** After laminectomy
C4 to C7 and opening of a markedly distended dura the hematoma is visible under the pia mater. **f** Part of the clot was removed after pial incision. **g** The spinal cord was decompressed
with a large Gore-Tex graft. Postoperatively, the patient could
be extubated 24 hours later and recovered function of her
upper extremities within a few weeks. **h** Three months after this
operation the T1-weighted MRI with gadolinium shows complete resolution of the hematomyelia and the grossly enlarged
subarachnoid space at the site of surgery. She eventually died
15 months later due to the widespread tumor disease

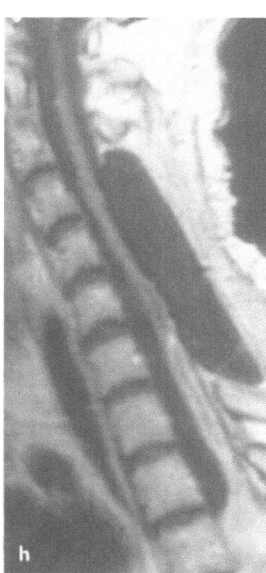

Fig. 4.36 h

method is very gentle to the cord. In other instances, the spinal cord may be very adherent to the tumor and even with a clear definition of a dissection plane preparation along this plane may be difficult. In such cases, sharp instruments like microscissors or diamond knifes have to be used to remove the tumor.

Of particular help to define a correct dissection plane may be an associated syrinx at the lower and/or the upper pole of the tumor. An associated syrinx not only clearly defines the limit of the tumorous process but also helps considerably to determine the lateral and anterior margins of the tumor [52]. Similarly, an elderly tumor hemorrhage may be helpful. However, a fresh intramedullary hemorrhage from an intramedullary tumor may make the determination of dissection planes impossible so that it may be wiser in such an instance to just remove the clot and to come back for removal of the tumor later when the area of bleeding has healed (Fig. 4.36). Again, no differences in terms of associated hemorrhages were found between tumors with or without syringomyelia (31% and 28%, respectively).

Once tissue planes are determined, the question arises whether to debulk the tumor (Fig. 4.34) or to remove it in toto (Fig. 4.35). The answer to this question depends on what puts the spinal cord under less stress, how clearly the dissection plane is defined, and how vascular the tumor is. With highly vascularized tumors, it is advisable to dissect around the tumor margin to avoid major bleeding and loss of the correct dissection plane with uncontrolled coagulation. With clearly defined tumors, removal in toto can generally be achieved. By often changing the area of dissection from left to right, we spread the stress we put on the cord during the removal. Particular attention has to

be paid to small arteries feeding the tumor from the anterior. They are encountered mainly in the midline and derived from the anterior spinal artery. They need to be dissected free before coagulation and sectioning in order to avoid injury to the anterior spinal artery itself.

In cases of tumors with an ill-defined margin, we proceed differently. The tumor is debulked from inside toward its lateral and anterior margin as long as one can be sure to be inside the tumor. This can be done with tumor forceps and microscissors or a cavitron ultrasonic aspirator (CUSA). Once some kind of a margin toward normal appearing cord tissue is reached, we stop. If normal cord tissue is intermingled with tumor, we do not attempt removal at all.

Once the tumor is removed, we check for adequate hemostasis. Inside the tumor bed, we use as little coagulation as possible and recommend small cotton paddies and simply taking some time to wait. To avoid adhesions between tumor bed and dura, we use a few 8-0 sutures for the pia mater to close the cord. Although recommended by some authors to prevent arachnoid scarring, we do not close the arachnoid. Finally, the dura is closed watertight. In cases with severe arachnoid adhesions or after incomplete removal of the tumor, we insert a Gore-Tex graft to enlarge the subarachnoid space. If appropriate, we reinsert the laminae after closure of the dura. They are fixated with miniplates. After incomplete removal of a tumor, we leave the laminae out. Fascia, subcutaneous tissue, and skin are closed in a conventional manner.

4.2.1.4
Postoperative Outcome

The majority of ependymomas, angioblastomas, and cavernomas could be removed completely in contrast to astrocytomas which were partially or subtotally resected in most instances [6, 8, 11, 14, 18, 19, 20, 27, 30, 31, 33, 34, 36, 38, 39, 40, 42, 45, 51, 54, 57, 58]. The amount of tumor removal for each of the different histologies is given in Table 4.17. As syringomyelia was associated more often with resectable tumor histologies, the rate of complete removal was significantly higher than with tumors without syringomyelia (62% and 35%, respectively; Chi-square test: $P=0.006$). Tumor removal alone was sufficient to decrease syrinx size, as confirmed for 91% of patients with adequate pre- and postoperative MRI scans.

Complications were encountered in 15% of patients (five wound infections, eight CSF leaks, two postoperative hematomas, two lamina dislocations after laminoplasty, two respiratory failures, one spinal instability, and one meningitis). Dislocations of laminae were observed only for patients in which laminae had

Table 4.17. Amount of tumor resection for intramedullary tumors

Histology	Complete	Subtotal	Partial	Biopsy
Ependymomas	79%	11%	8%	2%
Astrocytomas	16%	30%	41%	14%
Angioblastomas	86%	7%	7%	–
Cavernomas	80%	20%	–	–
Tumors with syringomyelia	62%	18%	15%	5%
Tumors without syringomyelia	35%	22%	27%	16%
All tumors	54%	18%	21%	6%

been inserted with sutures. With the introduction of miniplates, this complication no longer occurred. Surgical mortality was 3% for two patients with intramedullary metastases and one patient with a recurrent ependymoma.

For more than half of the patients (55%), the postoperative course was characterized by transient worsening of neurological symptoms for a few days or even months before functional recovery occurred. For one patient it took 21 months before he had achieved his preoperative level again. This may be attributed to edema or transient interference with spinal cord blood flow. Patients with a syrinx tended to recover a little bit earlier from operation (1.7±2.4 months and 2.3±4 months, respectively) be-

Table 4.18. Postoperative outcome for intramedullary tumors

Group	Preop.	Postop.	3 months	6 months	1 year
Sensory deficits					
Syrinx	3.0±1.2	2.1±1.3	2.3±1.3	2.3±1.4	2.3±1.4
No syrinx	3.1±1.0	2.3±1.2	2.3±1.2	2.4±1.2	2.4±1.2
Dysesthesias					
Syrinx	4.0±0.9	4.0±0.9	4.0±0.9	4.0±0.9	4.0±0.9
No syrinx	3.9±1.0	4.0±1.1	3.9±1.0	3.9±1.0	3.9±1.0
Pain					
Syrinx	4.0±1.1	3.9±1.0	4.3±0.8	4.4±0.9	4.4±0.9
No syrinx	4.1±1.0	4.0±1.1	4.2±0.9	4.4±0.8	4.4±0.8
Motor power					
Syrinx	3.4±1.4	2.7±1.6	3.0±1.5	3.2±1.5	3.3±1.5
No syrinx	3.2±1.3	2.9±1.4	3.3±1.3	3.4±1.4	3.4±1.5
Gait ataxia					
Syrinx	3.2±1.3	2.4±1.4	2.8±1.5	3.1±1.5	3.0±1.5
No syrinx	3.3±1.5	2.7±1.5	3.0±1.5	3.1±1.7	3.1±1.8
Bladder function					
Syrinx	4.1±1.3	3.6±1.9	4.0±1.5	4.1±1.4	4.1±1.4
No syrinx	4.1±1.7	3.4±2.0	3.7±1.8	3.7±1.8	3.8±1.7
Bowel function					
Syrinx	4.3±1.3	4.0±1.5	4.2±1.3	4.2±1.2	4.3±1.2
No syrinx	4.2±1.6	3.7±1.9	3.9±1.7	4.0±1.6	4.1±1.4
Karnofsky score					
Syrinx	66±17	58±18	63±18	66±17	66±18
No syrinx	65±19	57±18	61±20	64±20	64±21

Preop., preoperatively, *Postop.,* postoperatively

cause the proportion of resectable tumors was higher and the syrinx may have caused some of the preoperative symptoms in addition to the tumor. The combination of tumor resection and decrease of the syrinx may explain their faster recovery. Table 4.18 gives an overview on the postoperative results for individual symptoms in the first postoperative year for patients with and without a syrinx. After 1 year, no significant difference was detectable between groups for any symptom.

Permanent surgical morbidity was mainly related to the preoperative neurological status, the spinal level of the tumor, and the surgeon's experience. The major factor determining long-term outcome was the preoperative neurological status [11, 20, 22, 27, 30, 31, 34, 39, 52]. We observed marked differences in surgical morbidity depending on the preoperative Karnofsky score. For patients with a score above 70, who were able to live independently without assistance, this figure was 9%. For patients with scores between 40 and 70, who needed some assistance but were not dependent on a wheel chair, the figure rose to 38%. For pa-

tients with scores below 40, who were dependent on a wheel chair, surgical morbidity was also 38%. The corresponding rates of subsequent recurrence were 15%, 27%, and 16%, respectively. This trend was seen for all types of tumors. It indicates that 76% of patients with a score of 70 or better experienced a long-term benefit from surgery compared with 36% and 46% of patients with scores below 70 and 40, respectively (log-rank test: $P=0.0003$). Moreover, a new postoperative deficit had considerably more serious functional consequences for those patients who were already significantly disabled before surgery (Fig. 4.37).

A similarly strong factor for permanent surgical morbidity was the spinal level of the tumor. Cervical tumors were associated with a surgical morbidity of 10%, while thoracic tumors 19% and conus tumors 41% of patients demonstrated a permanent neurological deterioration after surgery [16, 33]. The subsequent recurrence rates also differed markedly (3% for cervical, 21% for thoracic, 25% for conus tumors, respectively; log-rank test: $P=0.0019$) (Figure 4.38).

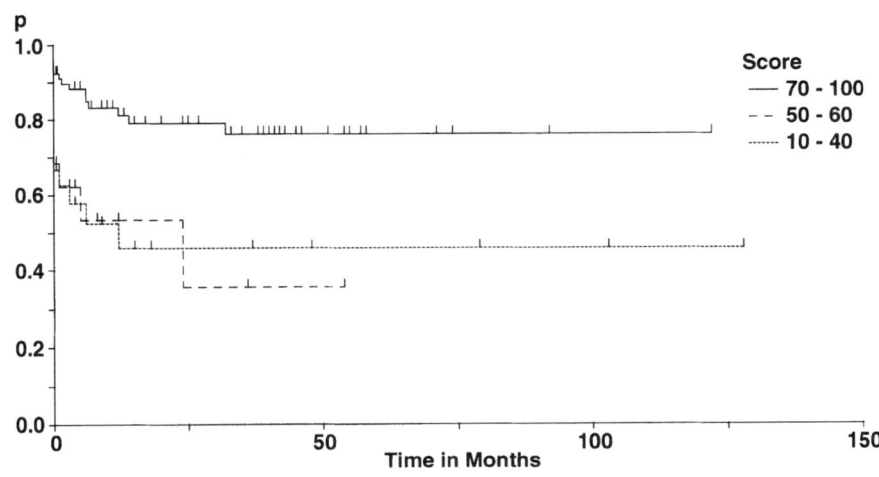

Fig. 4.37. Kaplan-Meier analysis of clinical recurrences for intramedullary tumors according to the preoperative Karnofsky score (log-rank test: $P=0.0003$)

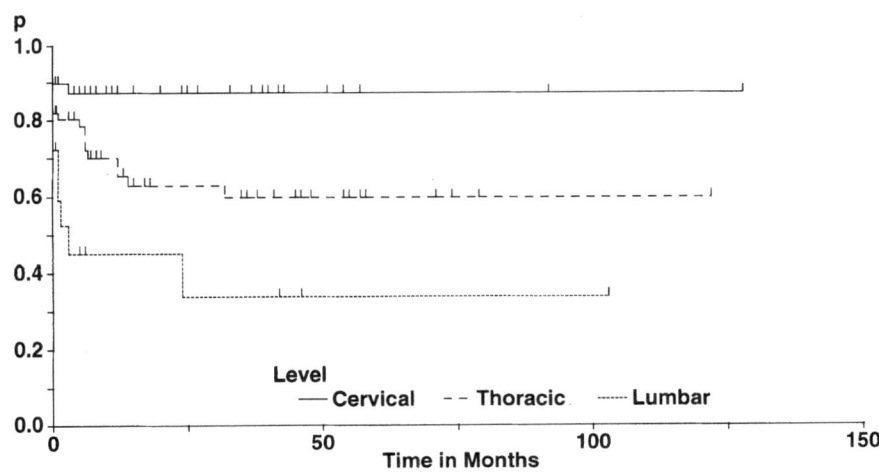

Fig. 4.38. Kaplan-Meier analysis of clinical recurrence rates for intramedullary tumors according to the spinal level of the tumor (log-rank test: $P=0.0019$)

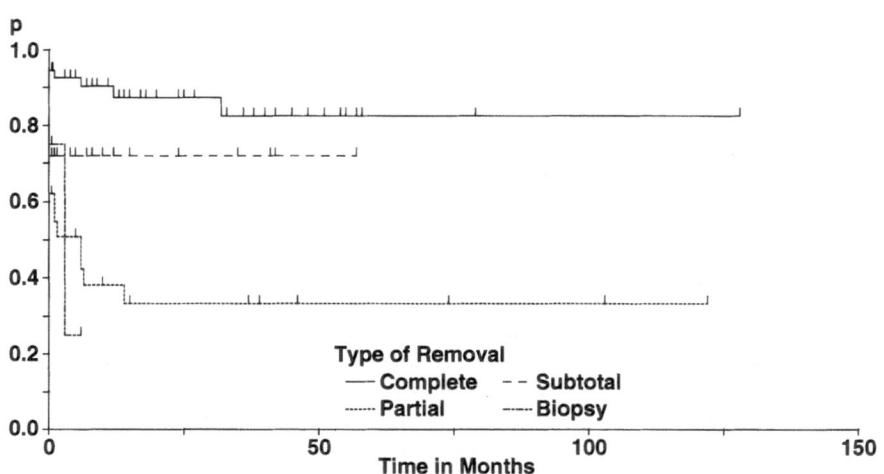

Fig. 4.39. Kaplan-Meier analysis of clinical recurrence rates for intramedullary tumors in relation to the amount of tumor resection (log-rank test: $P < 0.0001$)

Although complete tumor removal should be attempted, we emphasize not to force complete tumor removal, especially when a clear-cut cleavage plane cannot be identified – as in patients with astrocytomas, severe arachnoid scars are present – as in recurrent tumors, or the experience of the surgeon is limited. After complete or subtotal removal, permanent surgical morbidity was 7% and 28%, respectively. With tumor biopsy, morbidity was 25%. After partial removal, however, morbidity increased significantly to 45% (log-rank test: $P = < 0.0001$). This higher morbidity is a clear indicator of limited surgical experience which was the main factor leading to an incomplete removal (Figure 4.39).

Arachnoid scarring at the level of the tumor affected 25% of all patients [10]. It increased surgical morbidity only slightly from 16% to 24% [10, 24, 39, 52] and was not associated with a higher recurrence rate than cases without such arachnoid adhesions (16% and 19%, respectively) [24].

Except for ependymomas [20, 49, 55], the extent of tumor removal had only a minor influence on post-operative clinical outcome [2, 12, 29, 39], even though such a correlation was found by other authors [11, 21]. A correlation between amount of tumor resected and probability of a recurrence was not as clear-cut as might be expected. Between complete and subtotal removals, we could not determine significant differences in postoperative outcome. For patients harboring solitary angioblastomas, the prognosis is excellent after complete resection of the tumor. With von Hippel-Lindau disease, however, the local recurrence rate is higher and further angioblastomas may appear anytime [19].

Postoperative arachnoid scarring, i.e., a postoperative tethered cord, tended to increase postoperative long-term morbidity and the subsequent rate of clinical recurrence in patients after complete tumor resection (Fig. 4.40) (log-rank test: not significant). Patients with a postoperative tethered cord complained about dysesthesias, pain or progressive neurological symptoms even though the tumor had been completely removed [39, 52]. With suture of the pia mater to close the cord after tumor removal (Fig. 4.34), we were able to decrease the rate of postoperative tethering sig-

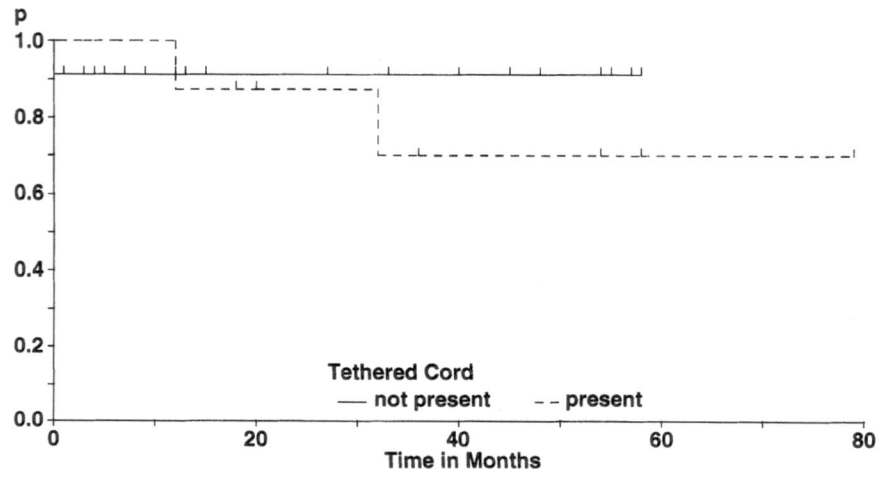

Fig. 4.40. Kaplan-Meier analysis of clinical recurrence rates after complete tumor resection comparing patients with and without postoperative arachnoid scarring leading to a tethered cord (log-rank test: not significant)

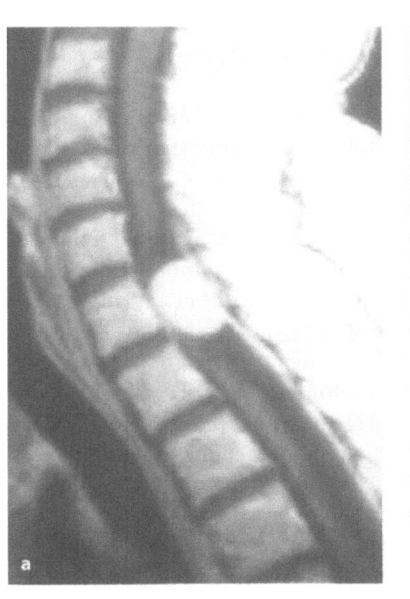
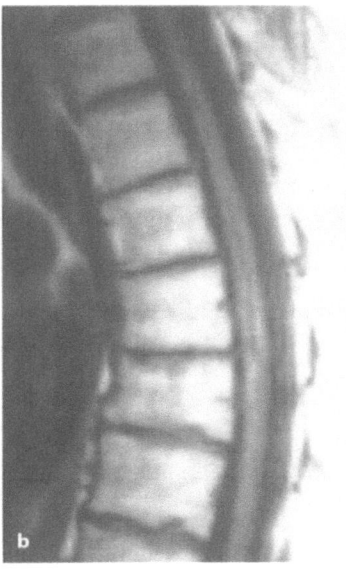

Fig. 4.41 a–e. This 66-year-old woman demonstrated a 3-year history of progressive gait ataxia and weakness of her right leg. The T1-weighted MRI scan with gadolinium disclosed a meningioma at the level of Th1 (a) with a small syrinx below the tumor (b, c). After complete resection of the tumor (d) the syrinx has disappeared (e)

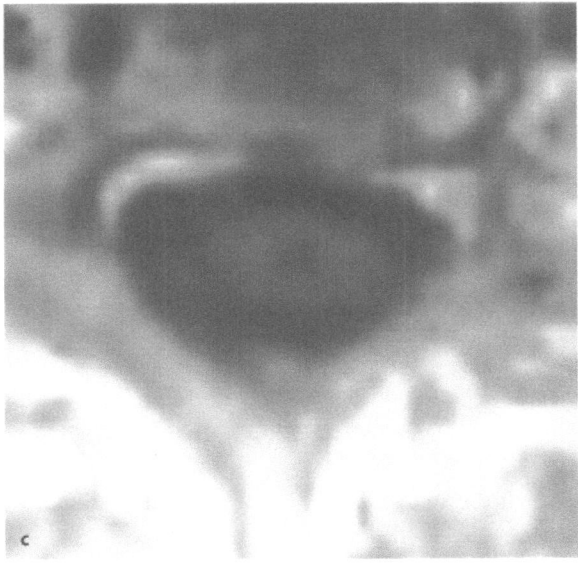
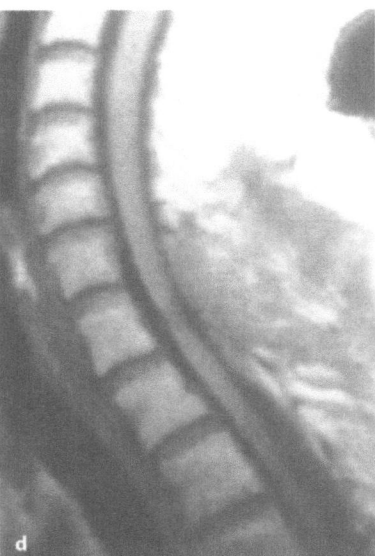

nificantly (22% with and 57% without suture, respectively; Chi-square test: $P=0.0012$). To limit the extent of postoperative arachnoid scarring further, we suggest decompression of the area of surgery using a Gore-Tex dura graft to maintain patency of the subarachnoid space, in particular, if the tumor is very vascularized or arachnoid scars had to be dissected.

In conclusion, intramedullary tumors should be operated on as soon as neurological symptoms have appeared. Waiting for further neurological progression raises the risk of surgery dramatically. If a syrinx accompanies the tumor, this should be interpreted as a favorable prognostic sign as it indicates a displacing rather than infiltrating tumor and thus suggests re-

sectability of the mass. It is sufficient to operate on the solid tumor part. The accompanying syrinx will decrease automatically if the tumor has been removed.

Complete tumor removal should not be attempted at any cost – in particular with infiltrating tumors. According to our experience, the rate of recurrence depends on the biology of the tumor rather than the amount of tumor resected – with the exception of ependymomas and angioblastomas. To minimize the risk of postoperative arachnoid scarring with its considerable morbidity, we suggest closing the cord with a pia suture after tumor removal and decompressing the subarachnoid space with a dural graft if appropriate.

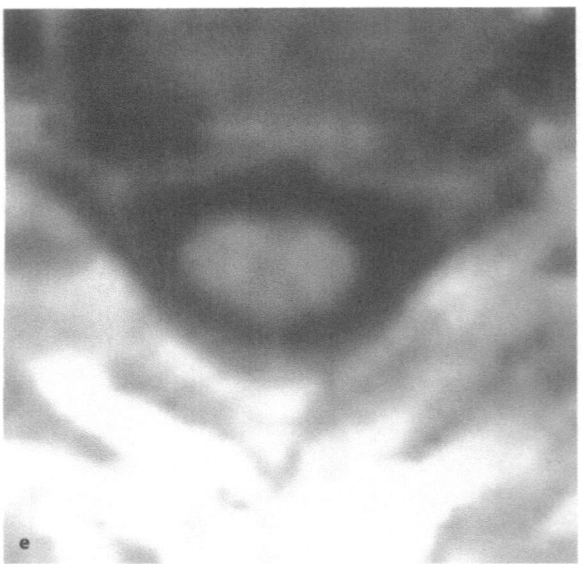

Fig. 4.41 e

4.2.2
Extramedullary and Epidural Tumors

Several case reports on extramedullary tumors associated with syringomyelia have appeared in the literature [1, 3, 4, 7, 9, 17, 25, 28, 32, 35, 41, 44, 46, 48, 50, 53]. 1.8% of 339 extramedullary and none among 322 epidural tumors, were associated with a syrinx in our series. Patients with extramedullary tumors and a syrinx were younger than those without syringomyelia (30±26 years and 49±17 years, respectively; *t*-test: *P*=0.008). In each of the five patients, the accompanying syrinx was asymptomatic. We observed two meningiomas (Fig. 4.41) and one patient each with a neurinoma, an ependymoma, an arachnoid cyst (Fig. 4.42), and a medulloblastoma metastasis. One tumor was located in the upper cervical canal, the ependymoma was situated below the conus originating from the filum terminale, and the remainder were located in the cervicothoracic junction.

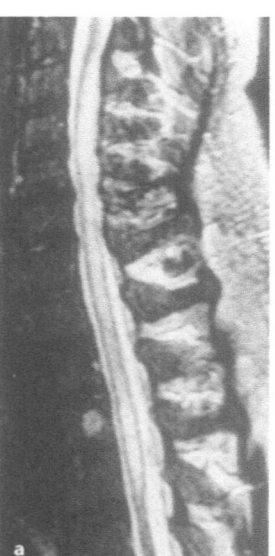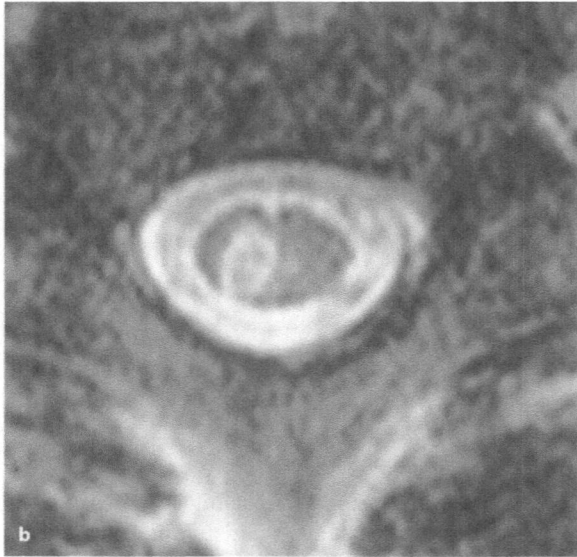

Fig. 4.42 a–j. This 35-year-old man complained about burning type dysesthesias in his right arm for the past 3 months. On examination, he demonstrated slight motor weakness and gait ataxia. **a** The T2-weighted MRI scan shows a syrinx between C2 and Th4 without evidence of a Chiari Malformation. **b** The axial scan at C7 displays the syrinx in the right half of the cord. **c** At the level of Th4/5, the cord appears compressed from posterior. **d, e** The phase contrast cine-MRI scans at the level of Th4/5 reveals a CSF flow obstruction in the posterior subarachnoid space. **f** The intraoperative view after dura opening reveals the corresponding arachnoid pathology. **g** After arachnoid opening, an arachnoid cyst is visible. **h** The cyst is resected completely. **i** The cord has collapsed after resection of the lesion and establishment of a free CSF passage

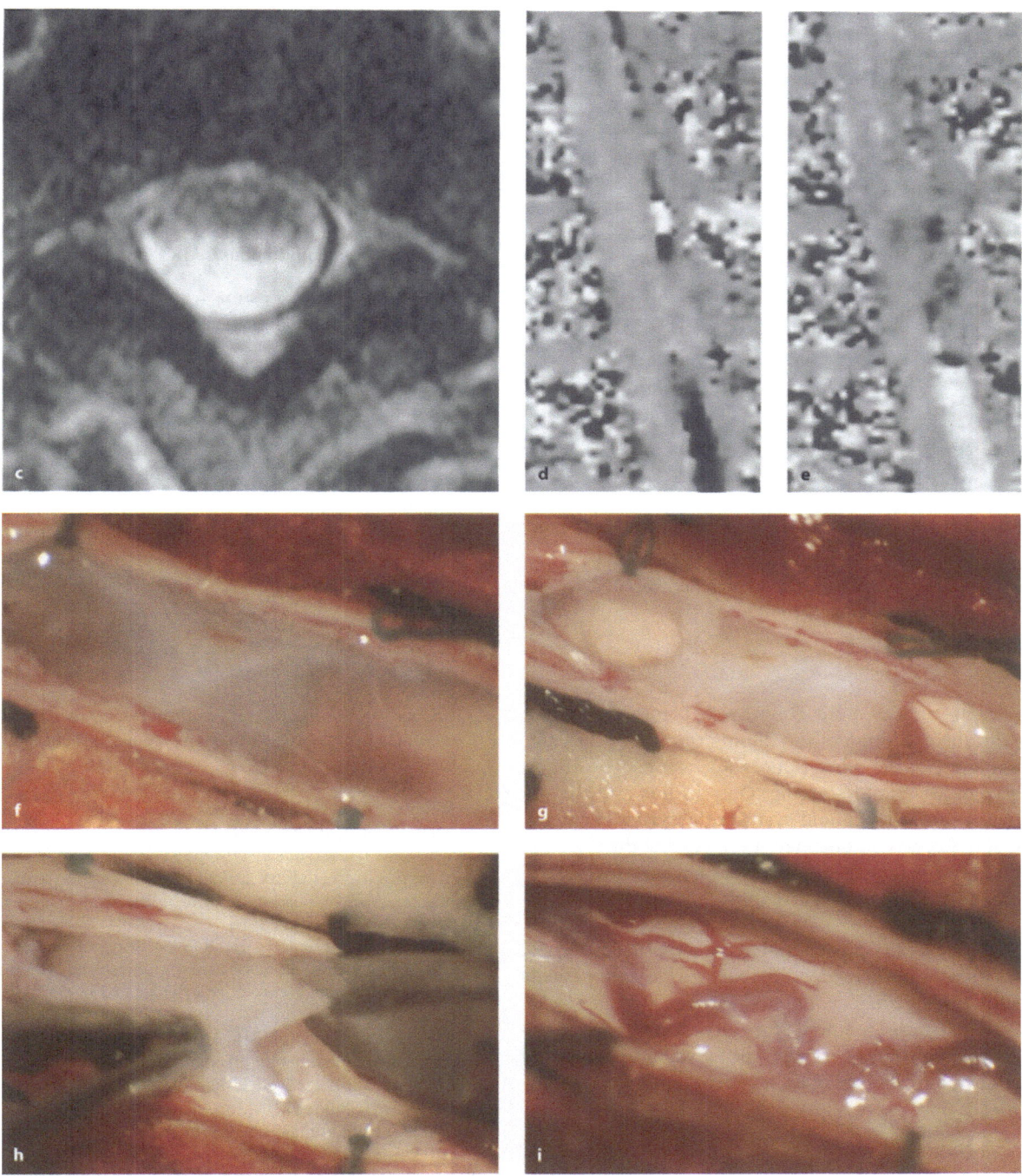

Fig. 4.42 c–i (continued on p. 172)

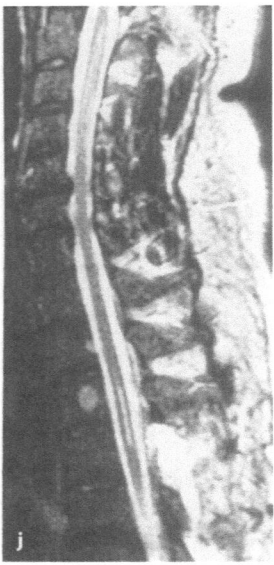

Fig. 4.42. j The postoperative T2-weighted MRI scan after 1 week shows already a marked decrease of the syrinx size. The patient improved in terms of motor power and gait. The burning type dysesthesias, however, were left unchanged

Four cavities were above, two below the tumor. With the exception of the filum terminale ependymoma, none of the other tumors was associated with an area of arachnoid scarring. Only in this and the patient with the arachnoid cyst was the syrinx of considerable size so that one may speculate that the syrinx in these two instances may have been caused by the arachnoid pathology rather than the space occupying tumor alone.

As far as the postoperative outcome is concerned, we did not observe any differences relative to patients with extramedullary tumors without syringomyelia. Patients were followed for an average period of 21±35 months. The syrinx regressed or disappeared after tumor removal in each patient.

References

1. Abe K, Sawada H, Fujiwara M, Mezaki T, Udaka F, Kitahara Y, Fujita M, Kameyama M (1988) MR imaging of syringobulbia with giant syrinx. Neuroradiology 30:442–443
2. Alvisi C, Cerisoli M, Giulioni M (1984) Intramedullary spinal gliomas: long-term results of surgical treatment. Acta Neurochir (Wien) 70:169–179
3. Barnett HJM, Rewcastle NB (1973) Syringomyelia and tumors of the nervous system. In: Barnett HJM, Foster JB, Hudgson P (eds) Syringomyelia. Major problems in neurology, vol 1. Saunders, London, pp 261–301
4. Blaylock RL (1981) Hydrosyringomyelia of the conus medullaris associated with a thoracic meningeoma. J Neurosurg 54:833–835
5. Braverman DL, Lachmann EA, Tunkel R, Nagler W (1997) Multiple sclerosis presenting as a spinal cord tumor. Arch Phys Med Rehabil 78:1274–1276
6. Canavero S, Pagni CA, Duca S, Bradac GB (1994) Spinal intramedullary cavernous angiomas: a literature meta-analysis. Surg Neurol 41:381–388
7. Castillo M, Quencer RM, Green BA, Montalvo BM (1988) Syringomyelia as a consequence of compressive extramedullary lesions: postoperative clinical and radiological manifestations. AJR Am J Roentgenol 150:391–396
8. Chandy MJ, Babu S (1999) Management of intramedullary spinal cord tumours: review of 68 patients. Neurol India 47:224–228
9. Chee CP, Tan CT, Nuruddin R (1990) Syringomyelia associated with a cauda equina meinigioma involving the conus medullaris. Br J Neurosurg 4:529–533
10. Chigasaki H, Pennybacker JB (1968) A long follow-up study of 128 cases of intramedullary spinal cord tumors. Neurol Med Chir 10:25–66
11. Constantini S, Miller DC, Allen JC, Rorke LB, Freed D, Epstein FJ (2000) Radical excision of intramedullary spinal cord tumors: surgical morbidity and long-term follow-up evaluation in 164 children and young adults. J Neurosurg 93:183–193
12. Cooper PR (1989) Outcome after operative treatment of intramedullary spinal cord tumors in adults: intermediate and long-term results in 51 patients. Neurosurgery 25:855–859
13. Cooper PR, Epstein F (1985) Radical resection of intramedullary spinal cord tumors in adults. J Neurosurg 63:492–499
14. Cosgrove GR, Bertrand G, Fontaine S, Robitaille Y, Melanson D (1988) Cavernous angiomas of the spinal cord. J Neurosurg 68:31–36
15. Cristante L, Herrmann HD (1994) Surgical management of intramedullary spinal cord tumors: functional outcome and sources of morbidity. Neurosurgery 35:69–74; discussion 74–76
16. Cristante L, Herrmann HD (1999) Surgical management of intramedullary hemangioblastoma of the spinal cord. Acta Neurochir (Wien) 141:333–339; discussion 339–340
17. De Buscher J, Scherer HJ, Thomas F (1938) Recklinghausen's neurofibromatosis combined with true syringomyelia. J Belge Neurol-Psychiat 38:788–802
18. Deutsch H, Jallo GI, Faktorovich A, Epstein F (2000) Spinal intramedullary cavernoma: clinical presentation and surgical outcome. J Neurosurg 93:65–70
19. Emery E, Hurth M, Lacroix-Jousselin C, David P, Richard S (1994) [Intraspinal hemangioblastoma. Apropos of a recent series of 20 cases]. Neurochirurgie 40:165–173
20. Epstein FJ, Epstein N (1982) Surgical treatment of spinal cord astrocytomas of childhood: a series of 19 patients. J Neurosurg 57:685–689
21. Epstein FJ, Farmer JP, Freed D (1992) Adult intramedullary astrocytomas of the spinal cord. J Neurosurg 77:355–359
22. Epstein FJ, Farmer JP, Freed D (1993) Adult intramedullary spinal cord ependymomas: the result of surgery in 38 patients. J Neurosurg 79:204–209

23. Ferry DJ, Hardman JM, Earle KM (1969) Syringomyelia and intramedullary neoplasms. Med Ann Distr Columbia 38:363–365

24. Fischer G, Mansuy L (1980) Total removal of intramedullary ependymomas: follow-up study of 16 cases. Surg Neurol 14:243–249

25. Gooding MR (1972) Syringomyelia in association with a neurofibroma of the filum terminale. J Neurol Neurosurg Psychiatry 35:560–564

26. Goy AM, Pinto RS, Raghavendra BN, Epstein FJ, Kricheff II (1986) Intramedullary spinal cord tumors: MR imaging with emphasis on associated cysts. Radiology 161:381–386

27. Guidetti B, Mercuri B, Vagnozzi R (1981) Long-term results of the surgical treatment of 129 intramedullary spinal gliomas. J Neurosurg 54:323–330

28. Harbitz F, Lossius E (1929) Extramedullary tumor. Arachnoiditis fibrosa cystica et ossificans. Gliosis of the medulla. Acta Psychiatr Neurol 4:51–64

29. Hardison HH, Packer RJ, Rorke LB, Schut L, Sutton LN, Bruce DA (1987) Outcome of children with primary intramedullary spinal cord tumors. Child's Nerv Syst 3:89–92

30. Hejazi N, Hassler W (1998) Microsurgical treatment of intramedullary spinal cord tumors. Neurol Med Chir (Tokyo) 38:266–271; discussion 271–273

31. Herrmann HD, Neuss M, Winkler D (1988) Intramedullary spinal cord tumors resected with CO2 Laser microsurgical technique: recent experience in fifteen patients. Neurosurgery 22:518–522

32. Hormigo A, Lobo-Antunes J, Bravo-Marques JM, Marques MS (1990) Syringomyelia secondary to compression of the cervical spinal cord by an extramedullary lymphoma. Neurosurgery 27:834–836

33. Hoshimaru M, Koyama T, Hashimoto N (2000) [Microsurgery of cervical intramedullary ependymomas extending into the medulla oblongata]. No Shinkei Geka 28:517–522

34. Innocenzi G, Raco A, Cantore G, Raimondi AJ (1996) Intramedullary astrocytomas and ependymomas in the pediatric age group: a retrospective study. Child's Nerv Syst 12:776–780

35. Jamjoon AB, Davies KG (1990) Syringomyelia associated with a spinal schwannoma: a case report. J Neurol Neurosurg Psychiatry 53:438–439

36. Kane PJ, el-Mahdy W, Singh A, Powell MP, Crockard HA (1999) Spinal intradural tumours. II. Intramedullary. Br J Neurosurg 13:558–563

37. Lee M, Epstein FJ, Rezai AR, Zagzag D (1998) Nonneoplastic intramedullary spinal cord lesions mimicking tumors. Neurosurgery 43:788–794; discussion 794–795

38. Malis LI (1978) Intramedullary spinal cord tumors. Clin Neurosurg 25:512–539

39. McCormick PC, Stein BM (1990) Intramedullary tumors in adults. In: Stein BM, McCormick PC (eds) Neurosurgery clinics in North America, vol 1. III. Intradural spinal surgery. Saunders, Philadelphia, pp 609–630

40. Mehdorn HM, Stolke D (1991) Cervical intramedullary cavernous angioma with MRI-proven haemorrhages. J Neurol 238:420–426

41. Milhorat TH, Johnson WD, Miller JI, Bergland RM, Hollenberg-Sher J (1992) Surgical treatment of syringomyelia based on magnetic resonance imaging criteria. Neurosurgery 31:231–245

42. Murota T, Symon L (1989) Surgical management of hemangioblastoma of the spinal cord: a report of 18 cases. Neurosurgery 25:699–708

43. Nadkarni TD, Rekate HL (1999) Pediatric intramedullary spinal cord tumors. Critical review of the literature [see comments]. Child's Nerv Syst 15:17–28

44. Nishiura I, Koyama T, Abe K, Kameyama M (1989) [An extramedullary spinal cord tumor associated with syringomyelia: a case report]. No Shinkei Geka 17:181–185

45. Park CK, Chung CK, Choe GY, Wang KC, Cho BK, Kim HJ (2000) Intramedullary spinal cord ganglioglioma: a report of five cases. Acta Neurochir (Wien) 142:547–552

46. Poser CM (1956) The relationship between syringomyelia and neoplasms. Charles C.Thomas, Springfield

47. Pullucino P, Kendall BE (1982) Computed tomography of cystic intramedullary lesions. Neuroradiology 23:117–121

48. Quencer RM, El Gammal T, Cohen G (1986) Syringomyelia associated with intradural extramedullary masses of the spinal canal. AJNR Am J Neuroradiol 7:143–148

49. Rawlings CE, Giangaspero F, Burger PC, Bullard DE (1988) Ependymomas: a clinicopathologic study. Surg Neurol 29:271–281

50. Rhyner PA, Hudgins RJ, Edwards MSB, Brant-Zawadzki M (1987) Magnetic resonance imaging of syringomyelia associated with an extramedullary spinal cord tumor: case report. Neurosurgery 21:233–235

51. Seifert V, Trost HA, Stolke D (1990) Mikrochirurgie spinaler Angioblastome. Neurochirurgia 33:100–105

52. Stein BM (1979) Surgery of intramedullary spinal cord tumours. Clin Neurosurg 26:529–542

53. Tokoro K, Chiba Y, Yagashita S, Kunimi Y (1989) Cordectomy for syringobulbo-myelia with sleep apnea secondary to a spinal extramedullary tumor: case report. Neurosurgery 24:118–124

54. Vaquero J, Salazar J, Martinez R, Martinez P, Bravo G (1987) Cavernomas of the central nervous system: clinical syndromes, CT scan diagnosis, and prognosis after surgical treatment in 25 cases. Acta Neurochir (Wien) 85:29–33

55. Vijayakumar S, Estes M, Hardy RW jr, Rosenblo SA, Thomas FJ (1988) Ependymoma of the spinal cord and cauda equina: a review. Cleve Clin J Med 55:163–170

56. Woltman HW, Kernohan JW, Adson AW, Craig WM (1951) Intramedullary tumors of spinal cord and gliomas of intradural portion of filum terminale. Fate of patients who have these tumors. Arch Neurol Psychiatr 65:378–393

57. Yasargil MG, Antic J, Laciga R, De Preux J, Fideler RW, Boone SC (1976) The microsurgical removal of intramedullary spinal hemangioblastomas. Report of twelve cases and a review of the literature. Surg Neurol 6:141–148

58. Zentner J, Hassler W, Gawehn J, Schroth G (1989) Intramedullary cavernous angiomas. Surg Neurol 31:64–68

4.3
Syringomyelia Related to Spinal Dysraphism

The association of dysraphic malformations with syringomyelia has already been described by Estienne [14] in the sixteenth and by Brunner [6] at the end of the seventeenth centuries. How often a syrinx accompanies spina bifida, however, has only been determined since MRI became available. Our experience with this entity is mainly confined to adult patients. In our series of 61 patients with dysraphic malformations, 23% showed an accompanying syrinx. Other reports gave various figures between 6% and 75% [4, 5, 7, 12, 22, 28, 29, 33, 43, 45, 50, 56, 57]. The pathophysiology of syringomyelia was rarely discussed in publications on spinal dysraphism as most authors considered the syrinx to be part of the malformation.

However, as outlined for malformations at the foramen magnum, syringomyelia is a secondary phenomenon. In the context of spinal dysraphism, it may be caused by CSF flow obstruction attributable to a hamartoma or arachnoid adhesions, which may accompany a dysraphic malformation primarily or as a result of previous surgeries [8, 13, 20, 21]. Alternatively, a syrinx may develop as a consequence of a tethered cord [29, 56]. In most instances, CSF flow obstruction and cord tethering act synergistically.

Spinal dysraphism affects the lumbosacral region in most instances [24] – 73% in our series. A various combination of bony anomalies, cord tethering, and a space-occupying hamartoma may be found. Each of these may cause a mechanism responsible for the patient's symptoms and each of these may be involved in the pathophysiology of an accompanying syrinx. The most common mechanism involved is a tethered cord [29, 32, 39, 43, 48, 55, 56]. A tethered cord does not require a low position of the conus medullaris [54] but describes a situation in which the conus is immobilized in the spinal canal [31, 38] due to a thick filum terminale, a hamartoma such as a lipoma, a diastematomyelia, or arachnoid adhesions. Even without an additional CSF flow obstruction, a tethered cord alone may cause syringomyelia. Levy [31] demonstrated impaired spinal cord motion in cine-MRI studies in patients with a tethered cord syndrome that recovered after release of the tethering. They even found a good correlation of their radiological findings with the clinical course of the patient: patients with disturbed spinal cord motion tended to develop progressive neurological deficits in contrast to patients with dysraphic lesions but preserved spinal cord motility.

Once a patient has been operated for spinal dysraphism, arachnoid adhesions and scars may become a considerable problem and are the most common cause of re-tethering [9, 29, 36, 56]. Of children with myelomeningocele, for instance, 78% [53] to 89% [25] develop radiological evidence of re-tethering of the cord at the site of the repair. About 15–20% of these may experience clinical symptoms of tethering requiring a second operation at that level [9, 37, 50].

Finally, all patients with a spinal hamartoma should undergo a complete evaluation of the entire neuraxis including the foramen magnum [3, 4, 25, 49]. The obligatory association of Chiari II malformation with spinal meningomyelocele was outlined in Chap. 3.1. Other forms of spinal dysraphism may be combined with a Chiari I malformation.

4.3.1
Clinical Presentation

In most patients with spinal dysraphism, an accompanying syrinx is clinically not apparent. The symptoms due to the malformation usually predominate. Quite often, minor traumatic incidents are reported by patients as having triggered a progressive course of events [39, 40]. Among 61 patients in our series, 46 operations were performed among 37 patients. Thirty-three percent were operated on more than once. Twenty-four patients were not operated on, as they did not present progressive neurological symptoms. This illustrates the enormous variety of the clinical course. Not every patient with spinal dysraphism will become symptomatic [10]. This fact is illustrated by patients who reach old age before the first symptoms start to appear [26].

When spinal dysraphism is suspected, the first step should be a thorough clinical examination to look for visible stigmata such as a dermal sinus or atypical hair growth at the site of the malformation. Comparing patients with and without an additional syrinx, differences in clinical presentation became apparent. With an associated syrinx, 38% of patients reported gait problems as the first clinical sign, 23% sensory deficits, 15% motor deficits or pain and 8% dysesthesias. Without an associated syrinx, the most common first clinical sign was pain (48%), which usually started at the spinal level of the malformation and extended in a radicular pattern. Gait problems were reported by 16%, motor deficits by 14%, and sphincter disturbances by 8%. Sensory deficits (2%), dysesthesias (2%), or hydrocephalus (2%) were rare initial complaints in the group without syringomyelia (Chi-square test: $P=0.0269$). The average history until admission for neurosurgical consultation was significantly shorter for patients with an additional syrinx (43 ± 52 months and 87 ± 121 months, respectively; t-test: $P=0.0332$). This may indicate a more dynamic clinical course in this group.

At the time of admission, those with a syrinx still mentioned gait disturbances as the most significant problem in 46% of cases, while 31% were mostly

Table 4.19. Clinical presentation of spinal dysraphism

Symptoms	With syringomyelia	Without syringomyelia
Gait ataxia	79%	71%
Motor weakness	71%	69%
Pain	50%	71%
Sensory deficits	86%	67%
Dysesthesias	57%	35%
Sphincter problems	43%	56%
Karnofsky score	70 ± 14	72 ± 14

troubled by pain. Eight percent each considered motor or sensory deficits and dysesthesias as the main symptom. Without a syrinx, 60% reported pain as the most distressing problem, 20% gait disturbances, 10% motor weakness, 8% cosmetic disfigurations, and 4% sphincter problems (Chi-square test: $P=0.0363$). Similar figures for adult patients have been presented in the literature [16, 17, 23].

In small children, sensorimotor deficits and sphincter problems predominate the clinical picture of spinal dysraphism irrespective of the presence or absence of syringomyelia [12, 24, 27, 42].

Table 4.19 gives an overview on the clinical presentation of patients with spinal dysraphism. Their Kar-

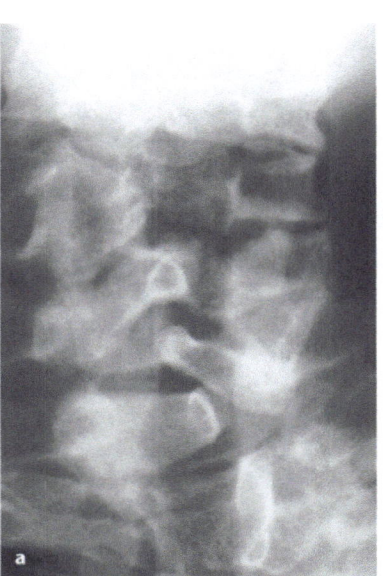
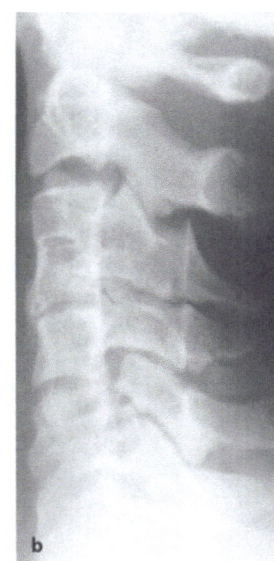

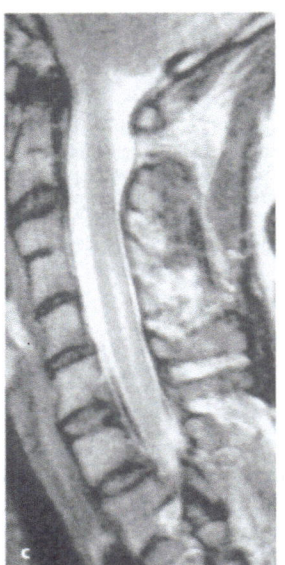
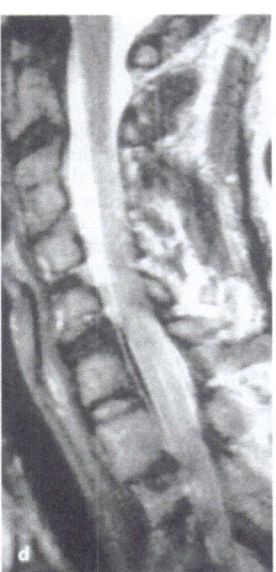
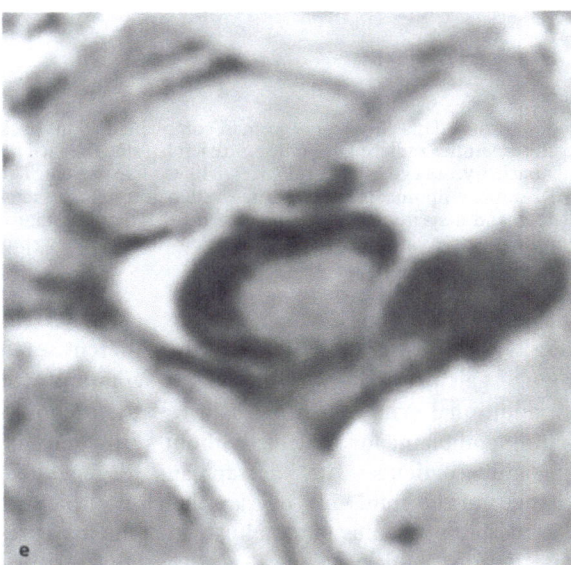

Fig. 4.43 a–e. This 43-year-old woman presented with slight neck pain, occasional dysesthesias in the C6 root on the left side and scoliosis. The X-ray studies (**a, b**) show a Klippel-Feil syndrome at C3/4 and a spina bifida at C5 to C7. **c, d** The T2-weighted sagittal MRI scans demonstrate a syrinx C4 to C7. **e** The axial scan at C5/6 indicates arachnoid adhesions at the C5/6 level. No surgery was recommended and the patient is followed clinically

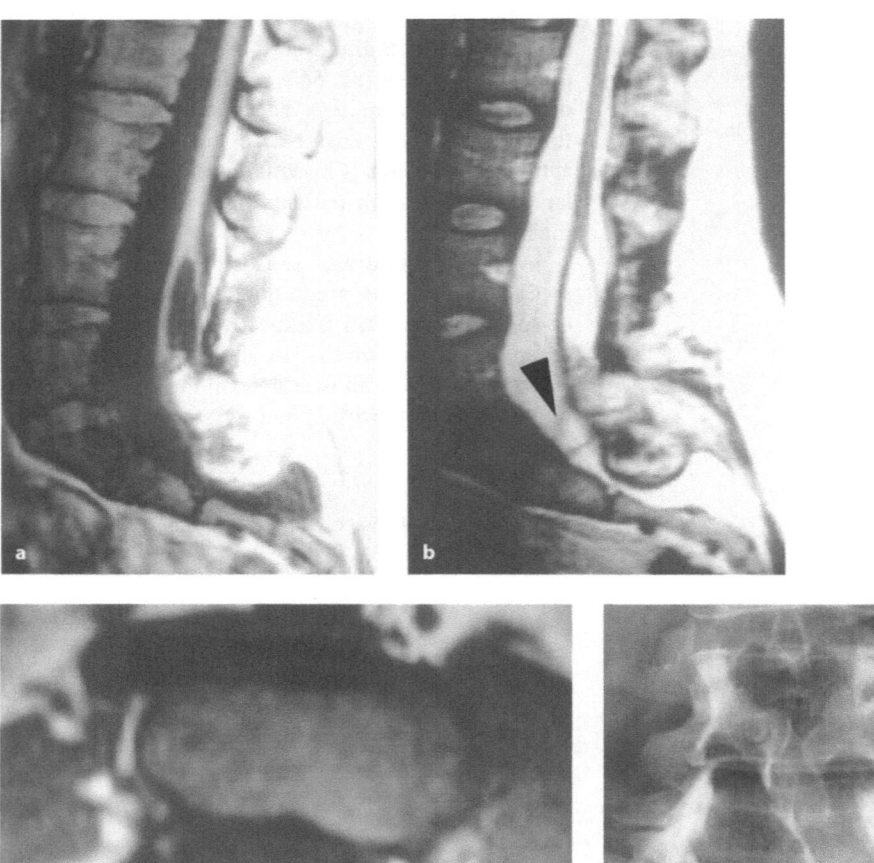

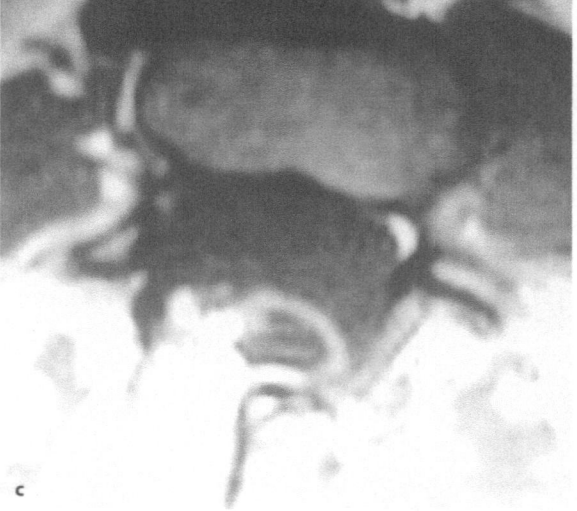

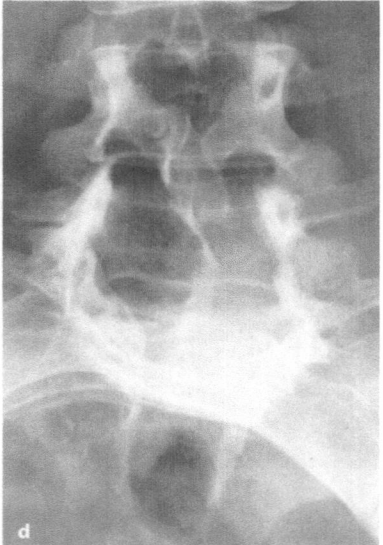

Fig. 4.44 a–d. This 60-year-old woman complained about back pain sometimes radiating into the entire left leg since she fell on her back 3 years ago. No neurological deficits were present. The MRI shows a lipoma, tethered cord, diastematomyelia, a sacral defect, and a syrinx in the left hemicord (**a**). The diastematomyelia is better visualized in T2. The *arrow* marks a bony spur dividing the cord at S1 (**b**). The axial T1-weighted image shows the connection of the left hemicord to a lipoma which penetrates the dura (**c**). **d** The X-ray study of her lower spine and sacrum displays the missing sacral roof. No surgery was recommended as the character and distribution of the pain did not suggest a correlation with the tethered cord

nofsky score was not significantly different even though gait problems were the major symptom with an additional symptom while pain was the predominating complaint for patients without syringomyelia. In adult patients with dysraphism, degenerative changes of the spine may overlap the clinical picture. Altered biomechanics of a malformed spine may predispose to secondary changes such as scoliosis, spinal stenosis, disc disease or spinal instability [56].

4.3.2
Neuroradiology

As a general rule, the entire neuraxis should be evaluated in patients with spinal dysraphism. If bony anomalies such as a spina bifida (Figs. 4.43, 4.44) or scalloping of vertebral bodies accompanies the malformation, functional studies should be undertaken if the possibility of instability has to be considered. The

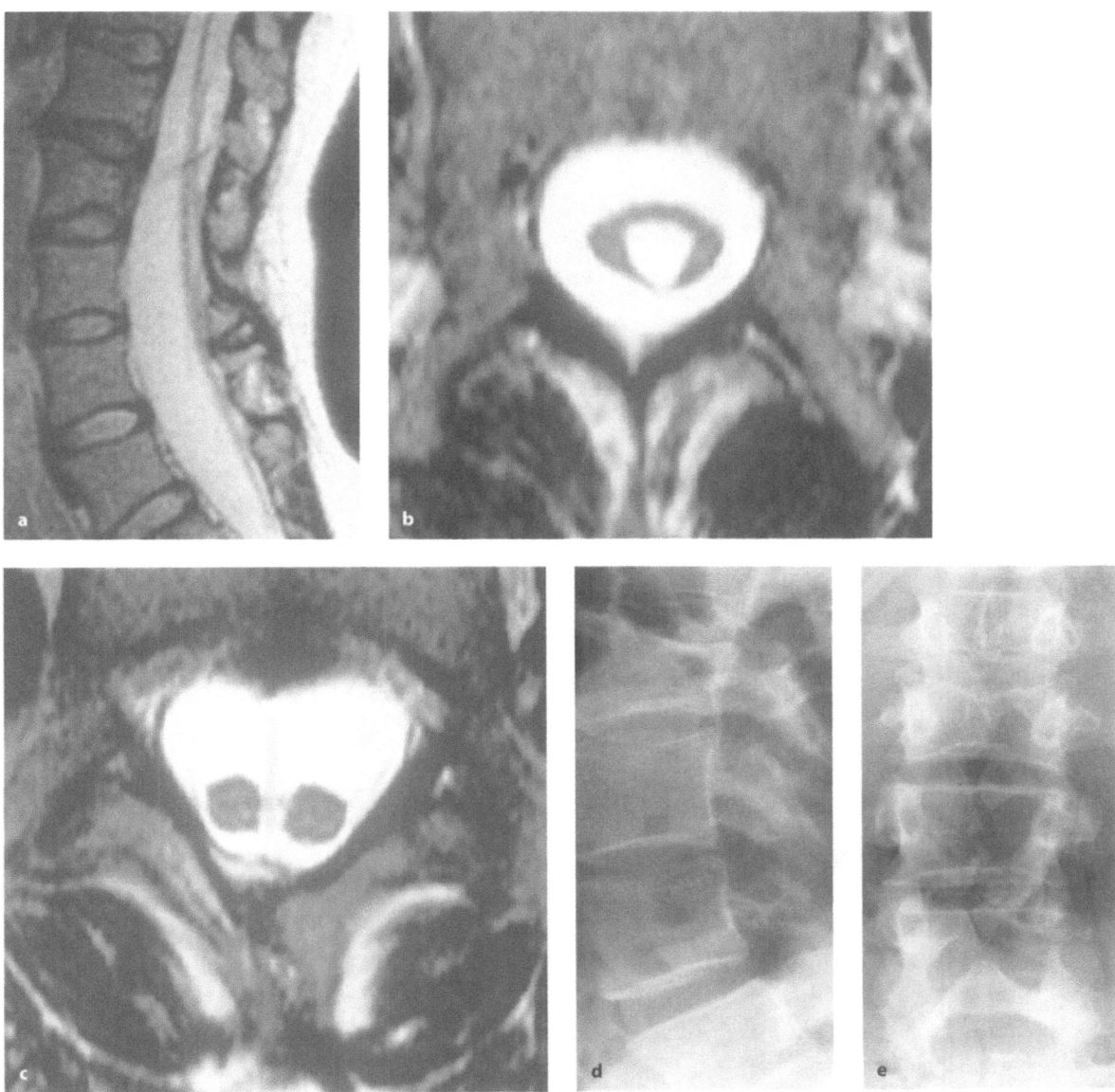

Fig. 4.45 a–s. This 35-year old woman presented with back pain radiating to the back of her right leg and hypesthesia of the right leg. She suffered from slight urinary incontinence but showed no motor weakness of her legs. **a** The T2-weighted MRI demonstrates a diastematomyelia with a fibrous band at L1/L2 and a small syrinx above (**b**). **c** This axial scan reveals the fibrous structure between both hemicords at L2. **d** The lateral X-ray demonstrates the malformed vertebral body of L2. **e** The a.p. view of the lumbar spine reveals a spina bifida of almost the entire lumbar spine (continued on next page)

most important study is a detailed MRI examination (Figs. 4.43–4.46). The position of the conus medullaris and the filum terminale are well outlined with this technique (Figs. 4.44, 4.45). Hamartomas such as a dermoid cyst, a neurenteric cyst, or a lipoma can be visualized accurately (Fig. 4.44). With lipomas, it is particularly important to study the spinal dura: is the lipoma strictly intradural, epidural or does it penetrate the dura (Fig. 4.44)? This is very important information for adequate surgical planning. However, for a sufficient visualization of bony anomalies, plain X-rays and CT are still required. In very complex malformations, a helical CT with 3D reconstruction can be very helpful for surgical planning (Fig. 4.45). In children, however, X-ray studies should be limited to minimize the amount of radiation.

Comparing patients with and without an associated syrinx, we were unable to identify significant differ-

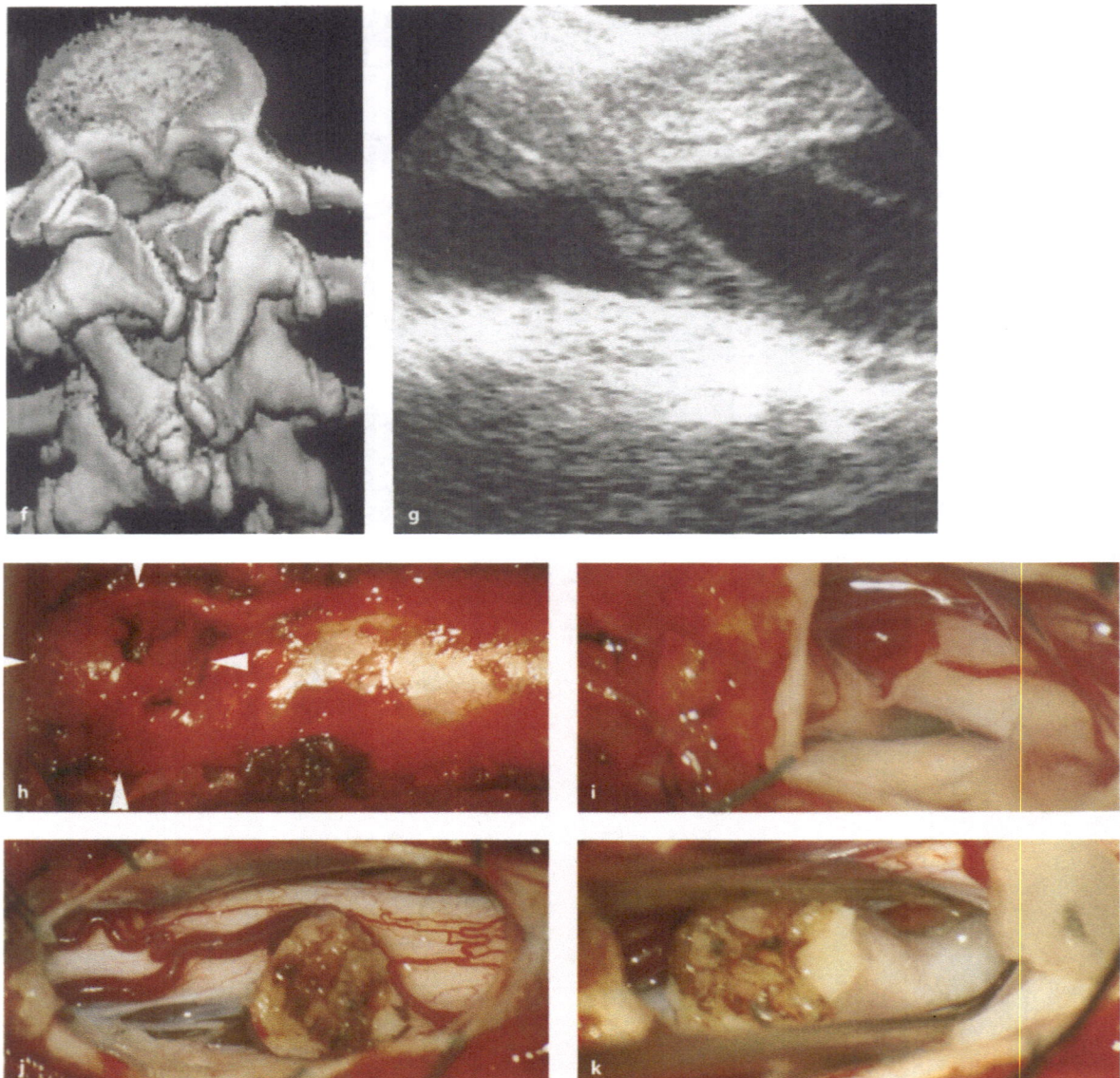

Fig. 4.45 f–k. f A 3D reconstruction model can provide good orientation for the intraoperative dissection. **g** After soft tissue dissection and removal of parts of laminae L1 and L2, this intraoperative sagittal ultrasound study shows the fibrous band clearly. **h** The intraoperative view of the dura demonstrates an abnormality on the left side (*arrow*). Here, the fibrous band penetrates the spinal canal surrounded by dura. **i** Dura opening is started from below and extended cranially to reveal the split cord malformation and the lower margin of the fibrous structure. **j** The dura is cut along the periphery of this dural sleeve to the cranial part of the exposure. **k** The anterior part of the dural sac is seen with the fibrous band penetrating the anterior border of the spinal canal. Here the structure is transected and hemostasis achieved with fibrin sponges. **l** The two hemicords are untethered completely. **m** A Gore-Tex duraplasty has been performed. Opening the spinal canal at S1 revealed the conus medullaris at this level. The exposure was slightly extended caudally until the filum terminale could be easily identified due to its fibrous and glossy texture (**n**). It is transected (**o**, **p**) and a second Gore-Tex duraplasty inserted (**q**). Postoperatively, symptoms improved for about 6 months when back pain and sensory problems reappeared. Since then the patient is in stable condition for 2 years. The sagittal (**r**) and axial (**s**) T2-weighted MRI scans show a completely untethered cord at both sites with no fibrous tissue between both hemicords

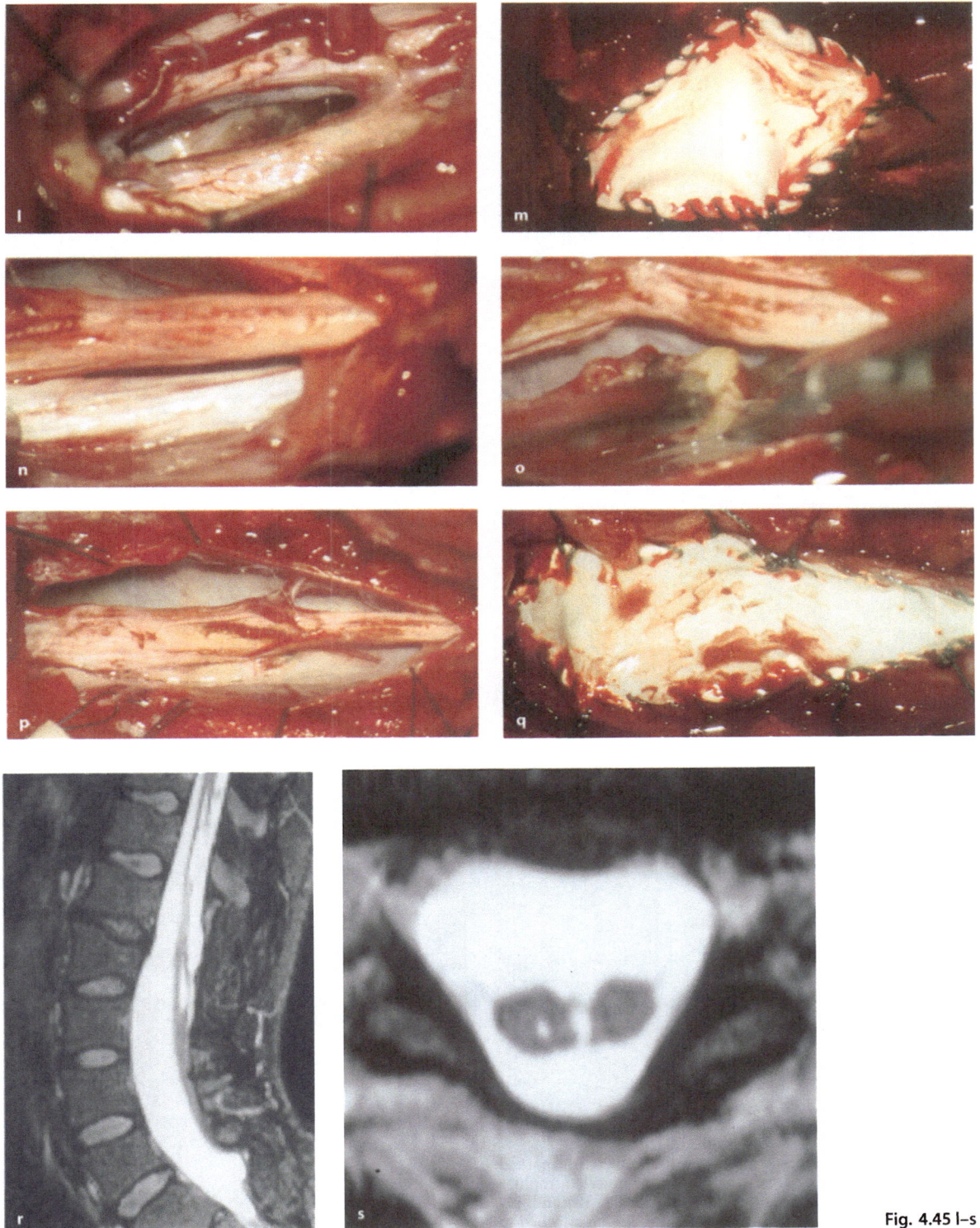

Fig. 4.45 l–s

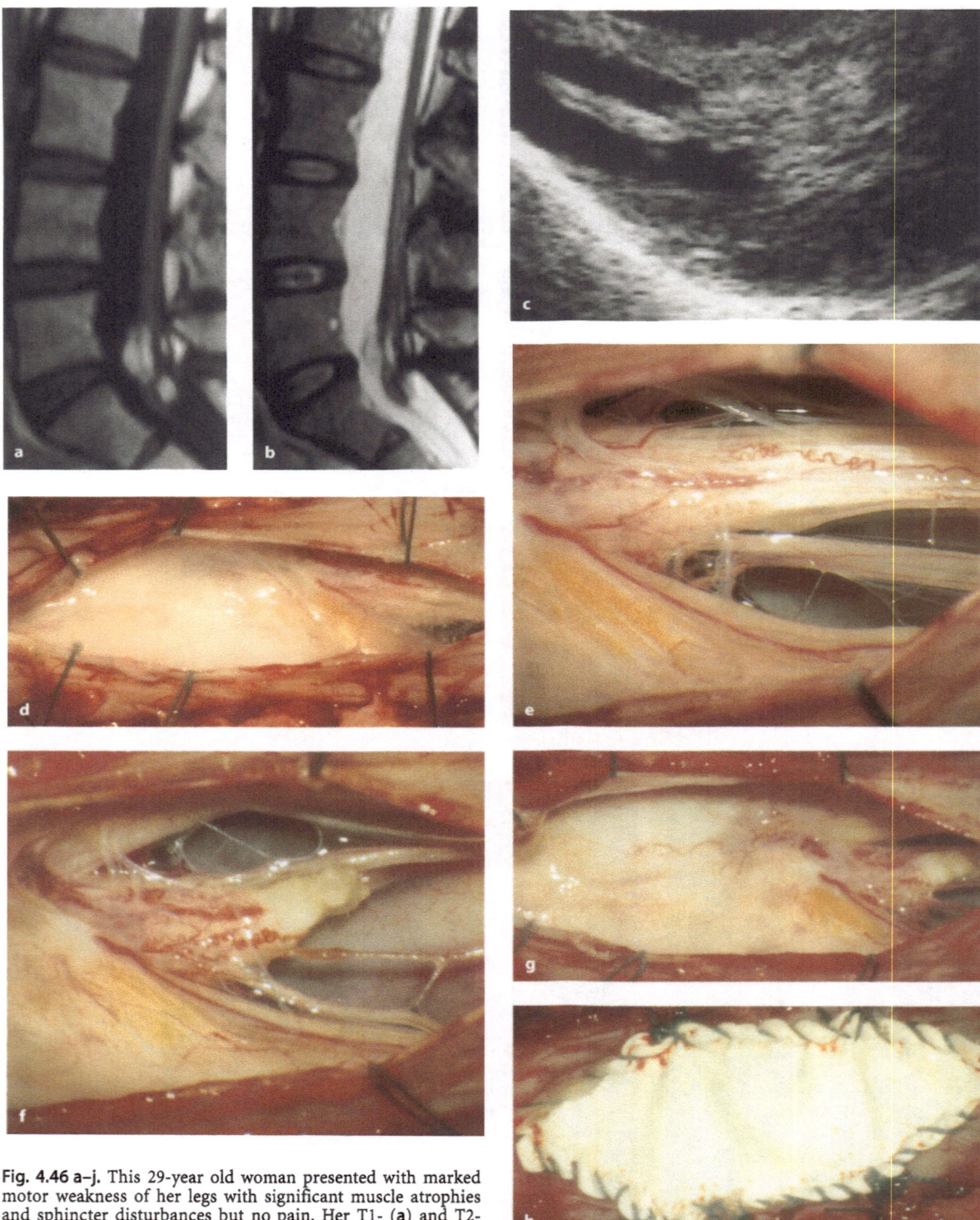

Fig. 4.46 a–j. This 29-year old woman presented with marked motor weakness of her legs with significant muscle atrophies and sphincter disturbances but no pain. Her T1- (**a**) and T2-weighted (**b**) MRI scans show an intradural lipoma attached to the conus medullaris at S1 and a thick filum terminale. **c** The intraoperative ultrasound shows the lipoma and spinal cord and provides information for safe entry to the subarachnoid space. **d** After dura opening, the lipoma is visible. The conus medullaris lies underneath. **e** Higher magnification of the lower part of the exposure displays the filum terminale with its characteristic texture. **f, g** After transsection of the filum, the cord is untethered in this case. No further dissection or resection of the lipoma is necessary. **h** A Gore-Tex duraplasty is performed. Postoperatively, she kept her neurological status with no progression for 3 years. The postoperative T1- (**i**) and T2-weighted (**j**) MRI scans demonstrate an untethered conus medullaris with no adhesions in the surgical area

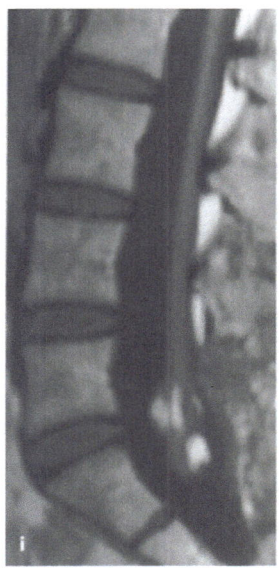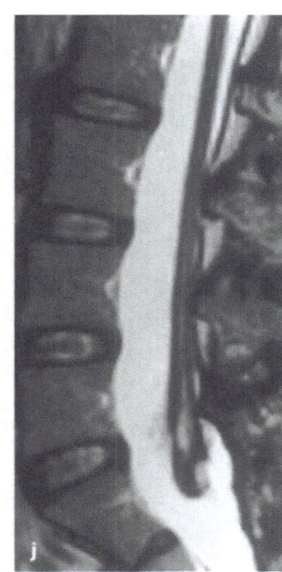

Fig. 4.46 i, j.

Table 4.20. Features of patients with spinal dysraphism

Feature	With syringomyelia	Without syringomyelia	P-value
Tethered cord	86%	63%	n.s.
Diastematomyelia	36%	16%	n.s.
Dermal sinus	–	28%	0.0196
Lumbosacral level	86%	88%	n.s.
Cervical or thoracic level	14%	12%	n.s.

ences in radiological features even though there was a trend for a higher proportion of patients with a tethered cord or a diastematomyelia in the syringomyelia group (Table 4.20).

4.3.3
Surgical Management

For appropriate surgical management, a number of points have to be considered:

1. Are spinal biomechanics altered due to the malformation?
2. Are degenerative problems part of the clinical picture?
3. Is there evidence of a tethered cord? If so, what contributes to the tethering?
4. Is a space occupying hamartoma present?
5. Is a Chiari malformation present?
6. Is hydrocephalus present?

Each of these aspects may have to be addressed for planning a successful surgical strategy. First, children and adults should be distinguished. In children, one may have to deal with a combination of Chiari II malformation and lumbosacral dysraphism. A syrinx may be caused by either of them. In adults, however, the spinal dysraphism is not combined with a craniocervical malformation in most cases but quite often with degenerative problems of the spine.

If syringomyelia is considered the major clinical problem in children with spinal dysraphism, the diag-

nostic evaluation should first establish whether hydrocephalus is present and adequately treated. A significant number of patients with spinal dysraphism and a large syrinx respond favorably to a revision of the ventriculoperitoneal shunt [29, 56]. If this has been ruled out or treated, the syringomyelia may be related to a Chiari II malformation or a tethered cord. The symptoms of the patient and the spinal distribution of the syrinx should guide the surgeon in the decision process whether to decompress a Chiari II malformation or perform an untethering operation [7, 29, 56]. The postoperative evaluation of the syrinx size is a good indicator as to whether untethering or decompression were adequate [12]. If such surgery fails to control the syringomyelia, we would recommend a shunt of the syrinx in accordance with other authors [7, 29, 52, 56]. Some authors insert a syringopleural or syringoperitoneal shunt initially when they operate on a tethered cord with an additional syrinx [12]. We would rather recommend restriction of the use of shunts to patients in whom the attempts to treat the cause of the syringomyelia have failed and prefer syringosubarachnoid shunts in such instances.

In adults, degenerative problems of the spine may cause clinical symptoms very similar to dysraphic lesions and pose considerable problems to plan adequate treatment [39, 47]. A patient with lumbar pain, a spina bifida occulta, and additional degenerative changes of the lumbar spine, for instance, may just require disc surgery for sufficient treatment. Surgery for dysraphic malformations in adults in particular is a rather complex issue and should only be undertaken if clinical progression is present and attributable to it.

If a hamartoma such as a dermoid cyst or a lipoma is present, spinal cord compression and cord tethering may be present alone or in combination (Fig. 4.46). A tethered cord may be caused by a hamartoma, a diastematomyelia (Fig. 4.45), a thick filum terminale (Figs. 4.45, 4.46), or arachnoid scars (Fig. 4.47). Each of these can again be active alone or in combination

Fig. 4.47 a–f

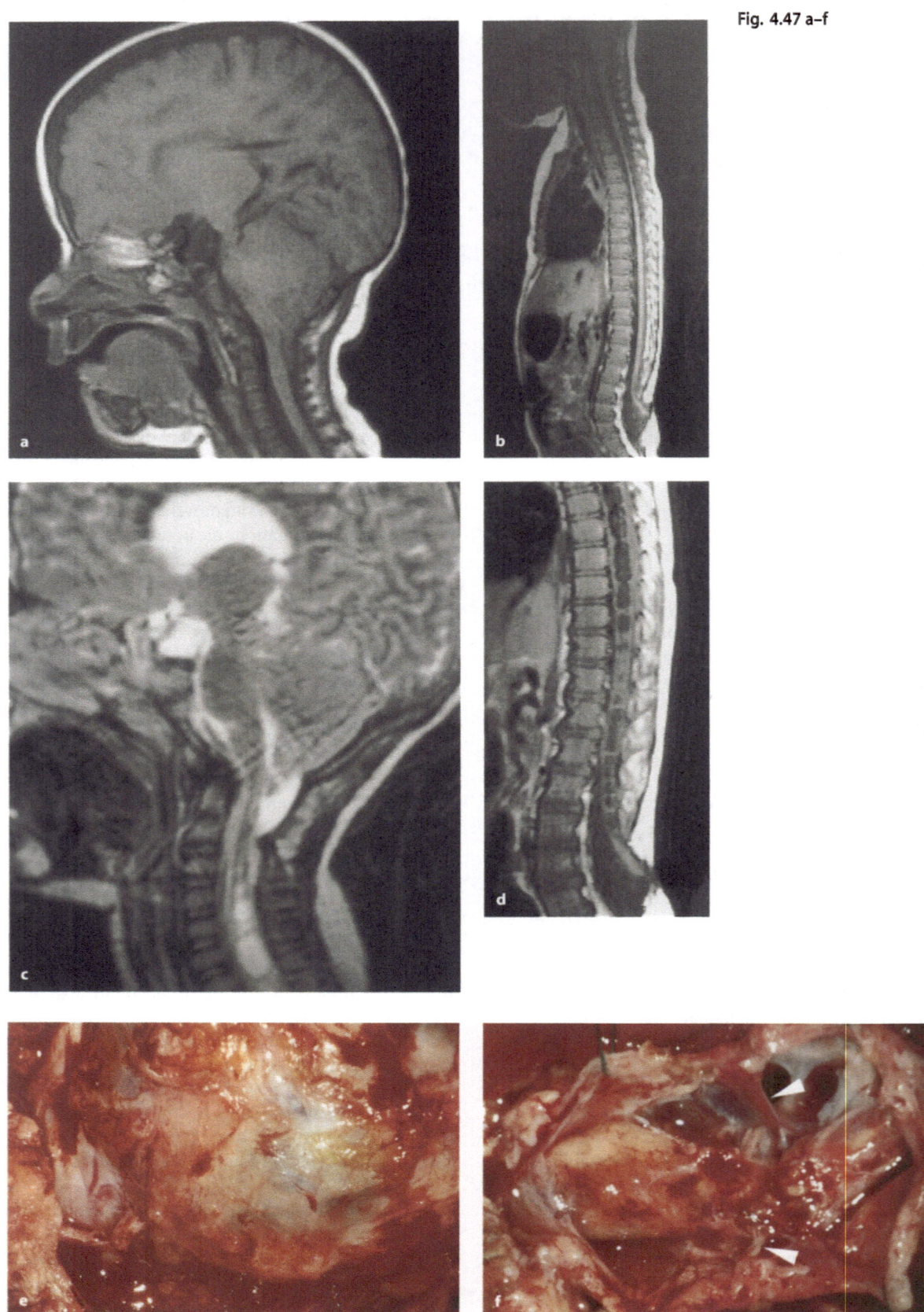

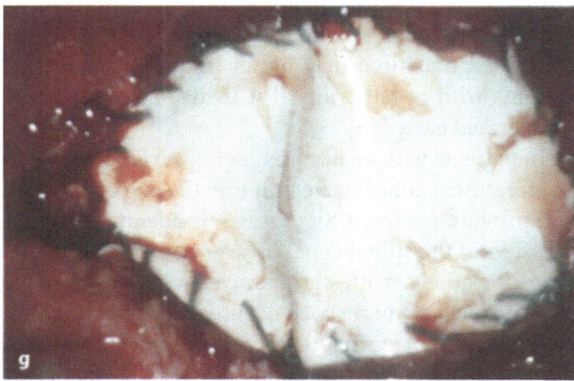

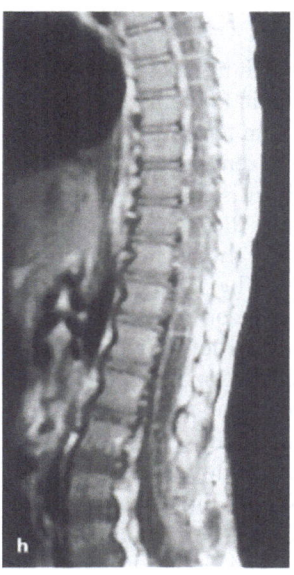

Fig. 4.47 a–h. This 5-year old boy was operated at birth for lumbar meningomyelocele and hydrocephalus. At the age of 13 months he underwent decompression of his Chiari II malformation (**a**) to improve apnea spells which have disappeared since then. At that time, no syringomyelia was present (**b**). Four and a half years later, despite a functioning ventriculoperitoneal shunt and free CSF passage at the cervical decompression (**c**), he presents with a large syrinx of his entire cord (**d**). Retethering at the site of the myelomeningocele repair was considered responsible. **e** This intraoperative view depicts the situation before dura incision. **f** The conus was adherent to the neighboring soft tissues. *Arrows* mark some of the nerve roots which provided an additional tethering effect. **g** A Gore-

Tex duraplasty was inserted. Postoperatively, the lower part of the syrinx appears slightly smaller 2 weeks after this partial untethering (**h**). No neurological deficits have appeared or worsened since the second operation

and at different spinal levels in a particular patient. Arachnoid adhesions or scars in particular may complicate surgery for spinal dysraphism even further [2].

Hamartomas can be separated into two groups: those that may grow and those that do not change their volume. Dermoid or epidermoid cysts may grow considerably as they contain tissue that produces a solid or fluid substance which then may accumulate in significant quantities to cause severe cord compression. If contents of the cyst contaminate the subarachnoid space, significant arachnoid scarring may be the result due to a local meningitis. The extraordinary rare event of intramedullary drainage of a spinal dermoid cyst has already been demonstrated in Chap. 2. However, lipomas do change their volume according to the remainder of the body fat [11]. Therefore, as a general rule, cystic hamartomas should be removed completely in order to decompress the cord and to limit the risk of a recurrence. For lipomas, however, untethering and decompression with a large duraplasty is sufficient (Fig. 4.46). Lipomas have a tendency to bleed considerably if the surgeon tries to resect them and they do not present a cleavage plane towards the spinal cord. Removal of an intradural lipoma, therefore, carries considerable risks.

Sufficient untethering of a spinal cord may just require simple transsection of a thick filum terminale. For other patients, it may be a very difficult and risky undertaking, require more than one operation, or even be impossible. Severe arachnoid scarring and

tethering by shortened but functional nerve roots have been the two major obstacles for successful untethering in our series (Fig. 4.47f). To take care of an additional syrinx, a free CSF passage and untethering of the cord are necessary. In other words, if space-occupying hamartomas and a tethered cord in a patient with a spinal dysraphic lesion can be treated successfully, the syrinx does not require any additional measures – similar to syringomyelia associated with intramedullary tumors. If, however, arachnoid adhesions are too severe or untethering cannot be achieved, a syringosubarachnoid shunt may be indicated if the syrinx does cause neurological symptoms.

The approach to a spinal dysraphic lesion is performed as outlined for other spinal pathologies. If a lipoma extending from the intradural compartment into the subcutaneous tissue has to be addressed, we do not recommend removing the subcutaneous part of the lipoma. This may cause problems with adequate wound closure and lead to profound subcutaneous seromas. In such cases, we rather detach the intraspinal from the extraspinal part of the lipoma and remove just the intraspinal epidural part of it right to the dural entry. Then the dura is incised under the microscope in the midline above and below that entry area to identify the position of the conus and nerve roots. Once the dura has been circumcised around the lipoma entering the dura, the lipoma no longer tethers the cord. We only remove intradural parts of a lipoma if this is necessary to visualize other intradural structures or to facilitate closure with a spacious dura graft.

Once the lipoma is dealt with in this manner, other pathologies possibly involved in the tethering process should be looked for. The filum terminale can usually be identified due to its different texture and color (Figs. 4.45 n, o and 4.46 e, f). It is coagulated and cut. With a low positioned conus, the unusual course of lumbar and sacral nerve roots should be considered. Sacral roots in particular may be shortened to a degree that even after transsection of the filum the cord is still tethered by such nerve roots (Fig. 4.47f). As these roots may still be of functional significance, a complete untethering in such a patient is not possible without risking neurological deficits.

In patients with a diastematomyelia, treatment has to concentrate on sufficient untethering of the cord. Either a fibrous band or a bony spur traverses both parts of the cord in a direction from posterior superior to anterior inferior. Whereas fibrous bands may be completely intradural, bony spurs are covered by dura. From both hemicords, fibrous connections representing aberrant nerve roots may be connected to the spur or band, respectively. To untether the cord in this area, the fibrous band or bony spur have to be resected as well as these aberrant nerve roots. Adequate hemostasis has to be achieved as blood vessels are encountered upon transsection of these fibrous or bony structures.

Dermoid cysts are removed with standard microsurgical techniques. If the cyst is opened, contents should be sucked out carefully while the surgical field is covered with cottonoids to avoid contamination of the subarachnoid space with a potentially irritating substance.

Arachnoid adhesions and scars may complicate the above-mentioned situations even further and to such a degree that they present the major problem as outlined in Chap. 4.1. No matter how large the spinal canal may appear at the end of the microsurgical dissection for spinal dysraphism, we recommend using a Gore-Tex patch for a spacious duraplasty to limit the chances of postoperative re-tethering.

4.3.4
Postoperative Outcome

For pediatric patients, favorable results are given in the literature with more than 80% of patients reported as improved or stabilized with surgery [24, 27]. For surgery of re-tethering at the site of the myelomeningocele repair, outcome is considerably worse. Colak et al. [9] reported a success rate of 6 of 19 children operated for re-tethering irrespective of the type of material used for duraplasty. Similar results are reported for the response of sphincter disturbances to surgery.

Postoperative improvements were much more likely for primary than secondary operations [15]. It was concluded that time may be an important factor for patients with re-tethering. If it is diagnosed it should be operated early [36].

In patients with an accompanying syrinx in our series, treatment concentrated on untethering of the cord and providing a free CSF passage by adequate decompression of the spinal canal in 56% of cases. The other 44% of patients with syringomyelia were treated by partial resection of a space occupying hamartoma. In patients without syringomyelia, a space-occupying hamartoma presented the major problem in most instances (87%). A complete resection was performed in 24%, a partial resection in 41%, and a decompression in 22%. Eleven percent underwent arachnolysis and duraplasty for cord tethering, one adult patient underwent closure of an untreated meningomyelocele. Untethering was successful in 86% of patients with syringomyelia and 68% of patients without a syrinx (Chisquare test: not significant). We observed a rate of 11% of postoperative CSF leaks but no other complications.

Table 4.21 gives an overview of the short-term results for patients with spinal dysraphism in relation to accompanying syringomyelia. With an associated syrinx, slight improvements were observed for dysesthesias, pain, gait, and sphincter functions. The Karnofsky score remained unchanged. Without syringomyelia, a good result was obtained for pain, which was the predominating problem in most patients of this group before surgery [16]. Slight improvements were obtained for dysesthesias and motor weakness. For sphincter functions, the postoperative result was variable. The Karnofsky score improved slightly. Overall, stabilization is the realistic goal of treatment [26, 44, 46, 57].

The long-term result was not influenced significantly by an additional syrinx even though the clinical recurrence rates tended to be lower for patients with syringomyelia (Fig. 4.48). This slight difference in long-term outcome may be attributable to the higher rate of successful untethering in this group.

The most significant factor for long-term outcome was the spinal level of the dysraphic lesion. Whereas no clinical recurrence was observed with thoracic processes, lumbosacral lesions were associated with a clinical recurrence rate of 48% within the first postoperative year (Fig. 4.49). The presence of a tethered cord associated with the dysraphic lesion tended to worsen the postoperative recurrence rate also relative to patients without a tethered cord (Fig. 4.50). However, this trend did not reach statistical significance.

If the group of lumbosacral dysraphism is separated into those patients without preoperative tethering or successful untethering on one side and patients with unsuccessful untethering on the other, the overall

Table 4.21. Postoperative clinical results for spinal dysraphism

Group	Preop.	Postop.	3 months	6 months
Sensory deficits				
With syrinx	3.6±0.9	3.8±0.8	3.8±0.8	3.8±0.8
Without syrinx	3.8±1.1	3.7±1.2	3.8±1.1	3.9±1.1
Dysesthesias				
With syrinx	4.0±1.0	4.2±0.8	4.2±0.8	4.2±0.8
Without syrinx	4.1±1.1	4.4±0.8	4.3±0.9	4.4±0.9
Pain				
With syrinx	4.6±0.9	4.8±0.5	4.8±0.5	4.8±0.5
Without syrinx	3.3±1.3	3.7±1.0	4.1±1.1	3.9±1.1
Motor power				
With syrinx	3.4±1.7	3.4±1.8	3.4±1.8	3.4±1.8
Without syrinx	3.6±1.2	3.8±1.0	3.9±1.0	3.9±1.0
Gait ataxia				
With syrinx	3.4±2.1	3.4±2.1	3.6±2.1	3.6±2.1
Without syrinx	4.1±0.9	4.1±0.9	4.1±0.9	4.1±0.9
Bladder function				
With syrinx	4.6±0.9	4.6±0.9	4.6±0.9	4.6±0.9
Without syrinx	3.8±1.0	3.4±1.3	4.0±1.0	3.9±1.0
Bowel function				
With syrinx	4.6±0.9	4.6±0.9	4.8±0.5	4.8±0.5
Without syrinx	4.2±1.0	3.6±1.4	3.9±1.1	4.0±1.1
Karnofsky score				
With syrinx	72±18	68±22	72±24	72±24
Without syrinx	71±12	71±12	75±11	75±12

Paired *t*-test: no significant differences between preoperative and postoperative scores after 6 months for any symptom in both groups

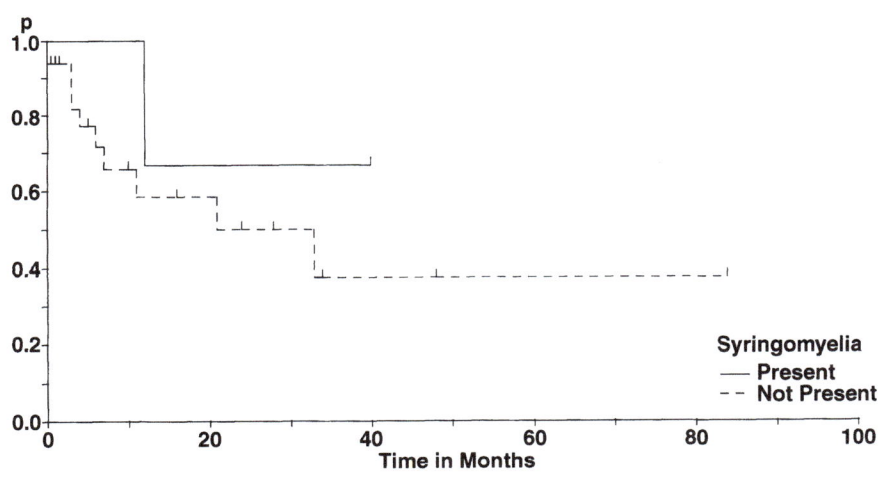

Fig. 4.48. Kaplan-Meier analysis of clinical recurrence rates for spinal dysraphism in relation to syringomyelia (log-rank test: not significant)

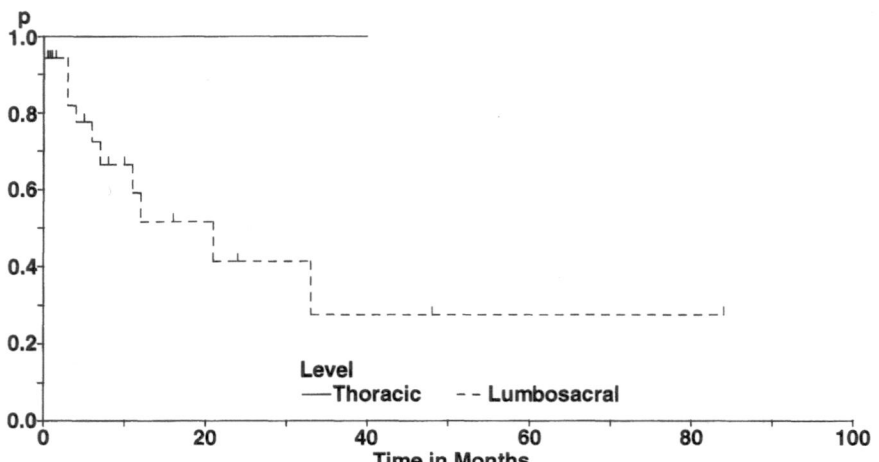

Fig. 4.49. Kaplan-Meier analysis of clinical recurrence rates for spinal dysraphism in relation to the spinal level (log-rank test: P=0.0357)

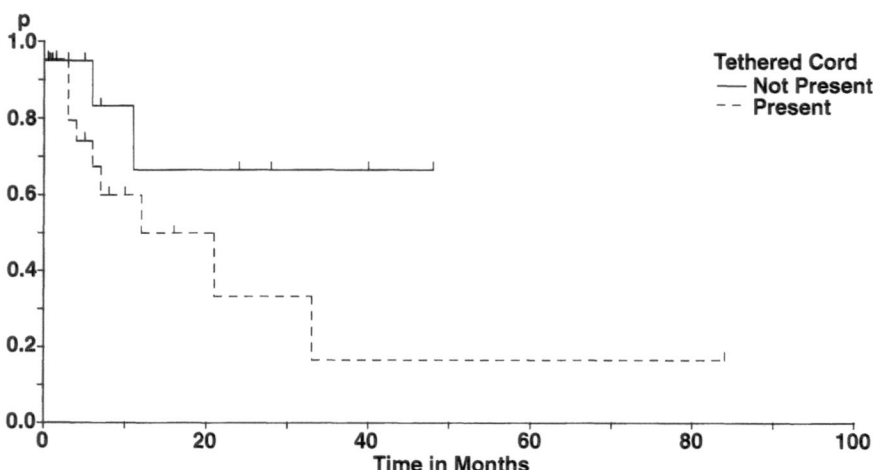

Fig. 4.50. Kaplan-Meier analysis of clinical recurrence rates for spinal dysraphism in relation to an additional tethered cord (log-rank test: not significant)

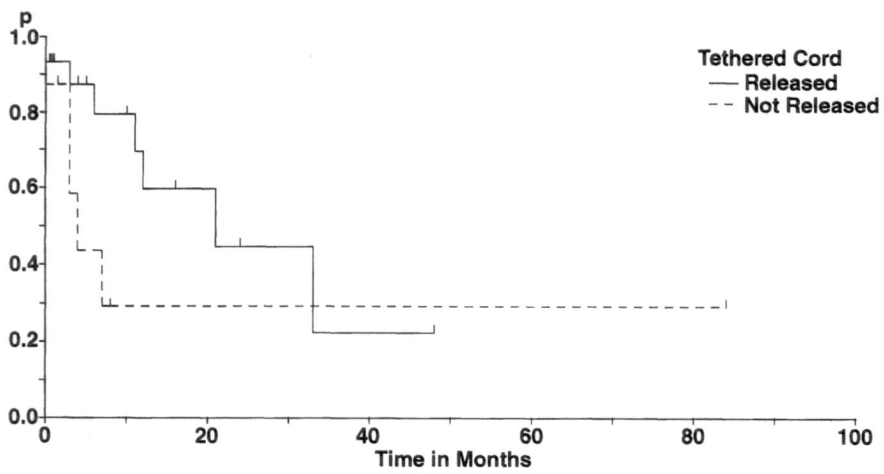

Fig. 4.51. Kaplan-Meier analysis for clinical recurrence rates of lumbosacral dysraphism comparing patients with successful release of a tethered cord or no cord tethering to those patients with unsuccessful untethering (log-rank test: not significant)

outcome did not differ much even though the clinical recurrences tended to occur later in the former group (Fig. 4.51). Despite some functional improvements [19, 30, 35, 55], as outlined in Table 4.21, the long-term prognosis is rather doubtful for lumbosacral dysraphism. The most likely explanations are arachnoid changes which complicated surgery for thoracic lesions in only 29% of patients but in 75% of lumbosacral pathologies (Chi-square test: $P=0.0263$) and the usually more complex malformations at the lumbosacral level [17, 42]. Looking at these results, we cannot substantiate the recommendation for prophylactic surgery for patients with lumbosacral dysraphism [18, 41, 48, 57]. Even if untethering was achieved and a duraplasty inserted to maintain a sufficient CSF pathway to minimize the risk of re-tethering [18, 20, 21, 34, 39], the analysis of clinical recurrence rates did not provide any evidence that progressive neurological symptoms can be improved or at least stabilized for the majority of patients if long-term results are considered [42, 51].

References

1. Aliredjo RP, de Vries J, Menovsky T, Grotenhuis JA, Merx J (1999) The use of Gore-Tex membrane for adhesion prevention in tethered spinal cord surgery: technical case reports. Neurosurgery 44:674–677; discussion 677–678
2. Anderson FM (1975) Occult spinal dysraphism: a series of 73 cases. Pediatrics 55:826–835
3. Assad A, Mansy A, Koto M, Hafez M (1989) Spinal dysraphism: experience with 250 cases operated upon. Child's Nerv Syst 5:324–329
4. Azimullah PC, Smit LMF, Rietveld-Knol E, Valk J (1991) Malformations of the spinal cord in 53 patients with spina bifida studied by magnetic resonance imaging. Child's Nerv Syst 7:63–66
5. Brophy JD, Sutton LN, Zimmerman RA, Bury E, Schut L (1989) Magnetic resonance imaging of lipomyelomeningocele and tethered cord. Neurosurgery 25:336–340
6. Brunner JC (1700) Hydrocephalo, sire hydrope capitis. In: Bonneti T (ed) Sepulchretum, Miscell. nat. curios. III. Dec. ann. I. 1688, Ed. II, Lib. I. Cramer and Perachon, Genf, p 394
7. Caldarelli M, Di Rocco C, La Marca F (1998) Treatment of hydromyelia in spina bifida. Surg Neurol 50:411–420
8. Chapman PH, Frim DM (1995) Symptomatic syringomyelia following surgery to treat retethering of lipomyelomeningoceles. J Neurosurg 82:752–755
9. Colak A, Pollack IF, Albright AL (1998) Recurrent tethering: a common long-term problem after lipomyelomeningocele repair. Pediatr Neurosurg 29:184–190
10. Cornette L, Verpoorten C, Lagae L, Van Calenbergh F, Plets C, Vereecken R, Casaer P (1998) Tethered cord syndrome in occult spinal dysraphism: timing and outcome of surgical release. Neurology 50:1761–1765
11. Endoh M, Iwasaki Y, Koyanagi I, Hida K, Abe H (1998) Spontaneous shrinkage of lumbosacral lipoma in conjunction with a general decrease in body fat: case report. Neurosurgery 43:150–151; discussion 151–152
12. Erkan K, Unal F, Kiris T (1999) Terminal syringomyelia in association with the tethered cord syndrome. Neurosurgery 45:1351–1359; discussion 1359–1360
13. Epstein F (1983) Meningomyelocele: "pitfalls" in early and late management. Clin Neurosurg 30:366–384
14. Estienne C (1546) La dissection des parties du corps humain divisée en trois livres. Book 3. Simon de Collines, Paris
15. Fone PD, Vapnek JM, Litwiller SE, Couillard DR, McDonald CM, Boggan JE, Stone AR (1997) Urodynamic findings in the tethered spinal cord syndrome: does surgical release improve bladder function? J Urol 157:604–609
16. Gupta SK, Khosla VK, Sharma BS, Mathuriya SN, Pathak A, Tewari MK (1999) Tethered cord syndrome in adults. Surg Neurol 52:362–369; discussion 370
17. Guyotat J, Bret P, Jouanneau E, Ricci AC, Lapras C (1998) [Tethered cord syndrome in adults]. Neurochirurgie 44:75–82
18. Hoffman HJ (1985) The tethered spinal cord. In: Holtzman RNN, Stein BM (eds) The tethered spinal cord. Thieme, Stuttgart, pp 91–98
19. Hoffman HJ, Hendrick EB, Humphreys RP (1976) The tethered spinal cord: its protean manifestations, diagnosis and surgical correction. Child's Brain 2:145–155
20. Hogenesch R, Zeilstra DJ, Breukers SME, Wiertsema GPA, Begeer JH, Ter Weeme CA (1990) Tethered cord syndrome following spina bifida aperta. Adv Neurosurg 18:158–162
21. Inoue HK, Kobayashi S, Ohbayashi K, Kohga H, Nakamura M (1994) Treatment and prevention of tethered and retethered spinal cord using a Gore-Tex surgical membrane. J Neurosurg 80:689–693
22. Iskandar BJ, Oakes WJ, McLaughlin C, Osumi AK, Tien RD (1994) Terminal syringohydromyelia and occult spinal dysraphism. J Neurosurg 81:513–519
23. Iskandar BJ, Fulmer BB, Hadley MN, Oakes WJ (1998) Congenital tethered spinal cord syndrome in adults. J Neurosurg 88:958–961
24. Jindal A, Mahapatra AK, Kamal R (1999) Spinal dysraphism. Indian J Pediatr 66:697–705
25. Just M, Schwarz M, Ludwig B, Ermert J, Thelen M (1990) Cerebral and spinal MR-findings in patients with postrepair myelomeningocele. Pediatr Radiol 20:262–266
26. Klekamp J, Raimondi AJ, Samii M (1994) Occult dysraphism in adulthood. Clinical course and management. Child's Nerv Syst 10:312–320
27. Koyanagi I, Iwasaki Y, Hida K, Abe H, Isu T, Akino M (1997) Surgical treatment supposed natural history of the tethered cord with occult spinal dysraphism. Child's Nerv Syst 13:268–274
28. Kuharik MA, Edwards MK, Grossman CB (1985) Magnetic resonance evaluation of pediatric spinal dysraphism. Pediatr Neurosci 12:213–218
29. La Marca F, Herman M, Grant JA, McLone DG (1997) Presentation and management of hydromyelia in children with Chiari type-II malformation. Pediatr Neurosurg 26:57–67
30. Lapras C, Patet JD, Huppert J, Bret P (1985) Syndrome

de traction du cone terminal ou syndrome de la moelle attachée. Lipomes lombo-sacres. Rev Neurol (Paris) 141:207–215

31. Levy LM (1999) MR imaging of cerebrospinal fluid flow and spinal cord motion in neurologic disorders of the spine. Magn Reson Imaging Clin N Am 7:573–587

32. Marin-Padilla M (1985) The tethered cord syndrome: developmental considerations. In: Holtzman RNN, Stein BM (eds) The tethered spinal cord. Thieme, Stuttgart, pp 3–13

33. McEnery G, Borzyskowski M, Cox TCS, Neville BGR (1992) The spinal cord in neurologically stable spina bifida: a clinical and MRI study. Dev Med Child Neurol 34:342–347

34. McLone DG, Naidich TP (1985) Spinal dysraphism: experimental and clinical. In: Holtzman RNN, Stein BM (eds) The tethered spinal cord. Thieme, Stuttgart, pp 14–28

35. Nakamura S, Camins MB, Hochwald GM (1983) Pressure-absorption responses to the infusion of fluid into the spinal cord central canal of kaolin-hydrocephalic cats. J Neurosurg 58:198–203

36. Ohe N, Futamura A, Kawada R, Minatsu H, Kohmura H, Hayashi K, Miwa K, Sakai N (2000) Secondary tethered cord syndrome in spinal dysraphism. Child's Nerv Syst 16:457–461

37. Oi S, Yamada H, Matsumoto S (1990) Tethered cord syndrome versus low-placed conus medullaris in an over-distended spinal cord following initial repair for myelodysplasia. Child's Nerv Syst 6:264–269

38. Ommaya AK (1968) Mechanical properties of tissues of the nervous system. J Biomech 1:127–138

39. Pang D (1985) Tethered cord syndrome in adults. In: Holtzman RNN, Stein BM (eds) The tethered cord syndrome. Thieme, Stuttgart, pp 99–115

40. Pang D, Wilberger JE Jr (1982) Tethered cord syndrome in adults. J Neurosurg 57:32–47

41. Pierre-Kahn A, Lacombe J, Pichon J, Giudicelli Y, Renier D, Sainte-Rose C, Perrigot M, Hirsch JF (1986) Intraspinal lipomas with spina bifida. Prognosis and treatment in 73 cases. J Neurosurg 65:756–761

42. Pierre-Kahn A, Zerah M, Renier D, Cinalli G, Saint-Rose C, Lellouch-Tubiana A, Brunelle F, Le Merrer M, Giudicelli Y, Pichon J, Kleinknecht B, Nataf F (1997) Congenital lumbosacral lipomas. Child's Nerv Syst 13:298–335

43. Raghavan N, Barkovich AJ, Edwards M, Norman D (1989) MR imaging in the tethered spinal cord syndrome. AJR Am J Roentgenol 152:843–852

44. Samuelsson L, Skoog M (1988) Ambulation in patients with myelomeningocele: a multivariate statistical analysis. J Pediatr Orthop 8:569–575

45. Scatliff JH, Kendall BE, Kingsley DPE, Britton J, Grant DN, Hayward RD (1989) Closed spinal dysraphism: analysis of clinical, radiological, and surgical findings in 104 consecutive patients. AJR Am J Roentgenol 152:1049–1057

46. Schmidt DM, Robinson B, Jones D (1990) The tethered spinal cord. Etiology and clinical manifestations. Orthop Rev 19:870–876

47. Sostrin RD, Thompson JR, Rouhe SA, Hasso AN (1977) Occult spinal dysraphism in the geriatric patient. Radiology 125:165–169

48. Stolke D, Zumkeller M, Seifert V (1988) Intraspinal li-

pomas in infancy and childhood causing a tethered cord syndrome. Neurosurg Rev 11:59–65

49. Szalay EA, Roach JW, Smith H, Maravilla K, Partain CL (1987) Magnetic resonance imaging of the spinal cord in spinal dysraphisms. J Pediatr Orthop 7:541–545

50. Tamaki N, Shirataki K, Kojima N, Shouse Y, Matsumoto S (1988) Tethered cord syndrome of delayed onset following repair of myelomeningocele. J Neurosurg 69:393–398

51. Van Calenbergh F, Vanvolsem S, Verpoorten C, Lagae L, Casaer P, Plets C (1999) Results after surgery for lumbosacral lipoma: the significance of early and late worsening. Child's Nerv Syst 15:439–442; discussion 443

52. Vernet O, Farmer JP, Montes JL (1996) Comparison of syringopleural and syringosubarachnoid shunting in the treatment of syringomyelia in children. J Neurosurg 84:624–628

53. Vogl D, Ring-Mrozik E, Baierl P, Vogl T, Zimmermann K (1987) Magnetic resonance imaging in children suffering from spina bifida. Z Kinderchir 42 [Suppl 1]:60–64

54. Warder DE, Oakes WJ (1994) Tethered cord syndrome: the low-lying and normally positioned conus. Neurosurgery 34:597–600

55. Yamada S, Knierim O, Yonekawa M, Schultz R, Maeda G (1983) Tethered cord syndrome. J Am Paraplegia Soc 6:58–61

56. Zerah M (1999) [Syringomyelia in children]. Neurochirurgie 45 [Suppl 1]:37–57

57. Zumkeller M, Stolke D, Dietz H (1990) Intraspinal lipomas with tethered cord syndrome – results of operative treatment in 30 children. Adv Neurosurg 18:164–169

4.4
Syringomyelia Related to Diseases of the Spine

4.4.1
Degenerative Diseases

The management of patients with syringomyelia and additional degenerative problems of the spine has already been discussed in each of the previous chapters. We also observed a few patients in whom degenerative diseases of the spine were thought to have caused syringomyelia in the absence of other pathologies. As with extramedullary and epidural tumors, this association is exceptionally rare [2, 10, 12, 21, 24]. Usually, such a syrinx is rather small and asymptomatic. Most authors interpreted these cysts as evidence of spinal cord hypoperfusion due to vascular compromise and spinal cord compression [10, 11, 16, 24]. Al-Mefty et al. [1] were able to substantiate this view experimentally. Interestingly, posterior compression of the spinal canal was not observed to be associated with intramedullary cysts even though a disease such as ossification of the posterior longitudinal ligament is a quite common disease in some parts of the world [12].

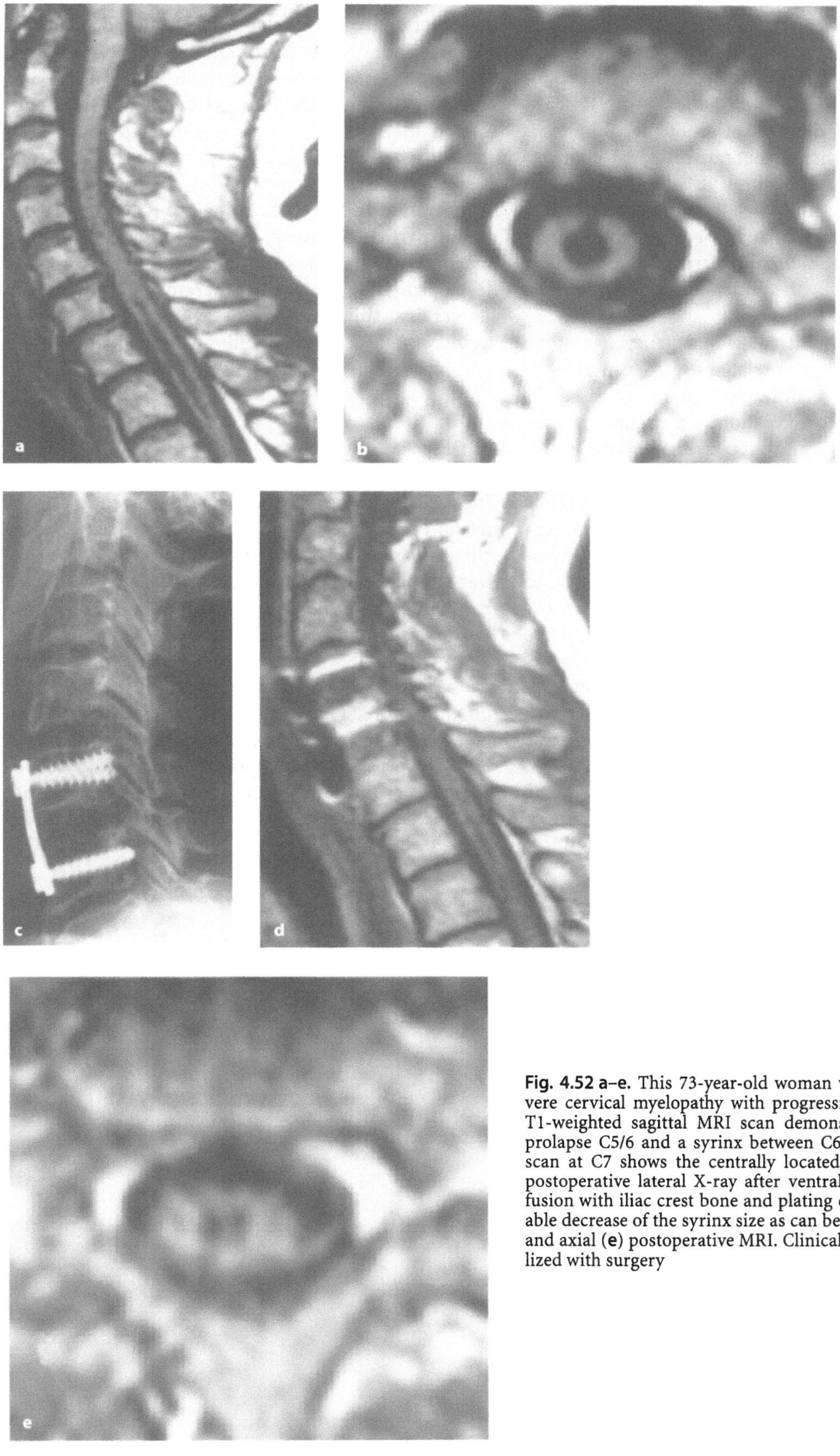

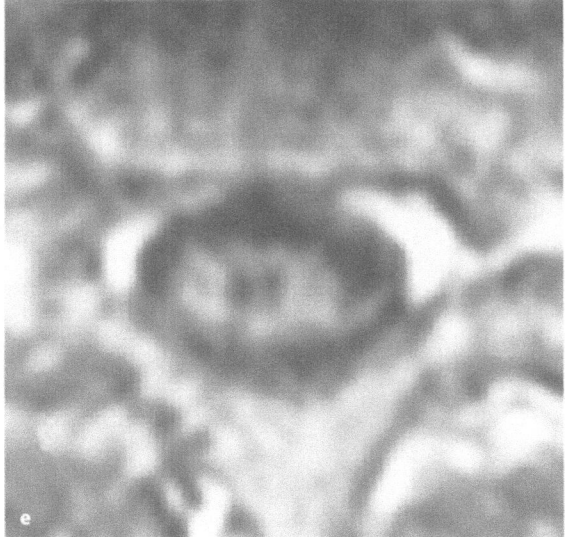

Fig. 4.52 a–e. This 73-year-old woman was suffering from severe cervical myelopathy with progressive tetraparesis. **a** The T1-weighted sagittal MRI scan demonstrates a cervical disc prolapse C5/6 and a syrinx between C6 and Th2. **b** The axial scan at C7 shows the centrally located syringomyelia. **c** The postoperative lateral X-ray after ventral discectomy C5/6 and fusion with iliac crest bone and plating did not cause a noticeable decrease of the syrinx size as can be seen in the sagittal (**d**) and axial (**e**) postoperative MRI. Clinical symptoms were stabilized with surgery

Apart from a vascular component in the pathophysiology of these cysts, alterations of CSF flow comparable with other diseases leading to syringomyelia could be demonstrated in this group as well [12]. A neuropathological study of four patients with cervical disc disease showed demyelination of the white matter, a loss of neurons, degenerative axonal changes, and arachnoid changes at the level of cord compression. Therefore, there may well be an overlap of myelomalacia caused by vascular compression and syringomyelia caused by arachnoid scarring and CSF flow obstruction similar to the situation in posttraumatic cases.

We observed 14 patients with degenerative spine disease and syringomyelia related to it. Seven of these were operated on, as clinical symptoms of radicular compression or myelopathy indicated surgical decompression. Figures 4.52 and 4.53 give an example of a cervical and a thoracic disc prolapse associated with syringomyelia, respectively. The other seven patients did not present such severe symptoms that surgery was required. Seven patients presented monosegmental disease, while three had two segments affected, and four patients three segments. Just two cavities extended for more than four spinal segments. Six were situated above and seven below the level of degenerative disease while one syrinx extended above and below. Twelve patients showed affections of the cervical spine, while just one thoracic and one lumbar disc was associated with a syrinx. A myelopathy was the predominating problem in five instances, while two patients complained about motor weakness and seven predominantly about pain due to radicular compression.

Postoperatively, one syrinx only decreased in size, the others were left unchanged despite adequate decompression of the subarachnoid space. However, clinical outcome was quite favorable with four patients reporting postoperative improvement while three considered their situation unchanged. This result indicates that an accompanying syrinx does not predispose to a worse postoperative result in patients with degenerative disease of the spine [2]. It does not represent a particular severe form of myelopathy unless myelomalacia, i.e., a necrotic lesion of the cord, has developed [11]. However, degenerative disc diseases of the cervical spine do become symptomatic earlier if syringomyelia associated with a Chiari malformation or spinal arachnoid scarring is present [25].

4.4.2
Spinal Scoliosis

The association between spinal scoliosis and syringomyelia [3, 4, 5, 6, 7, 8, 9, 14, 17, 19, 20, 22, 23, 26] or spinal dysraphism [18] is well documented. In children, in particular, any scoliosis associated with even the slightest neurological symptom should lead to a thorough radiological examination, including plain X-rays – which often demonstrate a dysraphic lesion already [19] – and MRIs of the spine, and craniocervical junction [3, 14, 19, 22, 26]. Most authors considered the scoliosis to be a consequence of the syrinx or the disease process underlying the syrinx, i.e., the scoliosis was interpreted as a symptom of the syrinx rather than the cause. Others, however, pointed out that scoliosis itself may cause syringomyelia due to the CSF

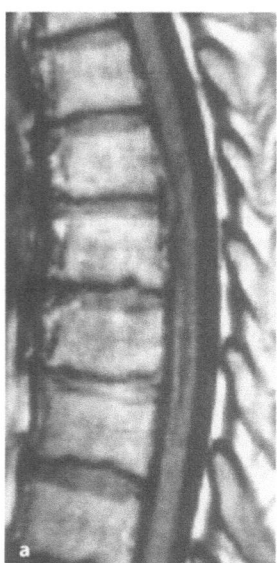
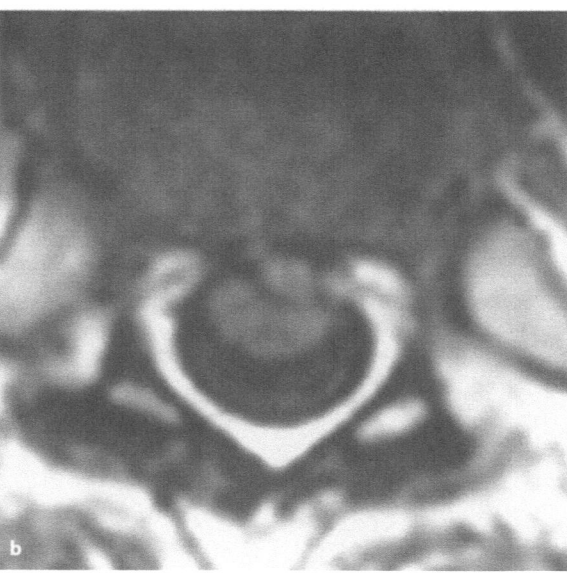

Fig. 4.53 a, b

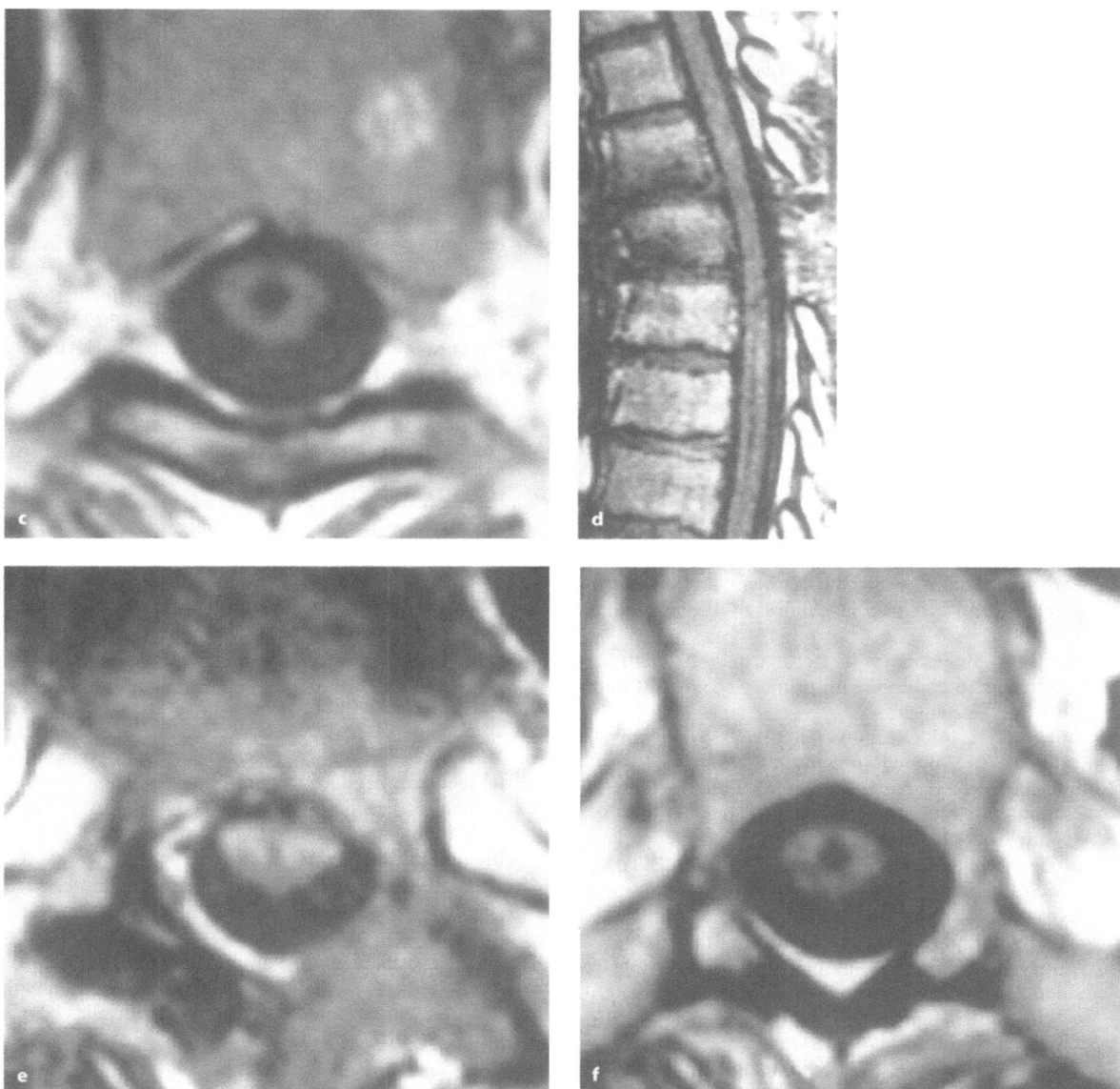

Fig. 4.53 a–f. This 57-year-old woman complained about severe back pain, gait ataxia and weakness of her left leg. **a** The T1-weighted MRI scan showed a thoracic disc prolapse Th6/7. A slit-like syrinx below the prolapse can be seen. **b, c** Axial scans demonstrate the left sided prolapse and the centrally located syrinx. **d** The postoperative sagittal MRI scan after removal of the disc Th6/7 shows no change of the syrinx caliber. **e, f** The axial scans confirm removal of the disc prolapse and the unchanged size of the syrinx. The patient improved considerably and is well 2 years after surgery

flow changes associated with it [20]. Even a myelomalacia may be induced by severe scoliosis, as considerable impairment of spinal cord blood flow may be observed in such instances [13]. Impaired coordination and weakness of back muscles is considered the major cause of scoliosis in patients with syringomyelia [6,

23]. This view is substantiated by observations that a scoliosis may improve with successful treatment of the syrinx [6, 8, 22] or the tethered cord [18] provided treatment is initiated early enough [22] before severe deformities have developed.

References

1. Al-Mefty O, Harkey HL, Marawi I, Haines DE, Peeler DF, Wilner HI, Smith RR, Holaday HR, Haining JL, Russell WF, Harrison B, Middleton TH (1993) Experimental chronic compressive cervical myelopathy. J Neurosurg 79:550–561

2. Albert FK, Aschoff A, Hampl J, Forstwig M, Kunze S (1993) Two cases of thoracic intervertebral disc herniation combined with circumscribed syringomyelia – coincidental or causative? Acta Neurochir 123:213–215

3. Arai S, Ohtsuka Y, Moriya H, Kitahara H, Minami S (1993) Scoliosis associated with syringomyelia. Spine 18:1591–1592

4. Bertrand SL, Drvaric DM, Roberts JM (1989) Scoliosis in syringomyelia. Orthopedics 12:335–337

5. Bindal AK, Dunsker SB, Tew JM (1995) Chiari I malformation: classification and management. Neurosurgery 37:1069–1074

6. Charry O, Koop S, Winter R, Lonstein J, Denis F, Bailey W. (1994) Syringomyelia and scoliosis: a review of twenty-five pediatric patients. J Pediatr Orthop 14:309–317

7. Farley FA, Song KM, Birch JG, Browne R (1995) Syringomyelia and scoliosis in children. J Pediatr Orthop 15:187–192

8. Hanieh A, Sutherland A, Foster B, Cundy P (2000) Syringomyelia in children with primary scoliosis. Child's Nerv Syst 16:200–202

9. Huebert HT, MacKinnon WB (1969) Syringomyelia and scoliosis. J Bone Joint Surg Br 51:338–343

10. Iwasaki Y, Abe H, Isu T, Miyasaka K (1985) CT myelography with intramedullary enhancement in cervical spondylosis. J Neurosurg 63:363–366

11. Jinkins JR, Bashir R, Al-Mefty O, Al-Kawi MZ, Fox JL (1986) Cystic necrosis of the spinal cord in compressive cervical myelopathy: demonstration by iopamidol CT-myelography. AJR Am J Roentgenol 147:767–775

12. Kameyama T, Ando T, Fukutsu H, Mizuno T, Takahashi A (1993) [Syringomyelia syndrome secondary to cervical canal stenosis and cervical spondylosis.] Rinsho Shinkeigaku 33:1179–1183

13. Keim HA, Hilal SK (1971) Spinal angiography in scoliosis patients. J Bone Joint Surg Am 53:904–912

14. Kim FM, Poussaint TY, Barnes PD (1999) Neuroimaging of scoliosis in childhood. Neuroimaging Clin N Am 9:195–221

15. Levy EI, Heiss JD, Kent MS, Riedel CJ, Oldfield EH (2000) Spinal cord swelling preceding syrinx development. Case report. J Neurosurg 92:93–97

16. Mimura F, Fujiwara K, Otake S, Miki Y, Kawakami K, Kuwata Y, Takada I, Masada T, Koyama M, Miyamoto S (1990) [MR imaging of compressive cervical myelopathy after surgery – high signal intensity of the spinal cord on T2 weighted images]. Nippon Igaku Hoshasen Gakkai Zasshi 50:567–576

17. Nohria V, Oakes WJ (9091) Chiari I malformation: a review of 43 patients. Pediatr Neurosurg 16:222–227

18. Pierz K, Banta J, Thomson J, Gahm N, Hartford J (2000) The effect of tethered cord release on scoliosis in myelomeningocele. J Pediatr Orthop 20:362–365

19. Prahinski JR, Polly DW Jr, McHale KA, Ellenbogen RG (2000) Occult intraspinal anomalies in congenital scoliosis. J Pediatr Orthop 20:59–63

20. Pravda J, Ghelman B, Levine DB (1992) Syringomyelia associated with congenital scoliosis. A case report. Spine 171:372–374

21. Ramanauskas WL, Wilner HI, Metes JJ, Lazo A, Kelly JK (1989) MR imaging of compressive myelomalacia. J Comput Assist Tomogr 13:399–404

22. Sengupta DK, Dorgan J, Findlay GF (2000) Can hindbrain decompression for syringomyelia lead to regression of scoliosis? Eur Spine J 9:198–201

23. Tomlinson RJ Jr, Wolfe MW, Nadall JM, Bennett JT, MacEwen GD (1994) Syringomyelia and developmental scoliosis. J Pediatr Orthop 14:580–585

24. Tumiati B, Casoli P (1991) Syringomyelia in a patient with rheumatoid subluxation of the cervical spine. J Rheumatol 18:1403–1405

25. Yu YL, Moseley IF (1987) Syringomyelia and cervical spondylosis: a clinicoradiological investigation. Neuroradiology 29:143–151

26. Zadeh HG, Sakha SA, Powell MP, Mehta MH (1995) Absent superficial abdominal reflexes in children with scoliosis. An early indicator of syringomyelia. J Bone Joint Surg Br 77:762–767

Subject Index